T0331003

Benjamin Rush, Civic Health, and Human Illness in the Early American Republic

Rochester Studies in Medical History

Series Editor: Christopher Crenner
Robert Hudson and Ralph Major Professor and Chair
Department of History and Philosophy of Medicine
University of Kansas School of Medicine

Additional Titles of Interest

Cancer, Research, and Educational Film at Midcentury: The Making of the Movie "Challenge: Science Against Cancer"
David Cantor

*Reimagining Psychiatric Epidemiology in a Global Frame:
Toward a Social and Conceptual History*
Edited by Anne M. Lovell and Gerald M. Oppenheimer

*Sickness in the Workhouse:
Poor Law Medical Care in Provincial England, 1834–1914*
Alistair Ritch

*Of Life and Limb:
Surgical Repair of the Arteries in War and Peace, 1880–1960*
Justin Barr

*The Hidden Affliction:
Sexually Transmitted Infections and Infertility in History*
Edited by Simon Szreter

China and the Globalization of Biomedicine
Edited by David Luesink, William H. Schneider, and Zhang Daqing

Explorations in Baltic Medical History, 1850–2015
Edited by Nils Hansson and Jonatan Wistrand

Health Education Films in the Twentieth Century
Edited by Christian Bonah, David Cantor, and Anja Laukötter

A complete list of titles in the Rochester Studies in Medical History series
may be found on our website, www.urpress.com.

Benjamin Rush, Civic Health, and Human Illness in the Early American Republic

Sarah E. Naramore

UNIVERSITY OF ROCHESTER PRESS

First published 2023

University of Rochester Press
668 Mt. Hope Avenue, Rochester, NY 14620, USA
www.urpress.com
and Boydell & Brewer Limited
PO Box 9, Woodbridge, Suffolk IP12 3DF, UK
www.boydellandbrewer.com

ISBN-13: 978-1-64825-069-9
ISSN: 1526-2715

Cataloging-in-publication data available from the Library of Congress

A catalogue record for this title is available from the British Library.

This publication is printed on acid-free paper.

Printed in the United States of America.

Cover image: *Dr. Benjamin Rush* by Charles Wilson Peale. Philadelphia, Pennsylvania, 1783–1786. Oil paint and canvas. 1959.0160A. Gift of Mrs. Julia B. Henry. Courtesy of Winterthur Museum.

Contents

Acknowledgments

No book comes into the world without a team of invested literary midwives. This one is no different.

My journey with Benjamin Rush began over a decade ago when he played a supporting role in my undergraduate thesis at Lafayette College. He took center stage during my first two semesters in the History and Philosophy of Science Program (HPS) at the University of Notre Dame. I owe a deep debt to Christopher Hamlin, advisor and mentor, who has now heard and read more about Rush than I suspect he imagined he ever would. To answer the question you had for me back in my first year: no, I am not bored with Rush yet. There is still plenty of Rush work out there, and I hope this book will be a jumping-off point for others as well as myself. I would also like to acknowledge my other early readers: Jon Coleman, Patrick Griffin, and Evan Ragland. Rush was a man of many interests and building up my expertise in environmental history, the American Revolution, and early modern science proved essential.

Thank you to the HPS program and department of history at Notre Dame. I had the privilege of spending several years with thoughtful and committed faculty and fellow graduate students across the history and philosophy departments, including Philip Sloan, Robert Goulding, Felipe Fernández-Armesto, Charles Pence, Richard Oosterhoff, Laura Bland, Michelle Marvin, Jeremy Steeger, Xiaoxing Jin, Jamee Elder, Mousa Mohammadian, Monica Solomon, John Slattery, Pablo Ruiz de Olano Altuna, Jessica Baron, and many others. Reading groups, the writing groups, and especially the HPS "Coffee and Cookies" helped me grow as a scholar and person. Your friendship and collegiality have been an important model for me going forward. To my fellow history of medicine colleagues—Nicholas Bonneau, Beatriz Carrillo, and Jonathan Riddle—you as much as anyone know what seeing this book in print means to me. Thank you for being in my corner.

Digging into Benjamin Rush of course meant having the pleasure of getting to know the City of Brotherly Love. Moving around Philadelphia's (and Northern Delaware's) libraries, archives, and universities was made possible with the generous support of the Consortium for the History of Science,

Technology, and Medicine, the College of Physicians of Philadelphia, and the Library Company of Philadelphia's Albert M. Greenfield Foundation Dissertation Fellowship. The time and resources provided allowed me to make vital connections with historians, archivists, librarians, and interested city residents who have all left their imprint on the final text. I would especially like to thank James N. Green, Cornelia King, Beth Lander, Charles B. Greifenstein, John Pollock, Adrianna Link, and Patrick Spero.

Parts of this book have also found their way into a variety of working groups, including the Humanities and Social Sciences Writing group at Northwest Missouri State University, Linda Hall Library Works in Progress Seminar, David Center for the American Revolution Seminar Series, Consortium Fellows Seminar, and Consortium Working Group on Medicine and Health, in addition to conference talks and invited talks. All have made an impact. I would also like to acknowledge colleagues who have read drafts of this work and been party to many a conversation about where this book would go. This text has greatly benefited from the careful insights of Suman Seth, David Barnes, Christopher Willoughby, Elaine LaFay, Cameron Strang, Sean Morey Smith, Emily Frazier, and my fellow Rush traveller, Stephen Fried.

Making the book ready for publication was certainly no simple task. I was very fortunate to work with an extremely supportive and patient editorial team. Thank you to my editor Sonia Kane, series editor Christopher Crenner, and those at University of Rochester Press who believed in this project. Through many drafts, reconfigurations, and moments of self-doubt, your belief in this book was the best pep talk an author could hope for. That included a complete restructuring of the chapters. The book is much the better for it. I also want to acknowledge the reviewers of this manuscript for their careful critiques and suggestions.

I would never have finished this work or believed it possible to finish without the support of the "Sarahs": Sarah Pickman, Sarah Qidway, and honorary Sarah, Kate Sheppard. What started out as a group chat has become a bedrock of support from three historians and humans who continue to amaze me. Your friendship has been invaluable in more ways than you know. If I can offer a piece of advice to anyone embarking on their own scholarly journey: find yourself some Sarahs, you won't regret it.

To my family, who have lived with Rush as long as I have. To my parents, Bruce and Sally Naramore—I failed miserably at rebelling and have followed you into history (even if I didn't follow you into museums). Your support, proofreading, and assistance through moves to at least three different states have been essential and deeply appreciated. Dad, without that conversation about historical medical records in 2011 at the local pub none of this would have happened. Thanks to my sister Susan Naramore for many long phone calls, surviving a year as roommates, and working through various historical puzzles. And lastly, to my husband and partner in all things, Nathan Gerth: You have endured late night talks about formatting and imposter syndrome and dinner chats about infectious disease (sorry again). Benjamin Rush's story would not have been understood or written half as well without your comments, critiques, and sharp analysis. Thank you.

Finally, I write this knowing that Benjamin Rush's first professional controversy emerged from his acknowledgments section. I am confident that my colleagues are less touchy about such things than were John Morgan and William Shippen Jr., but I apologize if anyone feels let down by their placement—no insults are intended.

Abbreviations

APS	American Philosophical Society
LCP	Library Company of Philadelphia
HSP	Historical Society of Pennsylvania

Introduction

"Truth Is a Unit"

In March 1787, Benjamin Rush sat in Benjamin Franklin's Philadelphia home discussing the nature of public punishments. The two Benjamins were not alone. Rush spoke to the newly formed Society for Promoting Political Inquiries of which he—as well as Franklin—was a founding member. The organization itself was dedicated not to the development of partisan politics, but to the study of politics as a science. Its members believed government could be understood, dismantled, and rebuilt with greater clarity. Just as the laws of motion or the nature of electricity yielded to inquiry, so too, they hoped, would the laws of human society and workings of the human mind. While a short walk away colleagues worked to construct the United States Constitution, these Philadelphians mused upon the basic framework of good governance at all levels. The group met most months between February 1787 and May 1789 at Franklin's home, with different members presenting each time. While short-lived, the society and its members represented the strong "improving" and "enlightened" impulse in post-Revolutionary American life and the extent to which "scientific" was an idealized adjective. After the war for independence, and in the midst of the development of a new constitution, members looked to science and scientific methods to guide them in developing national institutions and understanding political trends. Benjamin Rush took those lessons to heart in a variety of projects pre- and postdating his lecture in Franklin's home.

The Society counted among its members the leaders of Philadelphia's social, political, and scientific elite. Thomas Paine drafted their governing documents; local politicians George Clymer and William Bingham served as the first vice presidents. Franklin, at 81 the elder statesman of Philadelphia's intellectual society, acted as president. As a physician, Rush was joined by other men of science, including astronomer and naturalist

David Rittenhouse and his medical colleague Adam Kuhn.[1] Rush's oration on public punishments was one of the most influential and widely read documents to come out of the group and demonstrates his use of medical knowledge to craft social policy. As a physician, he focused in his talk on the ideal of medical progress and improvement. Health formed a foundation for personal and collective success in the new nation. When introducing his topic, Rush stated that "truth is a unit. It is the same thing in war—philosophy—medicine—morals—religion and government; and in proportion as we arrive at it in one science, we shall discover it in others."[2] This view underpinned not only Rush's worldview but that of his colleagues and friends gathered at Franklin's house. Expertise and knowledge in one domain could inform work in many others.

As he stood to speak in Franklin's home in 1787, Rush was entering the most productive and influential period of his professional life. Throughout the 1780s, he dedicated his thoughts on society to print and the public forum. Those same thoughts formed the foundation of medical theories that he made public in the 1790s and that directed his research for the remainder of his life. This book argues that for Rush this association between social and physical health went beyond analogy. The American medicine he created and instilled in his readers—medical students, colleagues, and lay readers—shaped the way they understood the country and its future, putting it on a path distinct from those of their European contemporaries.

When Rush considered the future of his country in the year of the Constitutional Convention—in the city that played host to this meeting as it had to two Continental Congresses—he may have been thinking just as much about the effects of the meeting on the physical constitutions of his fellow citizens. Rush stood up to speak not only on the specific topic of crime and appropriate punishments, but to make the case for a healthier, more socially stable future for his new polity. He made the case for medicine as a central profession in the creation of a republic. In his talk he urged some

---

1   Vinson, "The Society for Political Inquiries: The Limits of Republican Discourse in Philadelphia on the Eve of the Constitutional Convention, " 185–205; "News, February 19, 1787," The Daily Advertiser, February 19, 1787. Clymer was a patient and close friend of Rush as noted in the latter's commonplace book in the form of a eulogy, Rush and Biddle, *A Memorial Containing Travels Through Life Or Sundry Incidents in the Life of Dr. Benjamin Rush, Born Dec. 24, 1745 (Old Style) Died April 19, 1813*, 214.

2   Rush, *An Enquiry into the Effects of Public Punishments upon Criminals and upon Society*, 4.

of his city's most influential leaders to change the way they thought about punishment. Prior to the American Revolution long-term incarceration was practically unheard of. Those who committed crimes typically faced physical consequences ranging from the shame of the stocks to execution.

Some reformers suggested a move to labor as a punishment—forcing convicted criminals to clean city streets, for example. Rush, however, rejected both corporal and other forms of public punishment, claiming that they simply did not work and had never worked. On the contrary, they desensitized both punished and punisher. The 42-year-old boldly stated, "it is . . . to the combined operation of indolence, prejudice, ignorance—and the defect of culture of the human heart, alone, that we are to ascribe the continuation of public punishments, after such long and multiplied experience of their inefficacy to reform bad men."[3] Instead, he proposed a solution reminiscent of the strictures of hospital regulations. Rush wanted criminals cut off from their friends and family and put in the care of society to effect a "cure" to their behavior that would not inflame public emotions. Criminality—like so many things in Rush's gaze—acted like a disease. His emphasis on the good of society and the rightness of his views and plans may seem like overreach. It was certainly traumatic for those who encountered such systems.[4] It was also far from democratic. But Rush was not a democrat—he was a republican. The growth, balance, and good of the republic (and therefore society as a whole) motivated his actions.

Rush is a difficult figure to pin down in the history of American medicine. In the two centuries since his 1813 death, he has been alternately praised and reviled by physicians and historians. Some consider him a medical innovator and leader while others see him as unoriginal and ultimately harmful to a progressive historical narrative of American medicine. Both views limit Rush to his legacy rather than his significance during his lifetime. This is an oversight. Rush introduced to lay and medical audiences alike a view of the United States as a unique biological space that could not be untangled from its unusual political situation. His version of patriotism—defined by public service and private self-regulation—could not and should not be separated from his professional identity. In short, he was a figure who both shaped and

---

3   Rush, *An Enquiry into the Effects of Public Punishments upon Criminals and upon Society*, 10.

4   See Manion, *Liberty's Prisoners*; Meranze, *Laboratories of Virtue*; Frank, "Sympathy and Separation: Benjamin Rush and the Contagious Public," 27–57.

was shaped by the social and scientific world he inhabited, with lasting consequences for the development of American institutions.

Within his lifetime Rush was *the* American doctor. He was the man who not only signed the Declaration of Independence, but also declared a form of "medical independence" by pointing out the unique physical space and challenges of his country. This second independence claimed that European-descended bodies were indeed *American* rather than *British* bodies that inhabited a particular physical and social space created by the American Revolution. At a time in medicine when physicians and patients alike believed geography was destiny, biological independence meant that Americans not only faced different threats to health but were expected to respond to them differently. In this view future generations of American *citizens* would physically and psychologically differ from the British *subjects* who preceded them. To map the exact nature of this transformation required men of science trained in the United States to study the culture, geography, climate, and epidemiology of their nation. Rush asserted that American doctors needed to study and make sense out of their own situation for the good of the republic. The literal survival of the country rested in the kind of useful knowledge compiled by physicians.

In the years during and following the American Revolution, Rush's ideas and actions formed a unified program for national improvement that should be understood independent of the professionalization and specialization that was to come. This work takes a broad view of the American Revolution as a process that began in the 1760s and did not reach its end point until at least the 1790s with the establishment of social and political patterns that have continued to affect the course of public life in the United States.[5] Rush did not consider the Revolution finished in 1783. Rather, he continued to view himself as a revolutionary, moving the world of medicine and the public's health toward a more perfect future. He shifted a generation of medical minds to think of the citizens of the United States as *Americans* in need of a biological as well as political identity. Americans, in this sense, suffered from certain kinds of diseases, ate certain kinds of food, lived with unique

---

5　This builds on work by historians of the American Revolution and Early Republic, including Bradburn, *The Citizenship Revolution*; Branson, *These Fiery Frenchified Dames*; Greene, *Peripheries and Center*; Griffin, *America's Revolution*; Newman, *Fries's Rebellion*; Thompson et al., *State and Citizen*; Griffin, "Introduction: Imagining an American Imperial-Revolutionary History," 1–24.

mental stresses, and improved their situation through the action of public institutions. Rush as well as his colleagues, students, and fellow citizens would learn about themselves and shape their national and political identity through challenges to their own biology. Rush's American system of medicine promoted the primacy of local knowledge, rejected specific diseases, and emphasized connections between body, mind, and the natural, social, and political environment. Rush's work crossed nascent disciplinary boundaries rather than conformed to them. He was concerned with health in the broadest terms: that of the country. Rush's unique position as a physician, social reformer, educator, and political figure allows a historicist examination of early American medicine as a discipline deeply concerned with the social as well as physical well-being of the country. It also demonstrates that Rush was a foundational figure in the formation of an American medical profession that came to consider and continues to consider itself as distinct from the practices of other nations.

Benjamin Rush, Civic Health, and Human Illness in the Early American Republic is not a comprehensive analysis of all of Rush's work, nor does it aim to be a traditional biography. Rather, it explores key aspects of Rush's life and work to provide essential context for his contributions. Studying Rush's varied projects provides a window into the way medicine and human bodies directed his understanding of the world around him and the institutions required for American health. Some of this came from his experiences outside North America as a medical student in Scotland and London, as discussed in chapter 1. Like his colleagues and contemporaries at the University of Edinburgh, Rush understood his role as a physician to be a social one. As a young man he chose the medical profession in part because he believed that as a Christian it was his duty to use his intellectual talents to ease human suffering. This came to bear on some of his earlier career decisions. Rush was undecided between law and medicine after completing his studies at the College of New Jersey (Princeton). His former teacher, spiritual advisor, and surrogate father-figure Samuel Finley encouraged the young man to study medicine based on its ability to do real good in the world, while the law rewarded self-interest rather than self-sacrifice.

His initial inclination to work for the greater good of society rather than focus on narrower medical or scientific goals gained precision and refinement in the course of his experience at Edinburgh. There the young man engaged with the philosopher-physicians of the Scottish Common Sense school, especially the philosopher-physician John Gregory, who honed his views on ethics.[6] These mentors used medical systems based in physiological systems to explain human health, behavior, and environmental processes. Rush took these building blocks to develop a system of his own in that he found what he believed to be the basis of republican principles—division of power between coequal systems and regularity of action—within bodies. Moreover, Rush viewed his system as a guide to encouraging the public's health and nudging his fellow countrymen and women into "correct" behaviors. Building the institutions of the republic and grounding them in scientific principles *was* cutting-edge medical theory. To better understand Rush's world, historians must also eschew anachronistic boundaries between medicine, public health, and psychology.

This book sets out to answer the question of how and why Rush embarked on such an ambitious program of national improvement that echoed down through nineteenth-century medicine, especially the regional medicine of the South and Midwest. It responds not only to recent literature but to a long tradition of Rush scholarship. In 1946 historian of medicine Richard Shryock argued in his article "Benjamin Rush from the Perspective of the Twentieth Century" that Rush's legacy among physicians and historians of medicine had become more symbolic than substantive. As a remedy, he proposed a historicist reappraisal of Rush's work. By "historicist" Shryock suggested that historians consider Rush's work in the context of the late eighteenth century and the manner in which it addressed the medical needs (both theoretical and institutional) of the young nation. Shryock demonstrated this approach in the essay—highlighting Rush's career as primarily a medical one and discussing his mature (post-1793) system—but left the bulk of this work for his successors.[7]

Over seventy years later, Shryock's challenge remains largely unfulfilled. Historians and biographers often present Rush as either the "heroic" bleeder—obsessed with letting more blood from patients than they could tolerate in the name of health and thus responsible for the deaths of patients—or the hero-physician, a paradigm of professionalism who would not leave the city while an epidemic raged. Others emphasize Rush's political and

---

6   Barfoot, "James Gregory (1753–1821) and Scottish Scientific Metaphysics, 1750–1800"; Hamlin, "William Pulteney Alison, the Scottish Philosophy, and the Making of a Political Medicine," 144–86.

7   Shryock, "Benjamin Rush from the Perspective of the Twentieth Century" and "The Advent of Modern Medicine in Philadelphia, 1800–1850"; Shryock, "The Psychiatry of Benjamin Rush," 429.

reform activism, view him as the father of American psychiatry, or simply as a signer of the Declaration of Independence.[8] Historians of medicine have not fully grappled with the details of Rush's physiology and how contemporaries understood his views.

Meanwhile, from the perspective of scholarship on early American history, Rush has experienced something of a resurgence in recent years. His nonmedical achievements in particular have garnered interest from scholars as examples of American nation-building and nonpartisan reform movements of the early nineteenth century. A 2017 special issue of *Early American Studies* includes essays reflecting on his position as a political mediator between Federalist and Democratic-Republican factions, an antislavery advocate, and a promoter of common sense, both the pamphlet and the philosophy.[9] In the collection's introductory essay, Sari Altschuler and Christopher J. Bilodeau write that "[m]irroring Rush's jumbled legacy, Rush scholarship might be best characterized as a field in a state of energetic yet fractured engagement."[10] Work like that showcased in *Early American Studies* and this work is beginning to knit those fractures back together to form a clearer

---

8   Binger, *Revolutionary Doctor*; Brodsky, *Benjamin Rush: Patriot and Physician*; Starr, *The Social Transformation of American Medicine*; Bell, *The College of Physicians of Philadelphia: A Bicentennial History*; Estes et al., *A Melancholy Scene of Devastation: The Public Response to the 1793 Yellow Fever Epidemic*; Powell, *Bring Out Your Dead: The Great Plague of Yellow Fever in Philadelphia in 1793*; Marks and Beatty, *The Story of Medicine in America*; Myrsiades, *Medical Culture in Revolutionary America: Feuds, Duels, and a Court-Martial*; Rosenberg, *Our Present Complaint: American Medicine, Then and Now*, 46, 49; Breslaw, *Lotions, Potions, Pills, and Magic*; Hawke, *Benjamin Rush: Revolutionary Gadfly*; Woodbury, "Benjamin Rush: Patriot, Physician and Psychiator," 427–30.

9   Bell, "The Moral Thermometer: Rush, Republicanism, and Suicide," 308–31; Herschthal, "Antislavery Science in the Early Republic: The Case of Dr. Benjamin Rush," 274–307; King, "'Receive the Olive Branch': Benjamin Rush as Reconciler in the Early Republic," 352–81; Rosenfeld, "Benjamin Rush's Common Sense," 252–73. Elizabeth Webster, it should be noted, argues that Rush rejected many of the tenants of common sense philosophy, especially the concept that most people could be directed to moral and ethical behavior through it. Rush believed institutions and government programs were necessary to direct moral development. Webster, "American Science and the Pursuit of 'Useful Knowledge' in the Polite Eighteenth Century, 1750–1806" 147.

10   Altschuler and Bilodeau, "Ecce Homo!: The Figure of Benjamin Rush," 235.

picture of an influential, loquacious, but poorly understood intellectual leader of the Early Republic.

Additionally, Stephen Fried's 2018 biography, *Rush: Revolution, Madness, and the Visionary Doctor Who Became a Founding Father*, brings public attention to Rush and addresses the breadth of Rush's myriad interests.[11] The book delves into the details surrounding Rush's life, connecting his personal experiences to one of his most lasting achievements as a founding figure in American psychiatry. Fried presents an approachable and complicated Rush as a person driven by his work. While far from a perfect person, the Rush that emerges from the page is one who certainly *tried* to be the best version of himself. In some ways this reflects Fried's sources and method. The biography provides perhaps an unparalleled dive into Rush's mind and motivation, often referring to Rush's own autobiography, notes, and published work. As expected from a biography, Benjamin Rush is the main character. And Rush is an extremely compelling character as political figure, medical educator, and prolific writer and observer well-situated to witness the birth of the United States. Since the book's publication, Fried has continued to make Rush's work more accessible through the Rush Digital Portal hosted by the University of Pennsylvania. The Portal's homepage invites researchers and the interested public to "see the world through the eyes of America's Founding Physician."[12] If the project—and indeed Fried's biography—invite readers into Rush's worldview, this book invites readers to see Rush as his world understood him.

Amid this jumble of Rush's legacy—and perhaps because of it—Rush's work as a medical theorist is often overlooked. By the mid-twentieth century, historians of American medicine described the time period that encompassed Rush's professional life as an endpoint. Rush, in this narrative, concluded a mode of "traditional" Western medicine focused on humors, rational system-building, and ancient authority that preceded the "modern" skeptical medicine of the nineteenth century. That "modern" era was best exemplified by the Parisian clinical school of the early nineteenth century, which started to associate illness with particular sets of physical symptoms and treated bodies interchangeably. Essentially, by stressing the "modern," this view has been used to write Rush out as a serious figure in American medical history. Instead, he has become a foil used to show what "modern" medicine was not.

11   Fried, *Rush: Revolution, Madness, and the Visionary Doctor Who Became a Founding Father*.

12   "Benjamin Rush Portal – Home," *Benjamin Rush Portal*, https://guides.library. upenn.edu/benjamin-rush (accessed August 30, 2022).

John Harley Warner, for example, argues that Parisian-inspired empiricism and clinical pathology nullified appeals to rational systems like that of Rush, essentially erasing any long-term importance by the 1840s.[13]

Rather than assuming modern American medicine came only from a rejection of systems in the nineteenth century, this book argues that Rush played a critical role in the development of a self-identifying American medical community with specific needs and institutions designed for the United States. "Community" in this context refers to the collection of medical men who were educated in and/or practiced in the United States and recognized each other as legitimate practitioners of medicine. This excluded numerous other healers including family members, midwives, bleeders, bone-setters, and others who were more likely to be marginalized by race, class, and gender, as well as "irregular" medical practices. While far from central, these other medical people do appear on the edges of Rush's world. Within his narrow community, Rush's promotion of American education and local medical research strengthened connections and supported the creation of medical institutions and practices that turned community into profession. This book considers the late eighteenth century as an influential beginning for a homegrown American medicine. Rush's focus on physiology and the balance of the "animal oeconomy" necessitated local knowledge—both physical and sociological—which he believed could only be understood and appropriately synthesized by American practitioners.

This "American" medicine took for granted the uniqueness of American space—both physical and psychological—which required careful observation and original research by men of science (they were nearly always men). Medicine in this manner supported the growth of auxiliary sciences, especially botany, zoology, geology, and chemistry, which in turn provided additional information about American people, climates, animals, and places.

Medicine and the sciences that surrounded it shaped American identity. Rush's medicine argued that social situation and physical space impacted human constitutions and encouraged either regular (healthy) or irregular (unhealthy) actions. Understanding the American environment provided information about those powerful human-shaping forces and underscored Rush's arguments for Americans' physical uniqueness. In recent years, several historians have addressed the centrality of science in the creation of American identity. Lily Santoro's 2017 essay in *Pennsylvania History*, "Promoting the

---

13 Warner, *The Therapeutic Perspective: Medical Practice, Knowledge, and Identity in America, 1820–1885*; Warner, *Against the Spirit of System: The Impulse in Nineteenth-Century American Medicine.*

Book of Nature: Philadelphia's Role in Popularizing Science for Christian Citizens in the Early Republic," neatly summarizes the state of American science between 1776 and 1840. She argues that "the American context created uniquely American approaches to science" and that "Philadelphians promoting science for popular audiences emphasized the moral and civil benefits of studying the natural world."[14] Meanwhile other historians have noted the territorial nature of science. Natural knowledge was used at the turn of the nineteenth century to lay claim over vast and sparsely settled regions.[15] This project also, and more substantially, argues that Rush's emphasis on the importance of the American environment supported arguments for American medical research at the turn of the nineteenth century. This concept is indebted to Benjamin Park's work on Rush and Noah Webster. He addresses their view of the American nation as intimately tied to its geography and to physical alterations of the land. Jan Goliski and Katherine Arner likewise associate American self-fashioning and intellectual independence with the physical atmosphere and epidemic disease, respectively.[16]

In terms of methodology, this work shifts the primary source base away from published materials and toward manuscript collections. On the surface this may seem like an unnecessary difficulty. Rush was well-published and left numerous accounts in easy-to-read and often digitized print. They are, however, the polished work that Rush presented to the world rather than the somewhat messier versions of ideas in notebooks, letters, and lectures where

---

14 Santoro, "Promoting the Book of Nature: Philadelphia's Role in Popularizing Science for Christian Citizens in the Early Republic," 32.

15 Valencius et al., "Science in Early America: Print Culture and the Sciences of Territoriality," 73–123. See also Hindle, *The Pursuit of Science in Revolutionary America, 1735–1789*; Hindle, "The Underside of the Learned Society in New York, 1754–1854," 84–116; Greene, *American Science in the Age of Jefferson*; Ewan, "The Growth of Learned and Scientific Societies in the Southeastern United States to 1860," 208–18; Dupree, "The National Pattern of American Learned Societies, 1769–1863," 21–32.

16 Park, "The Bonds of Union: Benjamin Rush, Noah Webster, and Defining the Nation in the Early Republic," 382–408. Golinski, "Debating the Atmospheric Constitution: Yellow Fever and the American Climate," 149–65; Arner, "Making Yellow Fever American: The Early American Republic, the British Empire and the Geopolitics of Disease in the Atlantic World," 447–71. In some respects, this project provides an American complement to Mark Harrison's work in which he argues travel and variable colonial climates led to calls for rational and scientific medicine in Britain. Harrison, *Medicine in an Age of Commerce and Empire: Britian and Its Tropical Colonies*, 3.

he workshopped new ideas. I also relied heavily on what was said to Rush, to capture how the world viewed Rush rather than how Rush viewed the world. This book uses a sample of approximately 3,350 letters sent to Rush between 1768 and 1813 to better understand the networks he belonged to and his reputation with patients and colleagues while he was alive. This correspondence was donated with his personal library and that of his son James Rush to the Library Company of Philadelphia upon James's death in 1869. Most of those letters are in bound volumes in alphabetical order, prepared sometime during the nineteenth century. A few volumes were disbound and placed in boxes more recently. Some others specifically include the letters of especially noteworthy individuals like Joseph Priestley. The sample used for this project included 3,350 letters sent to Rush between 1765 and 1813. I estimate that this represents about half of the collection. The selection is mostly random; however, it does slightly privilege those with last names that start with letters early in the alphabet.

I also consciously chose volumes that were alphabetical rather than those associated with specific famous people. I did this for two reasons. First, to try and elevate the voices of ordinary students, patients, and patient family members over those of individuals well represented in the historiography. Second, this selection process hopefully provides a more accurate cross-section of what Rush's mailbox would have looked like. Yes, it contained notes from Thomas Jefferson and John Adams, but it also included people like Mrs. Mary, who gave Rush a chair supposedly made from Pennsylvania's Treaty Oak, or Thomas Pratt, a young doctor trying to start a new practice in South Carolina. This sample includes both the obviously relevant letters (like that of Pratt) but also the non sequiturs like that of Mrs. Mary to provide a better sense of how Rush interacted with the wider world. The figures below break down this sample in different ways to elucidate patterns of correspondence throughout Rush's life. About half of the letters were related to health and medicine. Others focused on his land investments, catching up with friends, and connections with family. In many cases letters do multiple things, moving seamlessly from conversations about the weather, to politics, to news about children, to disease outbreaks. This shift in focus opened new avenues for Rush research—including his views on gender, race, and his early reputation as an expert in diseases of the mind—and provides a strong base for analysis of professional as well as personal networks.

This work is a book in two parts. Part I, "Making an American System" examines the way in which Rush developed his ideas about health and society during and after the American Revolution. In this manner, it provides the foundation for the rest of the text and provides a quick review of eighteenth-century American medical thinking. Chapter 1 includes an early biography of Benjamin Rush with an emphasis on his educational experiences. Although Rush broke with some of his early mentors, he did stand on the shoulders of giants. He needed the ideas of his preceptors—especially William Cullen and John Gregory—in order to develop his own medical system. He also needed the social support of American mentors like John Morgan and financial support from Benjamin Franklin and his mother. The first chapter weaves the practical together with the theoretical in Rush's early life. Chapter 2 picks up where chapter 1 leaves off, around 1770, and argues that the crucible of revolution shifted Rush's priorities and ideas. It also addresses the key pillars of what became his American system of medicine. Chapters 3 and 4 break away from the chronological approach of the first two chapters and ask how and where Rush acquired his knowledge, the raw materials for a new system. Chapter 3 draws attention to the professional communities he belonged to and helped construct in the 1780s and 1790s. These organizations circulated information and lent professional creditability to physicians in the broader community. Chapter 4, meanwhile, returns to Rush's own work and his interactions with bodies. It considers his medical practice and how the categories of race and gender shaped his understanding of the world and ultimately his medical system.

Part II takes what Rush learned in Part I and demonstrates how he applied those ideas. As noted in this introduction, the application of Rush's system was varied and extensive. A comprehensive approach would take several books not one synthetic work. Instead, Part II looks at a few examples of how Rush applied his medical system and how it adjusted to the challenges of the American republic. Their order and content mirror the concerns of chapters in Part I. Chapter 5 continues the discussion of race and gender in Rush's published and private work and how medical theory came to bear on the roles prescribed for women and people of color in the American republic. It also considers how the American system understood and actively adapted non-American medical texts for the United States. Chapter 6 focuses on two characteristically American diseases: yellow fever and endemic goiter. In both cases, Rush looked to the environment and his network of colleagues to uncover causes and cures for diseases of specific geographies. Chapters 7 and 8 return to Rush's emphasis on organizations and institutions. The first, chapter 7, looks narrowly at medical institutions constructed at the turn of the nineteenth century. Chapter 8, meanwhile, concludes the book by focusing on Rush's image of the future through a medically informed system of education.

Part I

Making an American System

Overview

Historians of the American Revolution and Early Republic habitually remind us that the creation of a new nation did not occur in a day or even in the course of the War for Independence. The unfolding of a new identity, debate over the nature of the body politic, and psychological transition from subject to citizen all took time, to say nothing of violent conflict. In the field of medicine an analogous transformation took place from the late eighteenth century through the early years of the nineteenth century. A series of physicians tried to link health, illness, therapeutics, and physiology together into rational and self-contained "systems" of medicine. While they shared characteristics across time and space, the systems appeared to create a progressive trajectory for medicine, inching it from a focus on expertise rooted in tradition to one rooted in study and empiricism. While that progressive narrative appears false with hindsight it felt very real to medical men at the end of the eighteenth century. In the United States, these two transitions intersected and profoundly shaped early American medicine. Benjamin Rush and his contemporaries debated their new situation and the effect it would have on the bodies, minds, and spaces of their patients. This inspired Rush to become a systematist, one who eagerly compiled and organized information, striving to create comprehensive medical guidance for the new republic.

Rush believed American bodies needed a new medical system for the new nation. His efforts followed accepted thinking at the time that emphasized the interconnectedness of individuals, their society, and their physical surroundings. Revolution altered society and arguably the physical environment between urbanization in the East and American colonial conquest in the West. Rush saw an additional opportunity, however. A new society could also be molded to create a healthy population. Meanwhile, Rush and his fellow doctors underwent the same personal transformations as their patients. Coming of age as a physician and becoming an American were simultaneous events for Rush and his closest friends. While little of what Rush worked on would be considered modern public health there is no doubt that his work was designed to ensure the health of the public.

By the high point of his career in the 1790s, Rush had developed an American "system" of medicine that he viewed as antithetical to the one in which he had been trained and that proved remarkably flexible for his students. Rush followed the general pattern of systems and like his predecessors William Cullen, Herman Boerhaave, and Albrecht von Haller used observations in chemistry, physiology, and natural history to direct his theory of disease. Unlike earlier eighteenth-century medical theorists Rush actually used the term "system" to describe his approach to medicine, noting his dedication to a unified synthesis.[1] His work heavily emphasized the concept of unity and the reduction of the number of diagnosable diseases from hundreds to a handful of categories like "fever" and "mania."

Rush further described his system as "American," that is, designed to shape American bodies and heal them in cases of injury and illness. As discussed in the following chapters, the variable American climate and volatile American political system provided bodies with numerous sources of stimulus, both healthy and unhealthy. On the one hand, Rush saw the division of power in social and political systems as a good thing, modeled on the division of power among the body's organs and organ systems no single interest group could control the whole. On the other hand, variation could strike at an unfortunate moment and reverberate throughout the system. In the case of yellow fever, for example, the social and political failure to keep American cities cool and clean (from Rush's perspective) produced dangerous "miasmata" that interrupted regular organ function. For Rush, yellow fever in particular demonstrated the dire consequences of poorly managed physical space.[2] The consequences of yellow fever for American medicine have been

---

1   For more on the organization of medical systems see Barfoot, "James Gregory (1753–1821) and Scottish Scientific Metaphysics, 1750–1800"; Brown, "From Mechanism to Vitalism in Eighteenth Century English Physiology," 179–216; Emerson, "The Founding of the Edinburgh Medical School," 183–218; Guerrini, "Archibald Pitcairne and Newtonian Medicine," 70–83; Hall, *History of General Physiology: 600 B.C. to A.D. 1900*, 1969; Hamlin, *More Than Hot: A Short History of Fever*; King, *The Medical World of the Eighteenth Century*; Doig et al., *William Cullen and the 18th Century Medical World: A Bicentenary Exhibition and Symposium Arranged by the Royal College of Physicians of Edinburgh in 1990*.

2   Apel, "The Thucydidean Moment: History, Science, and the Yellow-Fever Controversy, 1793–1805," 315–47; Apel, *Feverish Bodies, Enlightened Minds: Science and the Yellow Fever Controversy in the Early American Republic*; Harrison, Contagion; Barnes, "Cargo, 'Infection,' and the Logic of

discussed from numerous perspectives and are outlined in chapter 6. Most agree that the fever was a foundational event in identifying an American medical profession.

The following chapters discuss Rush's medical education and the evolution of his "American System" of medicine. Chapter 1 focuses on his personal and educational background to explain why Rush became a physician and his early ambitions for a career. These early events created a foundation from which his system and ideas could grow. They also demonstrate that from his teen years Rush was primed to view the study of medicine as a useful profession for society that extended beyond individual health. Chapter 2 builds on this foundation and discusses how Rush's early career intersected with the American Revolution and War for Independence.

Chapters 3 and 4 move to the post-revolutionary era (1783–1813), the primary focus of the book, and show how connections with other scholars, teaching, and the everyday practice of a physician provided the raw material for Rush's medical theorizing. Chapter 3 emphasizes the role of network-building between colleagues, patients, and former students. This gave Rush a window into the anxieties and realities of living in the early United States from his vantage point in Philadelphia. Finally, chapter 4 addresses the material realities of treating patients and the connection between treatment and the new physiological theory Rush developed to explain American ills. This chapter pays special attention to the way Rush encountered and helped define race and gender roles at the turn of the nineteenth century.

Quarantine in the Nineteenth Century," 75–101; Coleman, Yellow Fever in the North: The Methods of Early Epidemiology; Pernick, "Politics, Parties, and Pestilence: Epidemic Yellow Fever in Philadelphia and the Rise of the First Party System," 559–86; Morman, "Guarding Against Alien Impurities: The Philadelphia Lazaretto 1854–1893," 131–51. Others have addressed the manner in which the disease confirmed the existence of a unique American environment. Arner, "Making Yellow Fever American: The Early American Republic, the British Empire and the Geopolitics of Disease in the Atlantic World"; Kornfeld, "Crisis in the Capital: The Cultural Significance of Philadelphia's Great Yellow Fever Epidemic," 189–205; Golinski, "Debating the Atmospheric Constitution: Yellow Fever and the American Climate."

Chapter One

The Education of Benjamin Rush

Benjamin Rush was both remarkable and ordinary as he began his medical practice in Philadelphia in 1769. The twenty-four-year-old son of a middling family returned to his hometown ambitious and fresh from the excitement of European capitals. He held a medical degree from the University of Edinburgh, visited London hospitals, and attended Parisian salons. Rush had come a long way in his short life. Before his departure, he already held a bachelor's degree from the College of New Jersey (Princeton University) and privately studied medicine under Dr. John Redman in Philadelphia. Such credentials proved more than sufficient to practice medicine in the American colonies. They did not, however, match the ambitions of the young Rush. He belonged to a generation of change that hoped to elevate medicine to a true, learned profession in colonial—soon independent—cities. As part of this promise, the Chair of Chemistry at the new Philadelphia medical school waited for him.

Over the course of the 1770s, the precocious young man successfully turned himself into a leading gentleman. His credentials placed Rush in a tiny minority of highly educated Americans before the Revolutionary War. The colonies boasted only a handful of colleges and no medical schools in the early 1760s when Rush arrived at Princeton's Nassau Hall. The individual lectures available from John Morgan and William Shippen Jr. at mid-decade did not yet add up to a medical school. Beyond his degrees and some personal charm, however, Rush lacked the kind of social standing he feared he needed to make it financially in Philadelphia. Degrees were one thing, but doctors needed patients. He had intellectual connections and proud mentors but limited family money. Additionally, as he began his career Rush knew his family saw him as an investment in their future. If he failed, he failed more than just himself but his mother, older sisters, and younger brother. Years later when completing his autobiography, middle-aged Rush looked back on his youth as one of economic struggle. He was the son of a gunsmith and farmer with a gentleman's degree; a Presbyterian in a Quaker and Anglican town.[1] Nevertheless, from an early age he wanted more than the financial stability his family craved. His ambitions took him first into the public sphere where he began to make a name for himself as a young man of strong opinions, both medical and political.

Rush worried about how he would make his mark and set out to be an exceptional physician *and* citizen in a revolutionary world. From the beginning of his career, he wanted to be part of the changes he believed were coming in science and society. In this way he modeled himself after the other famous Benjamin of Philadelphia: Benjamin Franklin. Franklin too climbed from the practical and artisanal "middling sort" to carve out a career as a man of letters. He also helped make Philadelphia the intellectual capital of the American provinces that could foster an ambition like young Rush's.[2] Indeed, Rush and Franklin met in London and continued to correspond and participate in the same organizations throughout the latter's life. But Franklin was far from Rush's only influence.

Understanding Rush's later medical and social projects requires a firm comprehension of his intellectual foundation. This chapter considers Rush's education and the way in which he absorbed and adapted medical and scientific knowledge for the creation of an American system and his own career. To understand Rush the famous professor and writer, this chapter goes back to the core of his intellectual development, in the early 1760s. Following his early education, Rush traveled to Scotland in 1766 and attended the University of Edinburgh, where he received a medical degree two years later. He completed his study abroad in London and Paris and returned home to Philadelphia in 1769 on the eve of revolution. Both in science and politics, his education left its mark on Rush's thinking and—more importantly—his actions.

Colonial Roots

On Christmas Eve, 1745, Susanna and John Rush of Byberry, Pennsylvania, welcomed their fourth child into the world. The Rushes were not especially wealthy or well-known people. John farmed, worked as a gunsmith, and

---

1   Rush and Biddle, *A Memorial Containing Travels Through Life Or Sundry Incidents in the Life of Dr. Benjamin Rush, Born Dec. 24, 1745 (Old Style) Died April 19, 1813*, 54.

2   Lyons, *The Society for Useful Knowledge: How Benjamin Franklin and Friends Brought the Enlightenment to America*; Wood, *The Americanization of Benjamin Franklin*.

owned a few properties in Philadelphia. He had a good reputation in business but was by no means part of the colonial elite.[3] Benjamin and his younger brother Jacob (born November 24, 1747) played in the gardens and woods near the farmhouse during the day. At night they may have been told the story of the "Old Trooper," their great-great-grandfather who commanded a mounted troop under Oliver Cromwell before becoming a Quaker and moving the family to Pennsylvania in 1683. The ancestor's sword eventually rested over Benjamin and Julia Rush's bed. In later years he pointed to it as a reminder of family history and lingering symbol of republicanism.[4] Despite their radical beginning, by the 1740s the Rushes were respectable Anglicans. By most accounts Rush's was an unremarkable early childhood. In the 1740s and 1750s the Rush children grew up the same as many provincial Britons during the Seven Years' War and enthusiastically supported the Crown and declared themselves British subjects. Susanna Rush, meanwhile, was from a Presbyterian family, the Halls, and eventually raised her children in that denomination with significant influence from the preachers of the First Great Awakening.

In his autobiography Benjamin Rush recorded little about his father, who died on July 3, 1751. Susanna Rush, however, survived John (who was her second husband) as well as a possibly abusive third husband to remain a dominant figure in her children's lives until her own death in 1795.[5] It was her guidance and resourcefulness that put her son in a position to attend college, apprentice with a physician, and travel to Europe. As a widowed shopkeeper in Philadelphia, Susanna Rush leveraged her family and religious connections to secure a good education for her younger sons (the eldest, James, died at sea when he was only twenty-one). In doing so she exercised what freedom she had as a woman without a husband and took the opportunities that she found to achieve some financial security, following a path relatively common for women of her situation and class.[6] They were also traits Benjamin found especially admirable and encouraged in other women and girls. Looking back at his childhood Benjamin wrote that his mother's "industry and uncommon talents and address in doing business commanded success, so that she was enabled, not only to educate her children agreeably

---

3   Rush, *The Autobiography of Benjamin Rush: His "Travels Through Life" Together with His Commonplace Book for 1789–1813*, 25.

4   Rush and Biddle, 223. As an adult Benjamin referenced the sword on occasion, and had it mounted over his bed.

5   Rush and Biddle, 228.

6   Wulf, *Not All Wives: Women of Colonial Philadelphia*.

to her wishes, but to save money."[7] Her younger sister Sarah Hall's marriage to scholar and minister Samuel Finley (1715–1766) proved especially important.[8] Susanna's ambitions and hard work paid off through investment in her sons. Both Benjamin and Jacob received a classical early education at Finley's West Nottingham Academy in northern Maryland, which started them on paths to the learned professions.[9]

Susanna's choice of West Nottingham reflects her careful management of her children's early influences and her commitment to her faith. Finley was a prominent figure on the "New Light" or revivalist side of the Presbyterian split during the First Great Awakening. He was also, of course, related by marriage. Educated at William Tennent's Log College, Finley eventually became the fifth president of its successor institution, the College of New Jersey.[10] Finley's religious qualifications were as important to Susanna Rush as his intellectual merits (which were also substantial) and kinship ties. By sending her sons to Finley, Susanna was setting them up to be well-educated, pious, and useful members of society. This blend of educated and evangelical thought was characteristic of the flavor of Presbyterian Enlightenment and eventually republicanism, outlined by historian Mark Noll. Rush grew up at the center of a new and increasingly "American" set of philosophies that embraced natural philosophy alongside religious commitments.[11]

As a sixteen-year-old college graduate, the next step on young Rush's journey was some sort of professional training. Despite spending formative years in the country, he did not have a future of gentleman farming ahead of him. Business, the law, the church, or medicine made up his main options in the mid-eighteenth century, and all required additional education, mentorship, or both. However, in one respect Rush was a typical college student, he did not know what to do with his future. Initially he arranged to study the law but was dissuaded by Finley. Finley (poised to take over the presidency at

---

7   Rush, *The Autobiography of Benjamin Rush: His "Travels Through Life" Together with His Commonplace Book for 1789–1813*, 27.

8   Fried, *Rush: Revolution, Madness, and the Visionary Doctor Who Became a Founding Father*, 22–23.

9   Manion, *Liberty's Prisoners: Carceral Culture in Early America*, 97; Rush and Biddle, 9.

10   The Log College was designed as a place to train Presbyterian clergy in the early days of revivalism. Bow, "Reforming Witherspoon's Legacy at Princeton: John Witherspoon, Samuel Stanhope Smith and James McCosh on Didactic Enlightenment, 1768–1888," 652–53.

11   Noll, *America's God*, 25–26, 65.

Princeton in the new academic year) suggested that his former pupil take up medicine instead of the law. The older man believed medicine was a more Christian profession and better suited his former pupil. Doctors tried to alleviate human suffering, thus doing God's work by caring for others. In this manner a good doctor had to be a selfless person who worked for the good of his (elite doctors were always men) fellow humans. Finley was less kind to lawyers, whom he considered too self-interested. The work of the law enriched the lawyer and elevated the wishes of the client above the community.[12]

Rush, therefore, began the study of medicine, not from a desire to advance science but to be of the greatest possible use to his community, follow a Christian vocation, and perhaps to please his surrogate father. Rush recounted the conversation in his autobiography:

> Before I took my leave of [Finley] . . . he called me to the end of the piazza and asked me whether I had chosen a profession. I told him I had, and that I expected to begin the study of the law as soon as I returned to Philadelphia. He said the practice of the bar was full of temptations and advised me by no means to think of it, but to study physic. "But before you determine on any thing [sic] (said he) set apart a day for fasting and prayer and ask God to direct you in the choice of a profession." I am sorry to say I neglected the latter part of his excellent advice, but yielded to the former, and accordingly obtained from Mr. Davies . . . a letter of recommendation to Dr. John Redman to become his pupil. On what slight circumstances do our destinies in life seem to depend![13]

Slight circumstances indeed! Rush's initial motivation is important. He was not drawn to medicine as a profession from a love of science or interest in the workings of specific human bodies. Nor did he think of it as an especially prestigious or lucrative calling (in both cases the law would have been better). He even reported an abhorrence of the sight of blood—not something one would expect from a man famous for bloodletting. From a young age Rush was interested in broader social issues and the role of his profession in the world. From the very beginning he saw medicine as more than the healing of individual bodies. Therefore, it should not be surprising that his professional and literary life wandered from topic to topic while remaining rooted in the experiences of human bodies and minds. Medicine could bring

---

12 Rush, *Travels Through Life, or An Account of Sundry Incidents and Events in the Life of Benjamin Rush born December 24, 1745 Old Style- Written for the Use of his Children*, APS, Manuscript Vol. I. Mss.B.R89t, 30.

13 Rush and Biddle, 18.

peace and comfort to others and model appropriate behavior. Both aspects spoke more to moral and social good than scientific advancement. Moreover, caring for the sick has a foundational association with Christianity harkening back to Christ's miracles. Rush's conviction that the practice of medicine could achieve larger goals only grew and took on additional secular meaning during his time in Scotland and participation in the American Revolution. Religion, and Finley's early advice, primed him to see medicine as a vocation worthy of a Christian gentleman and with implications that extended beyond individual bedsides.

Following Finley's advice, Rush returned home to Philadelphia, abandoned any aspirations to the bar, and began an apprenticeship under John Redman, a well-respected local physician who had graduated with a medical degree from the University of Leiden (one of Europe's premier medical institutions) in 1748 and attended lectures at the up-and-coming Edinburgh university.[14] Redman's professional history was grounded in extensive travel both in Europe and Britain's tropical colonies. Those experiences helped Redman stand out in an increasingly competitive medical marketplace of the mid-eighteenth century and gave him personal insights into how place shaped illness, a key interest of his pupil and many of their contemporaries. In addition to his medical credentials Redman was a particularly notable choice for Rush because they shared a religious background. As a fellow Presbyterian, Redman, like Finley, attended William Tennent's Log College prior to beginning his medical training, the first graduate of the institution to take his talents into medicine rather than the ministry.[15] Again, religion and duty to one's community were reinforced within medicine.

Like most young men before and after him, Redman started his career as a medical apprentice under an established physician. In his case John Kearsley—a respected Philadelphia physician—filled the role. After the completion of his studies Redman left the colony and began his career in Bermuda. While there, he gained experience with tropical diseases and learned to adapt his training to new circumstances, especially the violent appearance of seasonal fevers, which were gaining increased attention from

---

14   Reid-Maroney, *Philadelphia's Enlightenment*, 97.

15   Thacher, *American Medical Biography: Or Memoirs of Eminent Physicians Who Have Flourished in America to Which Is Prefixed a Succinct History of the Medical Science in the United States from the First Settlement of the Country, Vol. II.*, 16–17; Reid-Maroney, *Philadelphia's Enlightenment*, 97.

medical writers.[16] Decades later he leveraged this experience to treat the initially anomalous appearance of yellow fever in Philadelphia. Following his time in the Caribbean, Redman attended the University of Edinburgh and visited London and Paris in the 1740s before taking his degree in the Netherlands.

As a Presbyterian, Redman could not attend Oxford or Cambridge in the eighteenth century, a fact that may have been beneficial in the long run. He, along with other British dissenters (non-Anglican Protestants), looked to the rising (and religiously tolerant) star of Leiden for their medical training from the seventeenth century onward. Leiden, fortunately for those students, was at the cutting edge of Western medicine at the turn of the eighteenth century. A whole generation of Scottish medical professors—most of whom came from dissenting backgrounds—traced their intellectual lineage back to the Netherlands.[17] This genealogy entered the American profession, especially in the middle colonies through men like Redman and his students.

While in Leiden, Redman learned and adopted the medical system of Dutch physician Herman Boerhaave (1668–1738). Published lecture notes show that Boerhaave understood human bodies and complete systems that interacted with their surroundings mainly through their fluids. Malfunctions of that system caused disease and a restoration and maintenance of those systems created health. This general assumption was commonplace in the late seventeenth and early eighteenth centuries. In historian Lester King's words "it was Boerhaave's great virtue to fuse the old and the new into a well-organized complete system, blending fact and theory to satisfy the contemporary needs." That blending mixed the traditional four humors from ancient Mediterranean medicine—blood, black bile, yellow bile, phlegm— and a focus on the body's fluids as a source of balance with the new sciences of hydraulics, pulling from William Harvey's work on the circulation of the blood. Bodies required a healthy balance between the pressure of the fluids

---

16   Seth, *Difference and Disease: Medicine, Race, and the Eighteenth-Century British Empire*, 59–61.

17   Dingwall, *A History of Scottish Medicine: Themes and Influences*; Emerson, "The Founding of the Edinburgh Medical School"; Hamlin, "William Pulteney Alison, the Scottish Philosophy, and the Making of a Political Medicine," 170; Lawrence, "Medicine as Culture: Edinburgh and the Scottish Enlightenment"; Weidenhammer, "Patronage and Enlightened Medicine in the Eighteenth-Century British Military: The Rise and Fall of Dr John Pringle, 1707–1787," 21–43.

and the strength of the fibrous solids.[18] He also incorporated new chemical ideas into medicine, a path followed by Rush's Scottish preceptor William Cullen, discussed below, and eventually Rush himself.[19] All of this meant that Redman's teaching set Rush up to view modern medicine as a progression of one complete system to another as scientific knowledge increased overtime. At the same time, likely influenced by Redman's tropical experiences, he understood that locations had a strong influence on bodies and how they functioned. The unity of systems, philosophy, and religion set Rush up to look for that unity himself.

This transformation of medical knowledge fit well with the pupil-preceptor genealogy of eighteenth-century medical education. Apprenticeship formed a strong bond between mentor and mentee and provided important clinical experience and professional networking well into the nineteenth century. Young men depended on their preceptors to help them start careers of their own. Letters of recommendation and support stood in for more formal credentials like degrees and licensing, which did not appear until the early national period. Out of a sample of 3,350 letters sent to Rush in his lifetime, around 10 percent were letters of recommendation asking colleagues and friends to look kindly on former students just starting out.[20] This became all the more important as early nineteenth-century men moved farther and farther away from their own homes and personal networks to start a career, often in the South or West. Less directly, the reputation of a mentor rubbed off on students, either giving them a leg up in the world or a weight around their ankles. Physicians with generally good reputations like Redman, and Rush after him, could truly make or break their pupils. Additionally, some of the most valuable aspects of studying under someone like Redman in mid-eighteenth-century America were access to printed medical knowledge and practical experience with patients.

Rush's autobiography and letters detailing the experience of Rush's pupils show a bit of what apprenticeship entailed at the end of the eighteenth century. Medical apprentices remained under their instructor for several years learning the business and art of medicine. These young men lived with the families of their preceptor and were important contributors to systems of medical labor during the period. Apprentices mixed medicines, assisted their preceptor, and even saw patients (especially during epidemics when doctors

---

18   King, *The Medical World of the Eighteenth Century*, 60–68.

19   Christie, "Historiography of Chemistry in the Eighteenth Century: Hermann Boerhaave and William Cullen," 4–19.

20   LCP, Rush Family Papers, Benjamin Rush Correspondence.

were at a premium). During the 1793 yellow fever outbreak in Philadelphia, Rush's students treated not only patients but Rush himself. In a letter to his wife Julia, Benjamin spoke highly of Johnny Stall (who died of the fever) and John Redman Coxe, stating "when I add that as soon as I was seized with the fever, I committed myself wholly to their care and charged them if I should be unable to prescribed for myself, to prescribed exclusively for me."[21] Such trust—and hands-on experience—was the ideal form of interaction between preceptor and advanced pupil. Books could convey knowledge, but medicine was an embodied profession that required regular contact with ill patients to develop the skills and tacit knowledge required of doctors. Taking a pulse (with an emphasis on its quality and feel, not beats per minute), letting blood, negotiating prices, and gaining a patient's trust were just some of the skills that required actual time in a sick room. Rush spent six years under Redman living and working in the elder physician's home. All told, Rush spent more time working and living with Redman than he did in college and medical school combined.

In addition to learning by working at a preceptor's side, private pupils also attended to the business side of medical practice. Apprentices (both Rush himself and his own students thereafter) managed shops, filled prescriptions, and performed simple procedures like bloodletting in addition to their extensive reading. In his manuscript autobiography Rush wrote that "[i]n addition of preparing, & compounding medicines, visiting the sick, and performing many little offices of a nurse to them I took the exclusive charge of [Redman's] books & accounts."[22] A constant stream of seasonal fevers, injuries, influenza, gout, and smallpox inoculations kept Redman and his students busy. Rush remembered passing what down time he had in Redman's shop reading medical texts, especially Gerard van Swieten's (1700–1772) commentaries on Boerhaave's aphorisms and the works of Thomas Sydenham (1624–1689) on seasonal disease, especially the different atmospheric constitutions associated with plague in the seventeenth century.[23] Medicine was a vocation, scientific practice, and commercial business all rolled into one. These practices remained in place for years. A generation later, Frederick Augustus Hall

---

21   Benjamin Rush, "To Mrs. Rush (Philadelphia, September 23, 1793)" in *Letters of Benjamin Rush* Vol. II, 676–77.

22   Rush, *Travels Through Life*, APS.

23   Rush, *The Autobiography of Benjamin Rush: His "Travels Through Life" Together with His Commonplace Book for 1789–1813.*

Muhlenberg (1795–1867) agreed to study with Rush for at least four years and attend public medical lectures at the University of Pennsylvania.[24]

Rush's medical experience combined with his education (especially his familiarity with Latin) put him in the minority of colonial medical practitioners. At the end of his life, Rush's personal library contained several editions of publications by authors he read prior to his departure for Scotland. These included: Boerhaave's *Institutiones medicae, De viribus medicamentorum, Elements of Chemistry* (Latin, French, and English editions), *Libellus de materie medica, Dr. Boerhaave's Academical lectures on the theory of physic, Boerhaave's Medical Correspondence,* and *Boerhaave's Aphorisms*; and Sydenham's *Opera universa*.[25] With respect to the editions above, the

---

24 Rush died before Muhlenberg completed his education; however, letters between Rush and the young man's father Gotthilf Heinrich Ernst [Henry Ernst] Muhlenberg (1753–1815), the president of Franklin College in Lancaster, provide unusual details with respect to the educational experience.

25 Copies of the following editions can be found at the Library Company of Philadelphia as part of the Rush donation: Herman Boerhaave, *Institutiones Medicae* (Lugduni Batavorum: apud Johannem vander Linden, 1713); Herman Boerhaave, *De Viribus Medicamentorum* (London: printed for J. Wilcox, B. Creake, and John Sackfield, 1720); Herman Boerhaave, *Elementa Chemiae* (Paris, 1724); Herman Boerhaave, *Dr. Boerhaave's Elements of Chymistry* (London: printed for C. Rivington, 1737); Herman Boerhaave, *Elemens de Chymie* (Amsterdam: chez J. Wetstein, 1752); Herman Boerhaave, *Hermanni Boerhaave Libellus de Materie Medica* (Lugduni Batavorum: apud I. Severinum, 1740); Herman Boerhaave, *Dr. Boerhaave's Academical Lectures on the Theory of Physic: Being a Genuine Translation of His Institutes and Explanatory Comment, Collated and Adjusted to Each Other, as They Were Dictated to His Students at the University of Leyden ….* (London: W. Inny, 1744); Herman Boerhaave, *Boerhaave's Medical Correspondence* (London: printed for John Nourse, 1745); Herman Boerhaave, *Boerhaave's Aphorisms* (London: printed for W. Innys and J. Richardson, and C. Hitch and L. Hawes, 1755); Thomas Sydenham, *Thomae Sydenham, M.D. Opera Universa: In Quibus Non Solummodo Morborum Acutorum Historiae & Curationes, Nova & Exquisita Methodo, Diligentissime Traduntur; Verum Etiam Morborum Fere Omnium Chronicorum Curatio Brevissima, Pariter Ac Fidelissima, in Publici* (Lugduni Batavorum: Apud Joannem Heyligert, et Gaultherum Leffen, 1754). Curiously, Rush did not own a copy of van Swieten's commentaries from any date of publication. The only van Swieten publication included in James Rush's bequest to the Library Company in 1869 was a 1776 English edition of *The Diseases Incident to Armies.* He may have given the commentaries as a gift at some point or borrowed it from the Library Company, the College of

publication dates do not, of course, mean that Rush owned or had access to all of them prior to his study in Scotland. However, some would have graced Redman's bookshelves or those of accessible libraries in Philadelphia.

All the volumes mentioned above contained ideas that directed Anglo-American medical practice in the mid-eighteenth century. Medical texts, especially those attributed to Boerhaave and Sydenham, were common, even popular, in circles beyond the medical profession in mid-eighteenth-century Philadelphia. Private collections and lending libraries often included medical books on their shelves, which were accessed by literate men and women.[26] Boehaave's emphasis on the interactions of nerves and organs eclipsed ancient concepts of humors as central to human physiology. Sydenham's clinical observations of fever and epidemics, meanwhile, encouraged, and empowered doctors to make their own observations and conclusions.[27] Both approaches to medicine—the physiological system of Boerhaave and the epidemiology of Sydenham—had lasting effects on Rush's theory. He looked to the physiology of the blood vessels like Boerhaave and kept records of disease and weather conditions following Sydenham. But Rush had other experiences as well.

In 1760, no medical school existed in Britain's American colonies and few or no laws regulated the practice of medicine. This was starting to change in the larger colonial cities, like Philadelphia and New York, when physicians educated in European medical schools started to promote themselves as members of a self-regulating profession, preferable to the collection of other types of colonial healer. While a student of Redman, Rush borrowed money from his mother and attended some of the first medical lectures offered in Philadelphia—anatomy lectures from William Shippen Jr. (1736–1808) in 1762 and theory and practice from John Morgan (1735–1789) in 1765— the seed from which the city's first medical school grew. Rush struck up another important mentor-mentee relationship with Morgan. Morgan had also studied under Redman before leaving Philadelphia for the University of Edinburgh to attain a degree. At the time of their lectures, both Morgan and Shippen were fresh from European study and hoped to build a medical

---

Physicians (after 1787) or Pennsylvania Hospital library (after 1765) when necessary. It is also possible that James Rush donated, gave away, or lost books between 1813 and 1869. Books may also have been taken or gifted to friends and family during or after Rush's lifetime, a common practice in his circles.

26   Wolf, "Medical Books in Colonial Philadelphia," 73; Brandt, *Women Healers: Gender, Authority, and Medicine in Early Philadelphia*, 106–9.

27   Hamlin, *More Than Hot: A Short History of Fever*, 74–75, 82–83.

faculty similar to that at the University of Edinburgh.[28] Morgan in particular had grand ambitions for reforming medical education and practice in the colonies, as laid out in the 1765 publication *A Discourse upon the Institution of Medical Schools in America.*[29] However, with only two faculty members and scant resources in 1765, medical lectures were insufficient to help Rush stand out as a young physician wishing to start an urban practice.

With encouragement from Morgan, Shippen, and Redman—and some understanding of receiving a teaching position in the still-forming medical school—Rush made the decision to continue his education and earn an MD. Once again, Susanna invested in her son Benjamin and sent him to Scotland. To become the "American Sydenham"—as some called him—Rush needed to leave America.

Scottish Medicine, Colonial Student

As he prepared to depart for Scotland to take a medical degree on August 31, 1766, Benjamin Rush was steeped in medical theory from the end of the seventeenth century and the first half of the eighteenth century. He carried books by Boerhaave and Sydenham across the Atlantic and thought about physiological balance in terms of blood and hydraulics. Politically, he remained a loyal subject of King George III, although angered by Parliament's handling of the Stamp Act in 1765. Like his older colleague and countryman John Morgan, Rush returned to Philadelphia nearly three years later a different person. Scotland shaped his ambition and reinforced the idea that medical men could and should work to improve their whole communities, not only their patients. This early religious conviction would only be enflamed by the moral philosophy of Scotland's Enlightenment.[30] It also introduced him to new ideas about nervous physiology and disease nosology—organization of illness into genus and species—which he initially incorporated into his own thought but outright rejected by 1790. Whereas Morgan sought to formalize the colonial medical profession, Rush imported new physiology, politics, chemistry, and confidence in his own clinical observations.

In later years, Rush interpreted his education in Scotland as a political and personal turning point. With respect to both science and society he noted a

---

28 Rush, *Travels Through Life*, APS.

29 Morgan, *A Discourse upon the Institution of Medical Schools in America* (Philadelphia: Printed and sold by William Bradford, 1765).

30 Reid-Maroney, *Philadelphia's Enlightenment, 1740–1800*, 4.

shift in his attitude from privileging received knowledge to critical analysis, "this great and active truth became a ferment in my mind. I now suspected error in every thing [sic] I had been taught, or believed, and as far as I was able began to try the foundations of my opinions upon many other subjects."[31] Rush described an "Enlightenment" awakening of himself as a scholar and intellectual. This might sound like any twenty-something's political or philosophical awakening from living away from home for the first time or taking an especially thought-provoking college course. In part it was, but it also happened to take place during the Scottish Enlightenment, the beginning of the American Revolution, and with letters of introduction from Benjamin Franklin. Not your average twenty-something. Meanwhile, the "great and active truth" Rush referred to was that of republicanism. Despite a family history that included John "the old trooper" Rush of Oliver Cromwell's forces, the youthful Benjamin grew up respecting and admiring the British crown like most American subjects in the mid-eighteenth century.[32] Scotland, not America, could take credit for turning an apolitical medical student into a fervent supporter of liberty.[33] This context is important. Coming to republicanism in Scotland left Rush with strong convictions about the role of communities, patronage, and directing science for the common good. All broad aspects of the Scottish "Common Sense" school of the Enlightenment. Rush resonated with the broad project to better understand the world and human society through observation and use that shared knowledge to improve the human experience. In this form Enlightenment was almost a practical application of the scientific advances of the seventeenth century.

Of course, first he had to arrive in the Scottish capital and complete the required coursework in physic. Rush sailed with fellow student and friend Jonathan Potts (1745–1781) at the end of the summer of 1766. The two men arrived in Liverpool by mid-October and traveled overland to reach Edinburgh in time for the winter course of lectures. Rush and Potts were just two out of approximately two hundred American men who made a similar pilgrimage to the Scottish medical schools in Edinburgh and Glasgow during the eighteenth century. This migration in turn gave elite American

---

31   Rush, *The Autobiography of Benjamin Rush: His "Travels Through Life" Together with His Commonplace Book for 1789–1813*, 46.

32   For more on American support of the crown leading up to the revolution, see McConville, *The King's Three Faces: The Rise and Fall of Royal America, 1688–1776*.

33   Rush, *The Autobiography of Benjamin Rush: His "Travels Through Life" Together with His Commonplace Book for 1789–1813*, 43–46.

medical men (and the medical schools they established in Philadelphia and New York) a distinctly Scottish flavor.[34]

Rush tried to make the most out of his European experience by soaking up knowledge inside and outside the classroom. Between the autumn of 1766 and spring of 1769, he studied medicine, natural history, chemistry, languages, and politics in Edinburgh, London, and Paris. Philadelphia was an up-and-coming city in the mid-eighteenth century, but it lacked the institutions of the European capitals. The Pennsylvania Hospital, established in 1751 paled in comparison to the size and surgical expertise found in London. Meanwhile the handful of lectures Morgan and Shippen put together did not yet meet anyone's definition of a medical school. Rush's new experiences only enhanced the young man's commitment to a medical system tailored to the social and political realities in which bodies were embedded. Edinburgh may have moved on from Boerhaavian orthodoxy, but the systems that replaced it (discussed below) were designed by men with commitments to the association of bodies, minds, and spaces.

In terms of actual university attendance, Rush spent most of his time in Scotland sitting in formal lectures, preparing his thesis on digestion, and involving himself in the intellectual society of the Scottish capital. During his first winter he noted that he went to lectures in anatomy, chemistry, the institutes of medicine, natural philosophy, and the practice of medicine at the Edinburgh Infirmary. The following year he repeated each course and added one on *materia medica*—the common medicines used in eighteenth-century practice and precursor of pharmacology. Students like Rush repeated lectures in order to better retain information and fill out formal notebooks with gaps from previous years. The number of reptations varied from pupil to pupil. Historian Matthew Eddy has demonstrated that the manner of notetaking in Edinburgh was important as a means of recording, sharing, and transmitting information among students. Such notetaking typically involved students recording rough notes during class and later sharing recollections and committing them to more permanent bound notebooks.[35] Courses typically had printed lists of lecture topics (syllabi) but not textbooks, which

---

34   For more on the Scottish connections in American medical schools, see Rosner, "Thistle on the Delaware: Edinburgh Medical Education and Philadelphia Practice, 1800–1825," 19–42; Reid-Maroney, *Philadelphia's Enlightenment, 1740–1800.*

35   Eddy, "The Interactive Notebook: How Students Learned to Keep Notes during the Scottish Enlightenment," 86–131; Eddy, "The Nature of Notebooks: How Enlightenment Schoolchildren Transformed the Tabula Rasa," 275–307.

put additional emphasis on the importance of the individual and collective notetaking that monopolized student time.

Classes in Edinburgh certainly took more effort than the few independent lectures in Philadelphia. Recall that in Philadelphia, Rush only had the opportunity to attend lectures on anatomy and theory and practice with Shippen and Morgan. Meanwhile, during his time at Princeton, Rush would have focused on the classics and maybe some mathematics without any attention paid to the modern sciences. The breadth of the curriculum in Scotland expanded the subject matter that fell under the umbrella of "medicine" for Rush. The "allied sciences" of chemistry and botany were much more developed in Scotland than in Pennsylvania. In his future career Rush continued to consider medicine as a tool to address wide-ranging biological, social, and political issues branching out into educational theory, psychiatry, medical jurisprudence, antislavery, and temperance.

The short winter terms at the medical school were not Rush's only education. During the summer and early autumn of 1767 Rush furthered his studies in languages and auxiliary subjects. Despite his strong American education, he felt behind. After his time at Princeton Rush had let his Latin slide. In a 1765 letter to his friend and former classmate Ebenezer Hazard he apologized for writing in English after they agreed to correspond in Latin as a self-improvement exercise.[36] To remedy this perceived failure, he hired tutors in Latin and mathematics.[37] In Scotland, Rush claimed to enjoy his language work to a greater degree than he had in America and added to his study writing, "I likewise made myself master of the French language, and acquired so much knowledge of the Italian and Spanish languages as to be able to read them."[38] In later years, Rush championed the learning of modern languages, while downplaying the utility of Latin, and kept up international correspondence in both English and French. He also specifically argued against language instruction for young boys and claimed it was better suited to more advanced students as discussed below in chapter 8.

Rush entered the academic life of Edinburgh at an especially exciting time in the university and city's history. The mid-eighteenth century saw an impressive cast of characters hold court in Scotland's universities and salons. Edinburgh's medical faculty included John Gregory (1724–1773), Joseph Black (1728–1799), Alexander Monro, *secundus* (1733–1817), John Hope

---

36 Rush, "To Ebenezer Hazard (Philadelphia, July 27th, 1765)," *Letters of Benjamin Rush*, 16–17.

37 Rush and Biddle, 23.

38 Rush and Biddle, 23.

(1725–1786), and William Cullen (1710–1790). Cullen introduced the young provincial to new medical theories, an updated account of the nerves, and the theory of chemical affinities that set up modern chemical theory. Beyond the medical faculty proper Rush received an additional, informal education, in contemporary philosophy and politics. Like many American men of the revolutionary generation, Scottish Common Sense philosophy became central to his world view. Historian Mark Noll notes that with the rejection of tradition as an explanation for social and religious life, Scottish Philosophy—or the Scottish Enlightenment—formed an "intellectually respectable way for political leaders to reestablish public virtue and for religious leaders to defend Christian truth on the basis of a science unencumbered by tradition."[39] Scottish philosophy postulated that scientific work could provide the theoretical scaffolding for moral and virtuous society. For a young man seeking God's work in the temporal world, this approach must have been appealing. By the end of his life, Rush's library included works by influential Scottish philosophers, especially those with an interest in the human body and mind. Notable examples included Thomas Reid's (1710–1796) *Essays on the Powers of the Human Mind* and James Beattie's (1735–1803) *Elements of Moral Science.*[40] Both authors were key Scottish Enlightenment figures active during Rush's time in Edinburgh. He cited both men extensively in his psychiatric work.

Letters of recommendation from fellow Philadelphians Franklin and Morgan opened up crucial doors to the Edinburgh faculty and broader intellectual circles. In a letter home to Morgan, Rush wrote of the benefits derived from Morgan's letters of introduction noting, "[w]hen we [Rush and Potts] first waited upon Dr. Cullen and told him we had the honor of presenting him some letters from Philadelphia, he immediately answered, 'He hoped from his good friend Dr. Morgan.' After having read his letters he took each of us by the hand, [and] welcomed us to the College."[41] The wide-ranging interests of the city's intellectuals meant that the same societies and dinner tables might include medical faculty alongside economist Adam Smith (1723–1790) or philosopher David Hume (1711–1776),

---

39 Noll, "Common Sense Traditions and American Evangelical Thought," 218.

40 Rush's personal library included the following texts and editions: Beattie, *Essays: On Peotry and Music, as They Affect the Mind*; Beattie, *Elements of Moral Science*; Beattie, *Essai Sur La Poésie et Sur La Musique*; Reid, *Essays on the Powers of the Human Mind.*

41 Rush, "To John Morgan, November 16, 1766," in Letters of Benjamin Rush, 28.

with all participants comfortable in commenting on each other's work.[42] Occasionally, Cullen or Gregory extended an invitation to Rush and his fellow students where they were schooled by example in Enlightenment discourse. Rush found himself with additional invitations as well. Reminiscing on his time in Scotland he noted that he once had the pleasure of dining in the company of Hume at the home of Sir Alexander Dick. Of Hume, Rush simply wrote, "[h]e was civil in his manner and had no affectation of singularity about him."[43] In later years, Philadelphia developed a similar intellectual environment of societies and salons forming the intellectual capital of the new republic in the 1780s and 1790s. Rush was an early member to many of those new organizations.

Science, medicine, and politics in the eighteenth century relied on individual relationships, especially those with some power imbalance. Like the pupil-preceptor relationship discussed previously, established men often relied upon webs of influence and support from colleagues and especially from wealthy patrons. University appointments in Edinburgh were highly political. Although the Town Council ostensibly nominated and approved appointments, in reality, faculty were selected and promoted by strong patrons, usually from the nobility. Attaining a position at the university required familiarly and support of the establishment.[44] Hope, professor of *materia medica*, claimed to have secured his position with help from the Earl of Bute.[45] Cullen benefited from his close association with Lord Kames.[46]

As a result, Edinburgh professors were political and interested in questions of reform and the social role of medicine but were not radicals. This moderate approach that also believed in scientifically directed progress became foundational principles for Rush that shifted but did not break in later life. Rush emulated this approach to some extent and certainly took advantage of an introduction and summer spent with the Earl of Leven and his family in 1768. The acquaintance led to two significant friendships with

---

42 Golinski, *Science as Public Culture: Chemistry and Enlightenment in Britain, 1760–1820*, 12–13.

43 Rush and Biddle, 28.

44 Emerson, "The Founding of the Edinburgh Medical School," 184–86.

45 Emerson, 193.

46 Golinski, *Science as Public Culture: Chemistry and Enlightenment in Britain, 1760–1820*, 16; Weidenhammer, "Patronage and Enlightened Medicine in the Eighteenth-Century British Military: The Rise and Fall of Dr John Pringle, 1707–1787," 26; Jonsson, *Enlightenment's Frontier: The Scottish Highlands and the Origins of Environmentalism*.

the earl's children: Lady Jane Leslie (later Belches), with whom Rush had a flirtation, and second son Captain William Leslie.[47] The political situation surrounding the American revolution certainly altered relationships, but Rush did maintain some communication with the Leslie family and made sure Captain Leslie received a proper burial and headstone after his death at the Battle of Princeton in 1777 (Figure 1).

Rush also made time that summer to visit Rev. John Witherspoon (1722–1794) in Paisley, another important link between Rush's religion, politics, and profession. The beginning of Rush's association with Witherspoon was an education in itself. At the time the College of New Jersey was courting the Scottish clergyman to be the institution's next president after Finley's death in 1766. Richard Stockton (1730–1781), a fellow graduate of both the College of New Jersey and Finley's academy (and Rush's future father-in-law) unsuccessfully pressed the college's case to Witherspoon from his position as a trustee. Although interested in the position and feeling somewhat politically isolated in Scotland, Witherspoon hesitated to move his family (especially his unconvinced wife) across the Atlantic.[48] Rush credited himself with convincing Witherspoon to change his mind, in part by addressing Elizabeth Montgomery Witherspoon's concerns about the move while a guest at their home. It seems that unlike others Rush at least listened to her fears of moving, especially her fear of sailing so far. Beyond his attempt to make his alma mater proud, Rush greatly admired Witherspoon as a clergyman and a philosopher. He remembered the older man as one "of great and luminous mind. He seemed to arrive at truth, intuitively. He made use of his reasoning powers only to communicate it to others. His works will probably preserve his name to the end of time."[49] Witherspoon represented the merging of Rush's interests: a man of faith who also contributed to philosophy and encouraged the development of science.[50] Personal connections with leading figures of Scottish philosophy and medicine sparked Rush's transformation into an active and questioning participant in Atlantic Enlightenment on a scientific and political level.

---

47   Rush and Biddle, 30.

48   Rush and Biddle, 29.

49   Rush and Biddle, 29–30.

50   McCosh, *The Scottish Philosophy, Biographical, Expository, Critical, From Hutcheson to Hamilton*, 186–90; Noll, "Common Sense Traditions and American Evangelical Thought," 222–24, 227; Bow, "Reforming Witherspoon's Legacy at Princeton: John Witherspoon, Samuel Stanhope Smith and James McCosh on Didactic Enlightenment, 1768–1888," 652–55.

Rush as chemist is an important part of the puzzle as well. In a letter home to his friend Jonathan Baynard Smith in 1767, he described his chemistry course as "my favorite study, *Chemistry*. I know of no science in the world that affords more rational entertainment than this. It is not only a science of importance in itself but serves as a key to a thousand other sources of knowledge."[51] Rush the chemist is often lost in historical accounts of his life, and it is true that he published little of the subject specifically. However, chemistry never really disappeared from Rush's worldview after his student days in Edinburgh. One of his first published works was a chemical analysis of Pennsylvania mineral springs.[52] Meanwhile, the logic of chemistry and the search for fundamental characteristics of matter are evident in his physiology. His focus on the entity termed "excitement" is treated as a chemical characteristic, an affinity that bound all living tissues. It was the underlying property of all strong chemical interactions, and therefore all bodily reactions. Extreme cold, heat, acidity, or alkalinity could all be understood as possessing a large amount of "excitement." This was not a standard chemical theory, but it has the hallmarks of chemical thinking from the early "chemical revolution" Rush witnessed in Edinburgh. In a 1768 letter to Morgan, Cullen praised Rush and his prospects, stating "I expect that Dr. Rush is to be joined to your number [as a member of the medical faculty] & you will make a valuable acquisition. He has indeed applied to every Branch & study with great Diligence & Success, but Chemistry has always been a principal object & I am persuaded he may make a Figure in that Profession much to the credit of your College."[53]

Like Boerhaave and Cullen before him, Rush made the journey from chemistry professor to medical systematist, using his time spent on the building blocks of matter to understand their reaction in human bodies. Rush's time in Edinburgh expanded his knowledge of what might be called the "allied sciences" of medicine: chemistry, physiology, and natural history. In another letter to Morgan, Rush described American physicians as "8 to 10" years behind European theory, largely due to a lack of access to medical

51 Benjamin Rush "To Jonathan Baynard Smith," April 30, 1767, *Letters of Benjamin Rush*, 41.

52 Rush, *Experiments and Observations on the Mineral Waters of Philadelphia, Abington, and Bristol, in the Province of Pennsylvania.*

53 William Cullen to John Morgan (1768, copy), LCP, Rush Family Papers, Benjamin Rush Correspondence, Vol. XXIV.

society transactions from across the continent.[54] Indeed, lists of desired publications drawn up by the College of Physicians of Philadelphia in the 1780s
included requests for back issues of medical and scientific periodicals. This
need indicated the ongoing need for up-to-date information in the United
States and the difficulty of obtaining publications.[55]

The urgency Rush felt came from a profound sense of change within the
profession. Although Cullen and Boerhaave may seem like two representatives of the same tradition in hindsight, from Rush's perspective the change
of system from one to another was significant. He did not know a revolution
in clinical medicine would come in the nineteenth century, let alone germ
theory or bacteriology. What he did know was that his education felt dated,
and his Edinburgh professors seemed on the verge of a new medicine that
was undergoing constant revision and change. In the same letter to Baynard
Smith noted above Rush wrote that, "[t]he present era will be famous for a
revolution in physic. . . . The theory of physic is like our dress always changing, and we are always best pleased with that which is most fashionable."[56] It
appears from the letter and hindsight that the ambitious Rush had a fashion
change of his own in his sights, even if the theory did not yet exist. Medicine
was moving and he wanted to stay on top of it.

From Rush's vantage point the world did not look much like that of the
ancients, or even of his parents. When he was born, in 1745, physiological experiments, affinity-based chemistry, continued interest in climate and
health contributed to the growth of new medical systems.[57] While old books
could still be mined for useful observations the systems themselves could be
discarded and replaced. New medical "systems" competed in a marketplace
of scientific ideas and provided competing interpretations of physiological
observations. "System" is a slippery word in this period. Typically, it will
be used here as shorthand for a mode of medical practice rationally derived
from a set of physiological and ecological principles informed to a greater or
lesser extent by empirical observation and "pure" sciences like chemistry and

54 Benjamin Rush (1768), CPP, Scrapbook letters, Benjamin Rush to John
    Morgan.

55 Records of the College of Physicians [of Philadelphia], Vol. I (1787–1812),
    CPP, Manuscript Collections, Z10 227 v.1, 1787.

56 Rush, "To Jonathan Baynard Smith, April 30, 1767," in *Letters of Benjamin
    Rush*, , 41.

57 The best source to gain a sense of the rapid change (or feeling of rapid
    change) in Scottish medicine and society is Lawrence, "Medicine as Culture:
    Edinburgh and the Scottish Enlightenment."

physics. This fits most eighteenth-century approaches to medicine, but also those of twentieth century theorists, like Lawrence J. Henderson's biophysical system in 1914.[58] The idea of system was characteristic of the period. Although Rush and his teachers professed a dedication to Baconian experiment, they also adhered to the idea that bodies worked in accordance with clear rational rules.

Typically, a system was a mode of medical practice based on a set of physiological principles. By reasoning beyond the observable, medical systems took a physiological observation—for example, a muscle fiber contracting with the application of electricity—and used it to support a larger conclusion. In this case, because electricity caused the muscle to contract, a system might be implied by which living tissue is characterized by its innate ability to react to electrical stimulus and electrical therapy might make malfunctioning bodies work. Systems had the advantage of being logical and self-contained. Different interpretations of the same event, meanwhile, could spawn competing systems and encourage medical feuds. In other cases, physicians might borrow from multiple systems, adapting theory to what they saw on the ground. To make a mark in medicine ambitious physicians needed to contribute to its ongoing change.

Rush viewed himself within a version of medical history that positioned him at the cusp of a new medical world predicated on the hard-won progress of previous generations and healthy skepticism of past theory. This feeling impressed itself all the more on Rush given his own education. Boerhaave's work on fever, for example, exhibited a Baconian approach to understanding disease that American physicians adopted and used for nearly a century. The Dutch physician's study of fever located the defining symptom as a rapid pulse.[59] Rush continued to turn to the pulse as a source of information on fever even as he adapted a more complex view of the nervous system and allowed for a wider variety of chemical stimuli. Although he considered a greater number of states of the pulse to indicate fever than Boerhaave, Rush's focus on the arterial system and its alterations during illness do harken back to the system of his youth. It also included a Boerhaavian appeal to observation and simplicity. Boerhaave's definition of fever influenced Rush to claim that healthy activity could exhibit some traits of pathologies. Rapid pulse from exercise or emotion that resolved quickly was dubbed by Van Swieten a "true fever." Acute fevers, fevers that counted as diseases, arose when

---

58　Henderson, "The Functions of an Environment," 524–27.
59　King, *The Medical World of the Eighteenth Century*, 125.

accompanied by debility and could not be easily thrown off.[60] The "tables of fever" drawn by Rush's students demonstrate a similar principle. Despite the tabular name the diagrams look like two-dimensional thermometers with arrows indicating the cyclical movement of fever through various stages of illness. The "degrees" of the bodily system could correlate with the healthy course of the day or the pathological progress of fever.

When Rush arrived in Scotland, he learned the newer nervous physiology and chemistry practiced by Cullen held the potential to understand the body by bringing acidity, alkalinity, and affinities to the table alongside heat, pressure, and humidity. Often (as in the case of Rush) a synthesis of many ideas helped form a new system. He stood on the shoulders of giants, from Hippocrates to William Harvey and Isaac Newton, made all the more powerful with additional knowledge from Albrecht von Haller, David Hartley, Joseph Priestley, and Cullen. With colleagues on both sides of the Atlantic, he saw a bright future and a new medicine. As noted by historian Nina Reid-Maroney, this revolving door of new systems "caused no alarm" to Scottish and American physicians who readily embraced flexibility and uncertainty in their science.[61]

Cullen, provided a crash-course in the history of medicine in his textbook, *First Lines of the Practice of Physic*. This schematic of Cullen's history of medicine is not especially nuanced and lacks an acknowledgement of the work of nonphysicians and physicians in the periphery, whose work modern historians have recovered. Nevertheless, real or not, this is how Rush probably understood his own discipline's history at the edge of the American Revolution. Without an equivalent document from Rush, Cullen's history is the best representation of how Rush viewed himself within medical history in the 1760s and 1770s. In fact, Rush was so committed to Cullen's views that he arranged for the publication of *First Lines* in the United States in the midst of the Revolutionary War.[62] The history Cullen presented reflects a progressive and theory-centric view of the medical profession. In his description of the sixteenth and seventeenth centuries he derided both the Galenists for their reverence for the ancients and the Paracelcians for their overly empirical practice. Afterwards, he lauded the later seventeenth century as the dawn of scientific medicine alongside "science" itself.

---

60 King, 126.

61 Reid-Maroney, *Philadelphia's Enlightenment, 1740–1800: Kingdom of Christ, Empire of Reason,* 108.

62 Cullen and Rush, *First Lines of the Practice of Physic, for the Use of Students, in the University of Edinburgh, Vol. I.*

In Cullen's view, medicine came to the new philosophy slowly. Nevertheless, through the familiar narrative of William Harvey, Cullen brought medicine into the scientific fold. Nevertheless, from this short introduction to the history of medical science Cullen went on to critique some of his systemic predecessors. Of the numerous physiologists working in the seventeenth and eighteenth centuries, Cullen (and subsequently Rush in his own lectures) focused on three system-builders: Georg Ernst Stahl (1659–1734), Friedrich Hoffman (1660–1742), and Herman Boerhaave. Each of these physicians had an outsized influence on learned medicine of the century and, notably, can be associated with Dutch and German medicine, as can Edinburgh's medical school, which modeled itself on Leiden.

The first principle of Stahl's system (according to Cullen) was that the *vis medicatrix naturae* (propensity for living things to heal themselves) was "entirely in the rational soul."[63] This amounted to arguing that the soul was a characteristic of physical living things, essentially animism. Stahl's animism could claim to explain the workings of the body. However, its reliance on the concept of the soul eventually presented a problem both for physicians committed to more empirical investigation and for committed Christians like Rush who were uneasy about the theological implications of a fully material soul. Rush also rejected the idea that bodies were good at healing themselves.[64] Cullen agreed, writing, "*nature curing diseases . . .* has often had a very baneful influence on the practice of physic; as either leading physicians into, or continuing them in, a weak and feeble practice; and at the same time superseding or discouraging all the attempts of art.[65]

Hoffman was a different story. Cullen considered Hoffman a great observer of the animal oeconomy—physiological balance or metabolism—writing: "there can be no sort of doubt that the phenomena of the animal oeconomy in health and in sickness, can only be explained by *considering the state and affections of the primary moving powers in it . . .* we are therefore particularly indebted to *Dr Hoffman for putting us into the proper train of investigation.*"[66] Hoffman's focus on physiology, especially his descriptions of

63   Cullen, xxix.

64   Bassiri, "The Brain and the Unconscious Soul in Eighteenth-Century Nervous Physiology: Robert Whytt's Sensorium Commune," 425–48; Dyde, "Cullen, a Cautionary Tale," 226; Joseph Priestley, *Hartley's Theory of the Human Mind, on the Principle of the Association of Ideas; with Essays Relating to the Subject of It*, 37.

65   Emphasis from original, Cullen, *First Lines of the Practice of Physic, Vol. I*, xxxii.

66   Emphasis added, Cullen, xxxix–xl.

movement in terms of arterial spasm, became central concerns for Cullen.[67] Hoffman's definition of "fever" began with a dense consolidation of particles within the core of the body (like the center of a Cartesian vortex). That density resulted in the bursting of particles visible to the physician in the form of sudden heat and rapid pulse. Cullen left the physics behind but used the sudden action within the body, in his case the nerves based on predisposing debility, as the starting point for fever.[68] In terms of motion, Rush went even further than Cullen and adopted aspects of David Hartley's (1705–1757) theory of imperceptible vibrations throughout the body as the driving force in physiology, discussed further on.

Finally, Cullen discussed Boerhaave, the system Rush was most familiar with when he arrived in Scotland. It was also the system Cullen had learned and followed early in his career.[69] Cullen described Boerhaave's physiology as one that addressed the balance of bodies. Specifically, it focused on the state of solids (tense or lax) and the chemical composition of liquids (like blood). Rush emphasized the latter when he referred to Boerhaave's "unfortunate attachment to the fluids."[70] He called the fluid-based pathology "purely hypothetical."[71] This suggests that Cullen and Rush had a problem with Boerhaave's use of "lentor" and "viscosity" of blood and nervous fluid as an explanation for disease.[72] Cullen moved his attention to nervous spasm whereas Rush claimed that a disruption of regular bodily motions triggered fever. Both Rush and Cullen claimed numerous remote causes of fever including gaseous effluvia produced by putrefying matter.[73]

In addition to the systems of Stahl, Hoffman, Boerhaave, and Cullen, Rush incorporated the work of numerous other eighteenth-century physiologists into his own work, especially the concepts of Swiss physiologist Albrecht von Haller (1708–1777). Haller suggested that organs and tissues possessed properties of irritability (the power to respond to and create stimuli) and sensibility (the ability to respond to stimuli). Haller played a much bigger role in Rush's view of medical history. Rush used irritability and sensibility

---

67   King, *The Medical World of the Eighteenth Century*, 140.

68   Hamlin, *More Than Hot: A Short History of Fever*, 73, 128.

69   Cullen, *First Lines of the Practice of Physic, Vol. I*, xliii.

70   Hare Lecture Notes, Vol. I, KCRBM, Ms. Coll 225, Box 5, Item 9. Charles Greifenstein, "Benjamin Rush and the Medical Theorists of the 18th Century" (Philadelphia, n.d.).

71   Cullen, *First Lines of the Practice of Physic, Vol. I*, xlix.

72   King, *The Medical World of the Eighteenth Century*, 140–41.

73   King, 141.

as the basis for his own concepts of "excitement" and "excitability." He also relied on Haller's work on nerves to suggest that bodies were fundamentally excitable (moveable or living) entities. Haller's basic principles were widely accepted and adapted by medical theorists throughout Europe and European colonies.[74] In 1755 English physician Richard Brocklesby (1722–1797) replicated Haller's experiments for the Royal Society in London with success.[75] Nervous fibers and muscular reflex action or "irritability" pointed to an innate capacity for movement within bodies. Impulses sent from irritable tissues (especially the nerves) seemed to direct the actions of sensible organs. The eighteenth century saw the interest in the potential of the nervous system as an explanation for physiological function in Britain. Early in the century Robert Whytt (1714–1766) argued that the nerves helped unify the body and bring it into sympathy with itself.[76] Blood vessels conveyed sympathy while the nerves formed the seat of sensibility and formed connections with distant vessels and organs.[77]

The concept of sensibility and prevalence of nervous fevers permeated lay understanding of bodies by the end of the century. Outward displays of sensibility indicated a refined character. Hartley and Erasmus Darwin (1731–1802)—grandfather of the more famous Charles—hypothesized about unseen motions or vibrations in living bodies.[78] Both men inspired Rush in the United States to argue that such motions were responsible for sickness

---

74   For more on Haller and physiology of the mid-eighteenth-century more generally, see Cimino et al., *Vitalisms: From Haller to the Cell Theory*; Roe, *Matter, Life, and Generation: Eighteenth-Century Embryology and the Haller-Wolff Debate*; Reill, *Vitalizing Nature in the Enlightenment*; Mendelsohn, *Heat and Life: The Development of the Theory of Animal Heat*; Larson, *Interpreting Nature: The Science of Living Form from Linnaeus to Kant*; Larson, "Vital Forces: Regulative Principles or Constitutive Agents? A Strategy in German Physiology, 1786–1802," 235–49; Schofield, *Mechanism and Materialism: British Natural Philosophy in An Age of Reason*; Minter, "The Concept of Irritability and the Critique of Sensibility in Eighteenth-Century Germany," 463–76.

75   Brown, "From Mechanism to Vitalism in Eighteenth Century English Physiology," 180–81.

76   Bassiri, "The Brain and the Unconscious Soul in Eighteenth-Century Nervous Physiology: Robert Whytt's Sensorium Commune."

77   Whytt, *Observations on the Nature, Causes, and Cure of Those Disorders Which Have Been Commonly Called Nervous Hypochondirac, or Hysteric: To Which Are Prefixed Som Remarks on the Sympathy of the Nerves*, 33, 41, 82.

78   Priestley, *Hartley's Theory of the Human Mind, on the Principle of the Association of Ideas; with Essays Relating to the Subject of It*, 7.

and health although Rush reduced the power of the nerves themselves and argued that their primary goal was to perceive stimuli rather than to direct the actions of the body.[79] Rush was surrounded with ideas and inspiration for a physiology of balance. Where he began to differ from his British colleagues was in his dogged determination to see the stimulation of the system in the general excitement of the external environment as managed by a heterogeneous assortment of organs.

Systems and Cullen's history of medicine aside, Rush's Edinburgh education also exposed him to the work of John Gregory. Gregory's influence on his pupil was as much about the character of a good physician as it was about practice. The Scotsman's merging of moral and medical philosophy, in particular, appealed to Rush. As indicated above, Rush developed from student to professional during his time in Edinburgh. He expanded his knowledge but also his ability to question and think critically and philosophically. When he graduated in the Spring of 1768, after defending a thesis on theories of digestion, he was only 22 years old, still a very young man and not yet finished with his education. At the behest of his mentor Morgan, in September he and two companions began their overland journey to London.

Rush in the Capitals

According to his autobiography, Rush arrived in London in September 1768 and remained at lodgings in the Strand until February 1769.[80] With introductions from Franklin and John Fothergill (1712–1780), he attended dinners and meetings of philosophical figures and frequented the capital's salons. At these events, as in similar settings in Edinburgh, Rush absorbed new ideas about science and politics. Franklin became another substitute father-figure

---

79   D'Elia, "Benjamin Rush, David Hartley, and the Revolutionary Uses of Psychology," 109–18; Hartley, *Hartley's Theory of the Human Mind, on the Principle of the Association of Ideas*; Hartley, *Observations on Man, His Frame, His Duty, and His Expectations: In Two Parts. Part the Second: Containing Observation On The Duty and Expectations of Mankind*; Erasmus Darwin, *Zoonomia; Or, The Laws of Organic Life, Vol. 1*. The role of motion in a mechanical sense predated Hartley and Darwin, and theories like that of Archibald Pitcairn likely influenced the more "vitalist" motions of the late eighteenth century. Rush, in his magpie-like fashion, borrowed from across time and "schools." For the role of mechanical motions see Jackson, "Melancholia and Mechanical Explanation in Eighteenth-Century Medicine," 300–301.

80   Rush and Biddle, 42.

for Rush now that they had met. He even loaned the young man money for a trip to Paris and furnished him with additional letters of introduction for the French capital.[81] Fothergill, a prominent Quaker physician, maintained strong ties with Philadelphia and took an interest in the young man. Once a week, Rush had breakfast and conversation with Fothergill. The older doctor presented Rush with another example of how physicians fostered diverse interests.[82]

Rush followed Morgan's advice and furthered his education with hospital lectures in London, updating his knowledge of anatomy. Edinburgh may have been the center for formal medical education and theory, but the Scottish city simply wasn't big enough to support the size and variety of hospitals London offered. Anatomy lessons and clinical experience were best found in the imperial capital with thousands of available bodies for study. While in the city Rush attended William Hunter's (1718–1783) and William Hewson's (1739–1774) dissections, Richard Huck's (Saunders) (1720–1785) lectures at the Middlesex Hospital, and those of the physician-poet Mark Akenside (1721–1770) at St. Thomas's. Rush formed the warmest connection with Huck. The two maintained a mentor-mentee relationship for years, evidenced by their transatlantic correspondence. The elder physician critiqued some of the young American's early publications and tried (unsuccessfully) to find a politically opportune moment to put Rush's name up for election to the Royal Society in the early 1770s. Revolution and Franklin's fading star among some in London did not help Rush's case.[83]

Huck and Franklin also ushered Rush into London medical society by introducing him to Sir John Pringle (1707–1782). Pringle proved to be incredibly influential on Rush, especially in the way he leveraged military experience to promote medical improvement.[84] Pringle was also a physician closely associated with political power as a royal physician when Rush was

---

81 Rush and Biddle, 33, 42, 49.

82 Rush and Biddle, 33.

83 Richard Huck to Benjamin Rush (1771–1775), LCP, Rush Family Papers, Benjamin Rush Correspondence, Vol. VII. Delbourgo, *A Most Amazing Scene of Wonders: Electricity and Enlightenment in Early America*, 5–60; Lyons, *The Society for Useful Knoweldge: How Benjamin Franklin and Friends Brought the Enlightenment in America*, 132–33.

84 Rush, *The Autobiography of Benjamin Rush: His "Travels Through Life" Together with His Commonplace Book for 1789–1813*, 54. At another point Rush credited this introduction to Franklin, Pringle, and Rush, *Observations on the Diseases of the Army*, 305.

in England.[85] Both Huck and Pringle hosted "medical conversation" parties once a week in their homes, which the young man attended. At these conversations Rush heard more about the practice of medicine in Britain's tropical colonies, within the military, health challenges of cities, and ideas about the function of various organs and organ systems.[86]

Beyond medical circles Rush continued to involve himself in political and literary conversations as well. He attended historian Catherine Macaulay's weekly "literary coterie" and engaged her publicly in discussions of republicanism.[87] In 1769, when Rush prepared to return to Pennsylvania, she wrote that she would be sorry to lose his conversation from the "Senate" of her "republic"—high praise.[88] In an even more radical act, Rush attended a dinner served in Newgate prison for the detained politician John Wilkes (1725–1797). The dinner was arranged by Rush's friend and fellow American Arthur Lee of Virginia (1740–1792).[89] Rush was beginning to shed his monarchist sympathies and search for a more rational and divinely inspired form of government. As he would throughout his life he turned to bodies for answers. Rather than see hierarchy in natural systems, the balance and distribution of energy that characterized his medical system also provided an argument for republics in the book of nature. This idea even extended into bodies and the cooperation between organ systems in Rush's mature work.

In February 1769, Rush left London to visit Paris. He carried letters from Franklin that introduced him to the chemist Pierre-Joseph Macquer (1718–1784), the physicist Jean-Antoine Nollet (1700–1770), the philosopher Denis Diderot (1713–1784), and the physician Jacques Barbeu-Dubourg (1709–1779). Barbeu-Dubourg was one of the few physicians Rush spent time with while in Paris and continued to write to through the 1770s—although rarely on strictly medical topics. The short month-long visit was not particularly formative for the young man as a physician. He spent very little time in Parisian hospitals or working with French doctors. Rush had a conspicuous lack of interest in Parisian medicine even at the turn of the

---

85 For more on Pringle's association with the crown and political patronage, see Weidenhammer, "Patronage and Enlightened Medicine in the Eighteenth-Century British Military: The Rise and Fall of Dr John Pringle, 1707–1787."

86 Rush and Biddle, 32.

87 Rush and Biddle, 37; Rush, *Letters of Benjamin Rush*, 70.

88 Catherine Macaulay (1769), LCP, Rush Family Papers, Benjamin Rush Correspondence, Vol. XXIII.

89 Rush and Biddle, 38.

nineteenth century. Rather than being a time of medical improvement for him, Rush's time in Paris is notable for his absorption in political discourse, language acquisition, ethnographic observation, and chemical knowledge. With respect to politics Rush found himself in demand as an American during the imperial crisis. Barbeu-Dubourg introduced Rush to the economist Marquis de Mirabeau (1715–1789), who expressed his pleasure in meeting a friend of the great Dr. Franklin's and questioned the young man about John Dickinson's (1732–1808) recently translated *Letters from a Farmer in Pennsylvania* (1767–1768), which was making the rounds in Paris.[90]

With respect to medicine, Rush reported little of interest from Paris. While some hospitals were well-run by his reckoning, the Hotel Dieu was a comparative disgrace, "crowded and offensive. [He] saw four persons in one bed."[91] The absence of French, and especially Parisian medical thought, is glaring in Rush's later teaching and work. Moreover, his interest in the embodiment of individuals within their environment did not easily incorporate a view of bodies and body parts as primary units of medical analysis. In the end Edinburgh, and to a lesser extent London, set the tone for his teaching and professional pursuits. As noted previously, however, Rush's time in Paris emphasized not medicine, but other sciences, especially chemistry. He probably obtained his copies of Macquer's dictionary and Marie-Genevieve-Charlotte Thiroux d'Arconville's (1720–1805) work on putrefaction during his trip to Paris.[92] It is unclear if Rush met d'Arconville, however, he certainly shared a broad approach to the applications of chemistry with Macquer in the 1770s.[93] Both publications proved useful to Rush's chemistry lectures in Philadelphia and are cited in one of his first published works, a chemical analysis of Pennsylvania mineral waters.[94]

---

90 Rush and Biddle, 42–43.

91 Rush and Biddle, 44.

92 Rush's library contained the following volumes: Pierre Joseph Macquer, *Dictionnaire de Chyie, Tome Premiere* (Paris: Chez Lacombe, 1766); Pierre Joseph Macquer, *Dictionnaire de Chymie, Tome Second* (Paris: Chez Lacombe, 1766); Marie-Genevieve-Charlotte Thiroux d'Arconville, *Essai Pour Servier a l'histoire de La Putréfaction* (Paris: Chez P. Fr. Didot le jeune, 1766).

93 Lehman, "Pierre-Joseph Macquer: Chemistry in the French Enlightenment," 5–7.

94 Rush, *Experiments and Observations on the Mineral Waters of Philadelphia, Abington, and Bristol, in the Province of Pennsylvania*; Rush, *Directions for the Use of the Mineral Water and Cold Bath, at Harrogate near Philadelphia*.

Although Rush's European travels came to an end in May 1769, his work and research was only beginning. After a few months back in London he sailed to New York City and returned to Philadelphia overland. That winter he began teaching chemistry and based his lectures on the work of Cullen and Black. His mimicry, however, was not permanent. Like Redman, Rush incorporated his experiences into his medical philosophy and practice, but he also appreciated the difference between his situation and those of his Scottish and English teachers. America was as different from Europe as the tropical colonies. Rush's future endeavors sought to find the answer to the American medical puzzle.

The next chapter addresses the way Rush began to move from puzzlement to confidence. From his experiences in the American Revolution and the classroom, and as an increasingly prominent citizen, Rush built the tenants of what he believed to be a new system of medicine for the United States at a time when the term *United States* started to mean something.

Chapter Two

An American Physician

In 1785, Scottish physician and professor William Cullen wrote to his former pupil Benjamin Rush praising their continued friendship—and that of their respective universities—after the disruption of revolution and independence. Cullen noted, however, that he "must expect that the spirited exertions which have acquired your independence in politics will acquire the same in physic. The Medical School of Philadelphia as the chief of a great Empire must flourish more and more."[1] In other words, Cullen expected the medical men of the United States to strike out on their own and promote their research and profession independent of British concerns. Men like Rush wanted to make a name for themselves and their country, something Cullen understood. But it was more than just ambition that animated American science and medicine at the end of the eighteenth century. According to prevailing eighteenth-century medical theory, nations had peculiar interests, climates, characters, and therefore illnesses, which required experienced local and national physicians to interpret.

Cullen assumed medical and intellectual independence followed political independence. Just as the Scottish medical establishment worked for and within the structures of the state, so too, he thought, would the American. The two countries might participate as independent and equal members of the international scientific community and "republic of letters." Rush certainly tried to live up to that prediction through his extensive publishing, international correspondence, and unfailing self-identification as a republican. Nearly a decade later, on May 31, 1793, New York physician Valentine Seaman (1770–1817) addressed a letter to Rush referring to him as a "Republican in Medicine." Seaman further noted that with respect to the progress of medical publishing in New York, Rush would no doubt "be pleased with the . . . freedom of Thought [sic] & truly republican Spirit of

---

1   William Cullen (1785), LCP, Rush Family Papers, Benjamin Rush Correspondence, Vol. XXIV.

enquiry, upon a subject which perhaps has been too much fettered in the tyrannical trammels of great Authorities."[2]

What was this "republican spirit" that Seaman referred to? Both letter-writers used political language that leaches into medical discourse without serious concern or comment. Rather than fear the politization of medicine as we might now, Cullen, Seaman, and Rush expected independence and republicanism to alter their profession in the United States. For Rush, that republican form of medicine arrived in the form of stripped-down physiology focused on the regularity of a vague physiological entity he called excitement. This concept was easily adapted to the American climate and with an eye to checks and balances in organ systems. Rush saw republics in bodies as well as states. Following the book of nature, he focused his medical work accordingly.

In doing so, Rush and his colleagues modeled their language on the revolutionary rhetoric of the 1760s and 1770s and viewed themselves as an important component of the same project. Such a transformation, however, was not obvious. Rush began his career dedicated to Scottish medical models and anxious to be part of the broader British medical world. He ordered books from England, maintained European correspondence, and repeatedly sent papers to the Royal Society in hope of admission before the Revolutionary War. Disillusioned with his hometown early in his practice, he even contemplated returning to London in 1772 or moving south to the Carolinas in 1773.[3] Revolution and new medical challenges merged with his training, which saw medical history as progressive, slowly changed his mind.

This chapter demonstrates how and to what extent descriptions like Seamen's and Cullen's—which emphasized Rush's role as a creator of a new scientifically rigorous, republican, and American medicine—were warranted by looking at Rush's experience of revolution as well as his understanding of physiology, epidemiology, human variation, and American institutions. Rush's self-fashioning as a "republican" had scientific as well as political consequences in the years between the Revolutionary War and the War of 1812. To set the stage, this chapter discusses Rush's intellectual development before, during, and immediately after the American Revolutionary War, roughly the years 1761 to 1789. It considers his relationships with Scottish, English, and colonial medical authorities throughout the Anglophone world. Independence

---

2   Valentine Seamen (1793), LCP, Rush Family Papers, Benjamin Rush
     Correspondence, Vol. XV.

3   Richard Huck (Saunders) (1772–1773), LCP, Rush Family Papers Benjamin
     Rush Correspondence, Vol. VII.

did not mean isolation, but a careful adaptation and curation of political and scientific theories to fit an independent republic in the New World.

Rush and Revolution

After nearly three years of study in Europe, Rush arrived home in Philadelphia on July 18, 1769, and set up his medical practice. With the support of local mentors John Morgan and John Redman, he secured the position of chair of chemistry at the young medical school. By joining the new medical faculty Rush completed a group of professors and practitioners eager to bring the fundamentals of European (especially Scottish) medical training to the North American colonies. In addition to Rush in chemistry and Morgan in theory and practice, the initial faculty included William Shippen Jr. in anatomy and surgery, Adam Kuhn (1741–1817) in botany and *materia medica*, and Thomas Bond (1713–1784) who gave clinical lectures at the Pennsylvania Hospital. Bond was instrumental in establishing the hospital in the first place in the 1750s with Benjamin Franklin. All these men had some European training and all except Bond were in their twenties or early thirties. The youth of the faculty reflected the relative newness of such formal training in the American colonies. This collection of ambitious and competitive young men hoped to become leaders of provincial medicine in the early 1770s.

Young Benjamin Rush wanted to make a name for himself and build a reputation as a scientific practitioner. He did so carefully, fighting against long social odds as neither a wealthy man nor a member of a powerful religious group in Philadelphia like the Quakers or Anglicans.[4] Although Presbyterians like Rush were gaining a foothold in the city's intellectual and educational institutions, they did not (in Rush's view) have the legacy power and wealth to support one of many young doctors.[5] Despite this, by 1774 Rush could tell his friend Arthur Lee in London that his medical business "has exceeded the expectations with which I left London."[6] At the same time, his family still claimed his support and attention. For most of his extended Philadelphia bachelorhood Benjamin shared his lodgings with his younger

---

4   Rush and Biddle, *A Memorial Containing Travels Through Life Or Sundry Incidents in the Life of Dr. Benjamin Rush, Born Dec. 24, 1745 (Old Style) Died April 19, 1813*, 54.

5   Reid-Maroney, *Philadelphia's Enlightenment, 1740–1800*, 17.

6   Benjamin Rush "To Arthur Lee (Philadelphia, May 4th, 1774)," *Letters of Benjamin Rush, Vol. I*, 85.

brother Jacob (who was beginning a career in the law) in a household managed by his sister Rebecca Stamper. This system provided support for various family members, but also continued to delay his ability to marry and have children of his own.

In the absence of a small (or as it turned out, not so small) nuclear family, work became the focus of Rush's daily life. Like Morgan, he was impressed with the medical and scientific advances of European practice and missed the scholarly communities he had enjoyed in Edinburgh, London, and Paris. In this respect it is unsurprising that Rush became a frequent attendant at various societies and salons. After the revolution, he became a founding member of organizations like the College of Physicians of Philadelphia (1787) and Society for Promoting Political Inquiries (1787) in the city that acted as the intellectual and political capital of the nation. Unlike his colleague, however, Rush managed to avoid accusations of aloofness or charges of rocking the boat early in his career. While Morgan openly criticized American practice and professionalism, Rush busied himself by trying to carve out a space in the existing system despite his personal feelings.[7] In this respect Rush stuck with tradition. Throughout his career Rush and his private students continued to make and sell medicine as part of the wider medical business. Even when he moved away from producing his own medicine, his prescriptions influenced the work of local apothecaries. As a young man he certainly needed to establish a practice and make the living his family had helped him to achieve.

Rush needed a reputation as an effective and trustworthy healer as the first step to becoming a successful physician. Education helped, but so too did actions on the ground. It was one thing to have a degree but another thing to compete in an increasingly busy medical marketplace in a growing city. Without medical licensing or formal professionalization anyone could, in theory, set themselves up as a healer. Furthermore, not all ailments were considered sufficiently severe or appropriate to warrant a physician's attendance

---

7   In his 1765 *Discourse upon the Institution of Medical Schools in America,*
     Morgan argued (among other things) that American physicians should separate themselves from apothecaries and refuse to make or sell medication.
     This was the practice (and law) in London but had never been the case in
     the United States (or much of provincial Britain), where doctors often made
     more money selling drugs than dispensing advice. Hindle, *The Pursuit of
     Science in Revolutionary America, 1735–1789,* 111; Brunton, "The Transfer
     of Medical Education: Teaching at the Edinbrugh and Philadelphia Medical
     Schools," 242–58; Gelfand, "The Origins of a Modern Concept of Medical
     Specialization: John Morgan's Discourse of 1765," 511–35; Morgan, *A
     Discourse upon the Institution of Medical Schools in America.*

and cheaper bleeders, nurses, family members, and midwives filled in the gap.[8] Some benefited from belonging to medical families, like Shippen, but others needed to prove their value. Morgan spent several pages of his book recounting his background, education, and professional experience to demonstrate his value to the reading public.[9]

In his autobiography, Rush noted the importance of starting his practice among the poor (a tactic he also recommended to his students), which he claimed built his reputation and may have garnered some divine assistance. This harkens back to Finley's arguments about medicine being greater moral work than practicing law. By treating those who could not pay (or at least not pay well) Rush also gained experience that he sorely needed. He later helped formalize this kind of practice with the establishment of the Philadelphia Dispensary—a sort of charity outpatient clinic—in 1787.

Rush also relied on the recommendation of fellow medical practitioners, including both fellow physicians and nonphysician healers like midwives. In his autobiography Rush included a specific reference to his professional association with one midwife, Mrs. Patten.[10] He credited her with his early success—she referred him to her own patients—which is perhaps what led the mature scholar-physician to stress the importance of good relationships between doctors and women, if not midwives specifically. Ladies, he pointed out, frequently controlled which doctor attended ill family members and how often.[11] Midwives, presumably, had close and important connections with women and could become trusted sources of medical knowledge.[12]

Beyond the practicalities of running a medical business, Rush started down a path that would change the way medicine was taught and practiced in the United States. One path was through his role as an educator with the College of Philadelphia and its successor organization the University of Pennsylvania. Rush led the chair of chemistry from 1769 to 1789 and theory and practice of medicine from 1789 until his death in 1813. From its inception in the mid-1760s the medical faculty in Philadelphia had attempted to make medical education more accessible to American students and thereby

8   Brandt, *Women Healers: Gender, Authority, and Medicine in Early Philadelphia.*

9   Morgan, *A Discourse upon the Institution of Medical Schools in America,* x–xiv.

10   Rush, *The Autobiography of Benjamin Rush: His "Travels Through Life" Together with His Commonplace Book for 1789–1813,* 79–81.

11   Henry Powell, Lecture Notes (1809), KCRBM, Mss. Coll. 225, Item 7.

12   This is certainly evident in the social medicine practiced by contemporary Maine midwife, Martha Ballard. Ulrich, *A Midwife's Tale: The Life of Martha Ballard, Based on Her Diary, 1785–1812.*

improve colonial (later national) medical practice. While there, over 3,000 students attended Rush's lectures (with class sizes ranging from 29 to 370 according to Rush's ledgers), the majority of whom did so in order to practice medicine. The lectures, however, also attracted a small number of lawyers and members of the clergy according to Rush's personal account books. Medical lectures were "public" in the sense that any man could purchase a ticket and sit in on the classes. The fact that they occasionally did so is indicative of the broader interest in medicine and science in Philadelphia as well as the budding subfield of medical jurisprudence.[13]

Each year, Rush spent part of his days between November and April standing in front of a lecture hall filled with men attempting to gain medical knowledge. As in Scotland, medical education at this time was almost all lecture-based and involved a limited amount of basic scientific instruction. Those who did attain a MD needed to spend two years in theory and practice lectures (the same set of lectures repeated), a collection of other courses, oral examination, and completion of a thesis. During Rush's lifetime most of the College of Philadelphia/University of Pennsylvania students came from the Mid-Atlantic and Upper South, with the largest proportion from Pennsylvania and Virginia. However, by the early nineteenth century most of the United States and neighboring regions—including Canada and the British West Indies—were represented in medical school classes. This geographic diversity provided a shared medical language for American doctors early in the nineteenth century. It also reinforced the idea that American medicine needed to be adaptable. Men from Massachusetts, Georgia, and Ohio needed to be able to use the same education in wildly different regions. With only a few exceptions the men of Rush's classroom were American and established their practices in the new United States, with most students settling in rural areas. These young physicians spread Rush's ideas, and some kept in touch with their preceptor as they moved from one region to another during their professional lives.[14]

Another way Rush attained professional standing was by becoming what we might now call a public intellectual. By the late 1760s Philadelphia was already developing a collection of salons and societies dedicated to intellectual debate, social reform, and scientific discourse, including the American

13 Benjamin Rush "List of Students 1788–1803, 1804–1813," LCP, Rush Family Papers, Benjamin Rush Professorship at University of Pennsylvania, Vol. 106.

14 Naramore, "'My Master and Friend': Social Networks and Professional Identity in American Medicine, 1789–1815," 1–24.

Philosophical Society initially founded in 1743. The American Philosophical Society anchored a distinctly American form of intellectual community. Its focus on "useful knowledge" reflected its roots as a society of gentlemen, artisan-scientists, merchants, and professional men. This would have been a familiar space to Rush who was already accustomed to the mixed social, political, and scientific spaces of mid-eighteenth-century Edinburgh. Science was becoming a leisure activity in which those outside the leisure class could participate.[15] Colonial science in the future United States shared characteristics with other colonial sciences, including the collection and export of minerals, plants, and animals to metropolitan collectors. By the end of Rush's life Philadelphia (and the APS) would itself become a scientific center pulling knowledge in from the periphery.[16] However, the story of Philadelphia learned societies and Rush's youthful involvement add to histories that push back against the older colonial science model. Rush and his fellows had local ambitions for their work that could improve the lives of settler-colonists through medicine, technology, and natural history.

In the 1770s, Rush actively participated as a member of the American Philosophical Society. One of his earliest public addresses examined questions that were starting to take on significant political and scientific importance in the colony, questions of identity and race. In his oration on American Indians and their medical practices, Rush presented his arguments about the applicability of Native American medicine to European American bodies. Almost all of his information was second- or thirdhand. The oration was really a synthesis of preexisting information and stereotypes. Nevertheless, in Rush's hands that information took on a new and broader meaning for bodies living in North America. In addition to recounting concepts about generic "Indian" health, he also compared the customs of Native Americans and Europeans, especially elite British people. The reprinted text of the oration is discussed in greater detail in chapter 4; however, it is worth noting here that Rush argued even before the revolution that European-descended Americans were not the same as Europeans in Europe or Indigenous Americans. Rush essentially started to make a medical case for the kind of national and biological

---

15 Delbourgo, *A Most Amazing Scene of Wonders: Electricity and Enlightenment in Early America*, 155–122.

16 Strang, *Frontiers of Science: Imperialism and Natural Knowledge in the Gulf South Borderlands, 1500-1850*; Bolton Valencius et al., "Science in Early America: Print Culture and the Sciences of Territoriality."

identity his colleagues were making politically in the early 1770s. The Rush that wrote this was starting to become a revolutionary.[17]

Rush the man of science and medical educator took a back seat as political events came to a head in the mid-1770s. While the ideological work of revolution was well underway in Rush's head by the time he returned from Scotland, independence was something altogether different. War even more so. But both were coming, with political and biological challenges in their wake. At the beginning of this chapter both William Cullen and Valentine Seamen referred to the republican nature of Rush's medicine and work. Rush himself argued that any good physician was a republican because nature was full of evidence of the correctness of shared power. In the 1770s the young Philadelphia physician was slowly making a name for himself as a healer, educator, and decent scientific orator. Politics, however, started to take over his thinking as the decade wore on. Before the war for independence was won Rush would make friends with some of the leading figures of the day, influenced the naming of Thomas Paine's *Common Sense*, and take his medical mind to the battlefield.

By the mid-1770s Philadelphia was the largest city in British North America, well-connected to the coastal maritime trade, and relatively centrally located. In short, a good choice for the First and Second Continental Congresses to meet and discuss the imperial crisis. At this point Rush was nearing thirty. He had a reasonably stable career but was still young and enthusiastic about the possibility of reform and even revolution. John Adams famously recounted his first meeting with Rush outside the city. Some Philadelphians intercepted the Massachusetts delegation to escort them into town and appraise them of the delicate political situation. Rush did not come off especially well. He was too chatty and energetic to put Adams at ease. Despite the rocky beginning however, that meeting marked the first encounter of a long friendship.[18] Both men respected the other, were passionate about their views, and did not suffer fools. Not ideal characteristics for politicians, nevertheless they were dedicated to making change in their country.

Sitting in the center of the new American political establishment Rush moved from observer to active participant in the revolution. He tried his

---

17   Rush, "An Inquiry into the Natural History of Medicine among the Indians of North-America; and a Comparative View of Their Diseases and Remedies with Those of Civilized Nations," 1–68.

18   Rush and Biddle, *A Memorial Containing Travels Through Life Or Sundry Incidents in the Life of Dr. Benjamin Rush, Born Dec. 24, 1745 (Old Style) Died April 19, 1813*, 80–81.

hand at politics and was a representative for Pennsylvania in Congress—he signed the Declaration of Independence even though his term had not yet begun—and briefly served in the Pennsylvania legislature. The specifics of Rush's political activities have been documented elsewhere and don't have much to bear on the practical politics of republican medicine. Rush's republicanism, as noted in the introduction, focused on shared governance and actions by citizens to promote the common good rather than the specifics of partisan politics. This may be why Rush is notoriously hard to pin down in one or another political party. Many of his thoughts and actions lean toward the Jeffersonian, but his associations with Adams and Noah Webster, and his (hypothetical) love of order have a somewhat more federalist flavor. Ultimately Rush is more important as a cultural republican, someone who looked for a balance of power and checks on autocratic behavior in government, religion, nature, and even in friendship.

We can see this commitment in—of all places—Rush's personal relationships during the revolution. At long last Benjamin Rush married in the revolutionary year of 1776. The relationship between Benjamin Rush and Julia Stockton certainly had a political element. The personal is, after all, political. Not only did Julia Rush come from a revolutionary family—her father Richard Stockton represented New Jersey in the Continental Congress and was later imprisoned by British forces in New York—but their marriage itself was relatively forward-thinking and the two shared quite a bit of domestic power, forming their own little republic. They became partners in business as well as life. Benjamin and Julia discussed literature, politics, medicine, and the more mundane but no less important issues of managing a growing urban household.

Despite friendships with numerous exceptional women, including British historian Catherine Macaulay and American women of letters like Elizabeth Graeme Ferguson, Abigail Adams, and his mother-in-law, poet Annis Boudinot Stockton, Rush considered his own wife as the exemplar for female behavior and education. Unfortunately, most of Julia's words are lost to history and only about twenty letters remain readily available to researchers at the American Philosophical Society.[19] Most impressions of her come from her husband and are typically full of admiration. In his autobiography he wrote of her, "she fulfilled every duty as a wife, mother and mistress with fidelity and integrity. To me she was always a sincere and honest friend. Had

---

19   All of Julia Rush's letters have been recently digitized and made freely available by the American Philosophical Society.

I yielded to her advice upon many occasions, I should have known less distress from various causes in my journey through life."[20]

This statement is essentially a description of the partnership model of marriage promoted at the end of the eighteenth century. It was further modified in the early United States as the basis of republican family life and especially "republican womanhood." In this view, married couples were expected to provide mutual support, friendship, and advice. This differed from the more hierarchical form of marriage common in the early eighteenth century.[21] This new view was especially appealing in a republic where relationships based on absolute power were unacceptable. Spouses were supposed to share power while fulfilling different and complimentary roles in a family. This is like the way different parts of government worked together in a society, citizens supported their communities, and organ systems supported human bodies. Writers like Rush in the United States and Gregory and Macaulay in Britain (both of whom Rush looked to for guidance) actively promoted the idea of women as being the moral core of families. The postrevolutionary period also saw a more radical political critique of bad marriages as the result of masculine tyranny, critiques increasingly written by women as well as men.[22]

Some of what Rush admired about his wife is demonstrated in her wedding portrait painted by Charles Willson Peale (Figure 2.1). The painting emphasizes the traits of refined and educated femininity. For example, she is holding an instrument, which points to musical accomplishment. In letters Benjamin Rush wrote about his new wife to friend and former crush Lady Jane Wishard Belsches, he noted how he was struck by the quality of Julia's singing voice (reputed to resemble that of Lady Jane).[23] In later years Rush largely approved of singing as a healthy and practical accomplishment

---

20 Rush and Biddle, 127.

21 Appleby, *Inheriting the Revolution: The First Generation of Americans*, 169–74; Branson, *These Fiery Frenchified Dames: Women and Political Culture in Early National Philadelphia*, 13; Manion, *Liberty's Prisoners: Carceral Culture in Early America*, 77; Nash, "Rethinking Republican Motherhood: Benjamin Rush and the Young Ladies' Academy of Philadelphia," 189–90. Wulf, *Not All Wives: Women of Colonial Philadelphia*, 35.

22 Gunther-Canada, "Cultivating Virtue: Catherine Macaulay and Mary Wollstonecraft on Civic Education," 47–70; Gregory, *A Father's Legacy to His Daughters*.

23 Benjamin Rush to Lady Jane Wishard Belsches (Philadelphia, July 4, 1785), Rush, *Letters of Benjamin Rush*, 357.

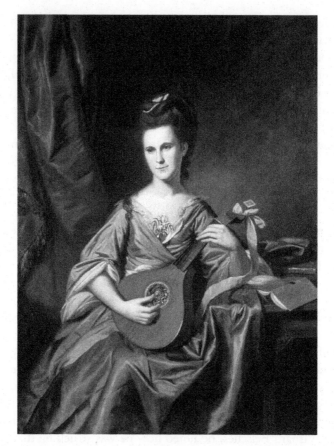

Figure 2.1 Julia Stockton Rush (Mrs. Benjamin Rush) by Charles Wilson Peale. Philadelphia, Pennsylvania 1776. Oil paint and canvas. 1960.0392A. Gift of Mrs. Julia B. Henry. Courtesy of Winterthur Museum.

for American women that exercised the lungs and could be practiced while completing other tasks.[24] To her left, however, we see books and paper, one book that looks like it has its place marked by being left open on the table. These items point to Julia Stockton Rush's education in literature and religion, which continued after her marriage. The family library was just that

---

24   Rush, "Thoughts upon Female Education, Accomodated to the Present State of Society, Manners, and Government, in the United States of America. Addressed to the Visitors of the Young Ladies' Academy in Philadelphia, 28th July, 1787," 80.

and Benjamin, Julia, and their children read widely and frequently. Such characteristics may have influenced Venezuelan revolutionary Francisco de Miranda's 1784 description of the young Mrs. Rush as "good looking and sensitive." While de Miranda used the appellation "good looking" frequently, Julia was the only Philadelphia lady noted for her sensitivity, a key marker of education for those considered enlightened and a trait increasingly associated with "good" wives and mothers.[25]

In a more sedate retelling of their first encounter, intended for his children, Rush claimed it was Julia's articulate admiration for a sermon by John Witherspoon and accomplished letter-writing that drew his attention to her.

> I had seen a letter of her writing to Mrs. [Elizabeth Graeme] Ferguson which gave me a favorable idea of her taste and understanding. It was much strengthened by an opinion I heard her give of Dr. Witherspoon's preaching. . . . She said he was the best preacher she had ever heard. Such a declaration I was sure could only proceed from a soundness of judgment and correctness of taste seldom to be met with in a person of her age [16 years old], for there was nothing in Dr. Witherspoon's sermons to recommend them, but their uncommon good sense and simplicity of style. From this moment I determined to offer her my hand.[26]

Both versions of their meeting, the one shared with friends and the one shared with their children, demonstrate the way Rush saw his wife as an ideal republican woman, an educated and pious partner, and an attractive healthy young woman. Until Benjamin's death in 1813 the two maintained a republican household, raised nine children to adulthood, and contributed to the intellectual community of Philadelphia as discussed in subsequent chapters. Their first few years of marriage, however, were characterized by war, uncertainty, separation, and loss. With British forces threatening Philadelphia, Julia gave birth for the first time in 1777 in Maryland, while among Benjamin's cousins, to a son named John (Jack or Jacky in the family). Meanwhile any joy must have been tainted by sadness. Julia's father, Richard Stockton, still suffered from ill health after his 1776–1777 imprisonment and Benjamin could spare only a few days with his young wife and son. Richard Stockton never fully recovered his health and died in 1781.

---

25 de Miranda, *The New Democracy in America: Travels of Francisco de Miranda in the United States, 1783–1784*, 49; Doyle, *Maternal Bodies: Redefining Motherhood in Early America*, 87–88.

26 Rush and Biddle, 86.

Politically, things were not going smoothly either. Rush's days as a politician were short when he found himself fighting against the more radical and even democratic trends in Pennsylvania politics. Rush was too sure of his views to move with the currents or compromise his feelings. Not long after his foray into politics and his marriage, Rush changed course and returned— for a time—to medical contributions, following his mentor John Morgan into the service of the Continental Army's medical department. Morgan had previous military experience from the Seven Years' War, but the realities of army camps and hospitals were new to Rush. Prior to his official posting, he took a keen interest in the organization and health of the army. Rush wrote to generals Anthony Wayne and Richard Henry Lee on multiple occasions about the role of officers in maintaining military health.[27] He also gained first-hand experience in January 1777 at the battlefield in Princeton where he treated patients, including the fatally wounded general Hugh Mercer.[28]

Starting in the spring of 1777, Rush served as surgeon-general in the medical department of the Continental Army supervising hospitals in Pennsylvania, New Jersey, and Maryland.[29] Rush continued his role as medical educator and private practitioner after his resignation from the Army in 1780. Although his military tenure was short—in part due to interpersonal squabbles between Morgan and Shippen in which Rush ended up on the wrong side and in part due to frustrations with the military itself—Rush looked back on his experiences often. Eighteenth-century wars could be won or lost based on health care. More soldiers died of disease in the American War for Independence (and in every other American military conflict before World War II) than from battle. Keeping the army as healthy as possible was a necessity and a never-ending task. Not only were army camps notoriously unhygienic, but the War for Independence also coincided with a massive smallpox epidemic that swept the whole continent from Mexico to Massachusetts to the Upper Missouri River.[30]

Despite these difficulties and the frustration caused by officers ignoring medical advice, Rush believed there were key advantages in military practice.

---

27 Benjamin Rush to Anthony Wayne, Philadelphia, September 29, 1776, *Letters of Benjamin Rush*, ed. L.H. Butterfield (Princeton, NJ: Published for the American Philosophical Society by Princeton University Press, 1951), 116–17.

28 Benjamin Rush to Richard Henry Lee, Philadelphia, January 7 and 14, 1777, *Letters of Benjamin Rush*, 125–26; 129–30.

29 Mitchell, *Historical Notes of Dr. Benjamin Rush 1777*.

30 Fenn, *Pox Americana: The Great Smallpox Epidemic of 1775–1782*.

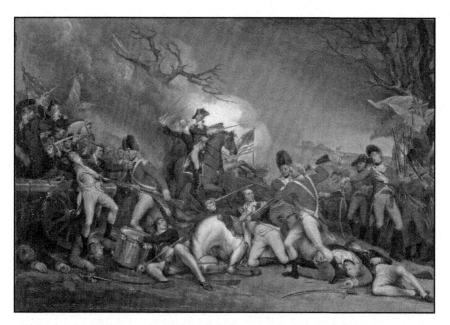

Figure 2.2 *Death of General Mercer* by John Trumbull. Courtesy of the Yale University Art Gallery.

Outside of hospital practice, military medicine was one of the only locations in which physicians were able to treat multiple patients at a time, see multiple cases of the same illness, and have more control over those bodies. Additionally, army camps, movement, and the stress of battle all acted as environmental causes of illness from the perspective of late-eighteenth-century medicine. This is especially evident in Pringle's work discussed in later chapters. As noted above, in-home care was a negotiated experience between physicians, patients, and patient family members. As head of the middle department of the Army medical establishment Rush was able to exert control over bodies, collect information, and attempted to standardize medical practice. He promoted the use of William Cullen's theories and even arranged for an American printing of *First Lines* as discussed at the top of this chapter. Perhaps most important, however, Rush met Americans from all parts of the country. His encounters with men from New England, New York, and the South left him with an appreciation for the variability of the country. Even small things, like Virginian's affinity for salted meat, found their way into lectures and publications focused on variability as a key

American characteristic.[31] After the revolution, Rush took what he learned from military and civilian practice and started to think about the brave new world of an independent and republican United States.

An American System of Medicine

Between 1780 and 1790, Rush's views on human physiology evolved. These alterations came out of his experiences with bodies and places as well as politics over the course of the 1770s and 1780s. The world had indeed been turned upside down and medicine along with it. Variation became the watchword of American medicine following the revolutionary war. The climate varied, form of government varied, and society seemed on the move. Regardless of how "revolutionary" or "radical" the events between 1765 and 1783 were or were not for Americans living through those years, the very foundations of their society shifted beneath them. Many aspects of social and political life were up for debate and examination from the institution of slavery, to voting rights, to the rights of women. It was a time both energizing and frightening in its possibility and medicine was not immune. Despite his education steeped in Boerhaave and Cullen, Rush hedged his devotion to any specific form of practice from as early as 1772. In his characteristic blending of science and religion the young chemistry professor wrote the following in his dedication of the short work *Sermons to the Rich and Studious, on Temperance and Exercise with a Dedication to Dr. Cadogan.*

> It is with pleasure we now see the same freedom of enquiry extending itself to medicine, which has long prevailed religion. While the common people reject infallibility in the head of the church, and a sovereign efficacy in a few rites and ceremonies, they have unhappily remained enslaved to the infallibility of medicine, or a few trifling prescriptions, which are as unequal to the expectations of the vulgar in curing diseases, as a wafer or extreme-unction are to expiate their sins.[32]

In this passage, Rush compares the over-devotion to any one medical system, or simply the authority of past practice, to the practices of the Catholic Church. As a dissenting Protestant, he viewed religious ritual and concepts

---

31   Rush, "The Result of Observations Made upon the Diseases Which Occurred in the Military Hospitals of the United States, during the Revolutionary War," 267–76.

32   Rush, *Sermons to the Rich and Studious, on Temperance and Exercise with a Dedication to Dr. Cadogan.*

like the infallibility of the Pope as dated, incorrect, and harmful. Likening medicine to such an institution was certainly an insult. Moreover, religion, politics, and health merged for Rush. In his discussion of Rush's religious views historian Mark Noll argues that for the Philadelphian religious and political faith "became one" during the revolutionary era.[33] Rush found support for republican values of balance, sobriety, and moderation in his Christian faith. He also found support in human bodies which maintain health via those same Protestant and republican values.

For an example, Rush referenced Cadogan's *Dissertation on the Gout, and all Chronic Diseases,* in which the British physician emphasized the role of temperate living and healthy labor in maintaining health. It is not a system-heavy text but presents its information in an accessible and direct manner. Cadogan also argued that all chronic diseases were alike and from the same cause writing, "the real original causes of all chronic diseases . . . may very fairly be reduced to these three: Indolence, Intemperance, and Vexation."[34] In style and in his search for the causes of disease Rush was similar to Cadogan. He argued that all fevers were ultimately the same and eventually all diseases from the same causes. Rush also looked to personal behavior and habit as a (although not *the*) determinant of health.[35] Despite the strong supporting language for Cadogan and condemnation of unnamed systems, this alone does not mean Rush broke with all prior medical knowledge. It does mean, however, that Rush saw himself as part of a profession defined by change both across time and space.

As noted in the previous chapter, to physicians of the late eighteenth century their profession did not feel static. New books, variations on past practices, and new locations continued to shift the profession from one system

---

33 Noll, *America's God: From Jonathan Edwards to Abraham Lincoln,* 65.

34 Cadogan, *Dissertation on the Gout, and All Chronic Diseases, Jointly Considered, As Proceeding from the Same Causes; What Those Causes Are; and A Rational and Natural Method of Cure Proposed,* 4.

35 The dedication to Cadogan—not a figure typically connected to Rush–shows that the American physician read multiple medical writers and from the 1770s onward comfortably borrowed ideas and attitudes that seemed to fit his own experiences. The same package from London bookseller Edward Dilly that brought Cadogan's work to Rush in 1771 also carried John Aikin's *Observations on the external use of preparation of Lead* (1771) and Donald Monro's *A Treatise on Mineral Waters, in two volumes* (1770). Edward and his brother Charles were acquaintances from London and became Rush's British publishers in later years. Fried, *Rush: Revolution, Madness, and the Visionary Doctor Who Became a Founding Father.*

of thought to another or none at all. This was especially the case in colonial practice. Mark Harrison has deftly identified the manner in which reform entered medical practice of the eighteenth century and how colonial practitioners were drivers of change in the profession. Rush's experiences and expressions of the need for a new system of practice demonstrate a similar tendency in the United States that Harrison identifies in the tropics.[36] Rush, like most of his colleagues and mentors, also adopted a neo-Hippocratic worldview acknowledging the connection between bodies and their physical and psychological environments. Reinforced by readings like Montesquieu's *Spirit of Laws*, revolution in society seemed like an obvious cause for revolution in medical education and care.[37]

Rush never set out a clear manifesto for his new system (which probably dates from the late 1780s based on student notes). However, he did mention his system at various points and several key characteristics are prevalent across his notes, student notebooks (from 1789–1813), and published texts (notably his lectures on animal life). Those key characteristics of Rush's view were: (1) bodies worked or malfunctioned based on the state of their environment, (2) all organs had distinctive roles to play in the maintenance of healthy balance, and (3) the American environment was unique and therefore provided unique challenges to human bodies. Together they reinforced a sense of natural republicanism. Nobody was isolated from its surroundings and within human bodies life and health relied upon different organ systems working together toward a common goal, not unlike the different states or branches of government that needed to function in a political republic. Meanwhile, he actively described other systems as monarchies. One student recorded Rush's argument against "monarchical" views of medicine, "Dr Cullen considered them [nerves] as Monarch to the System I conceive them acting a much more humble part they are only door-keepers or Messengers to the Bloodvessels, while the bloodvessels may be considered as the Centinels [sic] of the System."[38] Human bodies in Rush's view were the very model of good republics.

Rush described his work as a revolution in medicine, a self-conscious connection to the political and social aspects of the American Revolution. However, an evolution may be a more accurate term from the perspective of medical history. The idea that weather and bodies were linked had ancient

36 Harrison, *Medicine in an Age of Commerce and Empire: Britian and Its Tropical Colonies.*

37 Montésquieu, *The Spirit of Laws.*

38 Hare, Vol. I (1796), KCRBM, Ms. Coll. 225, Item 9.

roots and was ascendant during the eighteenth century.[39] In the new United States, however, these principles called medical men to trust their own observations and apply their knowledge to strengthening the republic.

Of course bodily republics, like political ones, required care, maintenance, and management. Like Cullen, Rush had a very dubious view of *vix medicatrix naturae*, the healing power of nature. Nature for Rush could be wrong, impotent, or even capricious. In short, the benevolence of God did not always extend to his creation even if his reason could be divined through it. Rush's vision of nature is often synonymous with wildness or wilderness. In nature the actions of living and nonliving entities were left without regulation or good management. The importance of improving or managing space had a long history in North America as a sign of use, ownership, and "civilization"; so too did a fear of the wilderness. Rush's view of nature as capricious, or a world out of sync with its own best interest reflects the Biblical concept of an imperfect world after the Fall in Genesis. Nature held within it the possibility of perfection (with intervention) but, left on its own, nature remained an untrustworthy ally. So too were one's own assumptions about the world. In his work on public punishments, Rush wrote, "in medicine . . . we perceive many instances of the want of relation between the apparent cause and effect . . . Cause and effect appear to be related in philosophy, like the objects of chymistry. Similar bodies often repel each other, while bodies that are dissimilar . . . often unite together . . . we can discover these chymical relations only by experiment."[40] In other words, things we might assume

---

39   Adamson, "'The Languor of the Hot Weather': Everyday Perspectives on Weather and Climate in Colonial Bombay, 1819–1828," 145; Chakrabarti, "'Neither of Meate nor Drinke, but What the Doctor Alloweth': Medicine amidst War and Commerce in Eighteenth-Century Madras.," 1–38; Chard, "Lassitude and Revival in the Warm South: Relaxing and Exciting Travel, 1750–1830"; Deacon, "The Politics of Medical Topograhy: Seeking Healthiness at the Cape during the Nineteenth Century," 279–97; Glacken, *Traces on the Rhodian Shore: Nature and Culture in Western Thought from Ancient Times to the End of the Eighteenth Century*; Harrison, *Medicine in an Age of Commerce and Empire: Britian and Its Tropical Colonies*; Harrison, *Climates & Constitutions: Health, Race, Environment and British Imperialism in India, 1600-1850*; Harrison, "'The Tender Frame of Man': Disease, Climate, and Racial Difference in India and the West Indies, 1760–1860," 68–93; Jepson, "Of Soil, Situation, and Salubrity: Medical Topography and Medical Officers in Early Nineteenth-Century British India," 137–55; Riley, *The Eighteenth-Century Campaign to Avoid Disease*.

40   Rush, *An Enquiry into the Effects of Public Punishments upon Criminals and upon Society: Read in the Society for Promoting Political Enquiries, Convened at*

(like the attraction of like particles) might be very wrong when subjected to experiment. So too, Rush reasoned, might proper treatments for disease. Symptoms could be tricky and appear in a location distant from the affected part as a result of internal circulations and sympathies.

To "improve" human bodies—a concept central to the Scottish Enlightenment theories he encountered as a medical student—Rush believed that he needed to understand their underlying principles and alter them to restore health. He concluded that bodies possessed a certain amount of "excitement," which required stimulus to keep up and maintain health. Rush was never specific about what excitement was or its source. Often it was described as a fluid that entered and moved around bodies analogous to electricity (in the late-eighteenth century understanding of the term).[41] At other times it acted more like a category under which various forms of chemical, physical, or psychological activity could be found. In this, he benefited from the work of another Cullen student, John Brown. The Brunonian system— as it came to be known—emphasized the use of stimulants like alcohol to treat most diseases and argued that bodies needed a constant supply of external stimulus.[42]

Rush actively distanced his system from that of Brown. On one hand, they shared a vocabulary and desire to simplify disease concepts. Both Brown and Rush set their views in opposition to the nosology—or disease classification—of Cullen and others. Rather than name diseases, Rush and Brown focused on broader categories of disease and fever generally. That, however, is where the similarities largely end. Therapeutically the two diverged over the use of stimulating versus depressing remedies. Brown's system usually called for the added stimulus of alcohol or opium (not to be confused with their classification as depressants in modern pharmacology). Rush, on the other hand, tended to favor treatments that would reduce excitement in bodies

---

the House of His Excellency Benjamin Franklin, Esquire in Philadelphia, March 9th, 1787, 3–4.

41   Delbourgo, A Most Amazing Scene of Wonders: Electricity and Enlightenment in Early America.

42   Barfoot, "Brunonianism under the Bed: An Alternative to University Medicine in Edinburgh in the 1780s," 22–45; Hinds, "Dr. Rush and Mr. Peale: The Figure of the Animal in Late Eighteenth-Century Medical Discourse," 645. King, The Medical World of the Eighteenth Century, 143–47; Neubauer, "Dr. John Brown (1735-88) and Early German Romanticism," 369. Brown's ideas were taken up by German Romantics, especially Schelling as discussed by Neubauer and Risse, "Schelling, 'Naturphilosophie' and John Brown's System of Medicine," 321–34.

like bloodletting, purges, and very low diets (food with little seasoning, little meat, and small portions). This was not because Rush believed bodies were overstimulated in a diseased state but because they were irregularly excited. By reducing the body's system, the physician could restore regular motions during convalescence. This focus on regularity or quality of stimulus over quantity is in large part derived from Rush's interpretation of David Hartley's psychology, which described imperceptible motions in the brain as the cause of its function. Rush argued that the action of the blood stimulated the arteries and heart into motion which in turn imparted "extensive and uniform impressions to every animal fibre."[43] Irregular motions in the nerves, but especially in blood and blood vessels, caused disease. An elevated pulse could be healthy if regular, as it might be after running, riding, or dancing. Irregular motion, on the other hand, indicated fever.[44]

For Rush, "excitement" acted as a common measure of stimuli generated by emotions, chemicals, and physical alterations in the environment. Even a political event, like a parade or election might bring high levels of excitement and stimulate the body. In the same manner, an alkaline water might carry high excitement and so too could a warm bath. So too a brisk walk on a warm day might cause the walker to become flushed and sweaty. Red cheeks and moisture also accompanied the emotional excitement induced by seeing the object of one's desire. A body unable to return to equilibrium exhibited disease, typically from some physical blockage, meaning that too much excitement to an already damaged body could trigger a fever. Love-sickness, to Rush and many of his contemporaries, could literally be a disease.[45]

Among his published works, Rush's essays on the causes of animal life come closest to laying out his theory. They were—for the most part—an edited and polished version of his lecture notes from the beginning of his course on the theory and practice of medicine (the first and second weeks). He began his lectures with three general propositions. First, "[e]very part of the human body . . . is endowed with sensibility," defined as "the power of having sensation excited by the action of impressions" and "excitability" as "that property in the human body, by which motion is excited." These definitions were nearly synonymous with irritability, contractility, mobility,

---

43 Rush, "An Inquiry into the Cause of Animal Life," 388.

44 Rush, *Medical Inquiries and Observations: Vol. 3*, 18.

45 Hamlin, *More Than Hot: A Short History of Fever*, 97–98, 131, 306–8. At one point, an anonymous student left Rush a letter asking for help with this particular disease after losing the lady he admired, LC, Rush Family Papers, Benjamin Rush Correspondence, Vol. I, Box 2, Folder 37.

and stimulability found in other eighteenth-century physiology texts.[46] Excitability included motions both visible and imperceptible in its expansive definition. The second proposition stated that bodies were "so formed and connected, that impressions made in the healthy state upon one part, excite motion, or sensation, or both, in every other part of the body. From this view, it [the body] appears to be a *unit, or a simple and indivisible quality.*"[47] Proposition three, deduced from propositions one and two that "[l]ife is the effect of certain stimuli acting upon the sensibility and excitability which are extended, in different degrees, over every external and internal part of the body" and that "stimuli are as necessary to its existence, as air is to flame."

Putting these three axioms together, Rush called life a "forced state," following a supposedly abandoned idea of Cullen's.[48] By *forced*, he argued that life could exist onlyin the presence of external sources of excitement acting upon human or animal bodies and moderated by social and physical conditions. The excitement spurred on the regular vibrations, which made organs function and sympathize (or work) with one another. Rush believed life was inseparable from the forces from which it was created. The "forced state" language appears repeatedly in Rush's publications and manuscript lectures and those of his students. In his published lectures on animal life, he used the concept to argue that bodies are not "self-moving machines" or automatons, but are moved by the external forces of heat, acidity/alkalinity, or mental stimulation.[49] Bodies, and their associated minds, bombarded with stimulation underwent changes in their physical motions and internal chemistry that induced life. Bodies in this sense could not be considered isolated from their surroundings. In doing so Rush not only showed his connection to his preceptor Cullen, and contemporary Brown, but to a much wider debate on the nature of living bodies and minds.

In the theory's mature state Rush moved beyond mechanism to use excitement as a bridge between chemical transformations, bodily motions, and human minds. Samuel Agnew, a student in 1810, recorded the following:

> *Do not the passions and Emotions of the mind, and the increased action of the nerves and arteries,* which are found to *have a great effect on the secretions act by creating motion which increase Fermentation?* Mr. Leibniz to account for it, has supposed, that there are but five original forms of matter in existence, and that all the different

---

46 Rush, "An Inquiry into the Cause of Animal Life," 375–76.
47 Emphasis added, Rush, 376.
48 Rush, 376–77.
49 Rush, 377.

properties and appearances [of] bodies are owing to different modifications.—This opinion appears improbable when we reflect on the *amazing number of forms which bodies put on as taught as by chemistry* the very airs which appear all similar, to be characterized by distinct properties.—And the late new discoveries concerning water, that it consists of two kinds of air in humid form.[50]

This passage again notes Rush's indebtedness to the science of chemistry and chemical affinity in his exploration of human bodies. The seemingly endless chemical substances that could be created with a few building blocks serves as an analogy for the reduction of life to a few simple stimuli. Furthermore, the body itself acted as a chemical laboratory, causing transformations like fermentation that could in turn help create health or sickness.

Rush worked within a physiology that appeared simple on the surface but quickly became complex. Combining different applications of excitement from different sources to create health or repair illness became the job of the physician. The fact that stimulation came from collective, even social, and political sources, as well as individual sources meant that the purview of the doctor was as expansive as society itself. Rush's focus on small motions and life as a collection of vibrations came in part from the work of Hartley and was fostered through his relationship with Joseph Priestley, who admired and commented on Hartley's work. Rush studied Hartley extensively in the 1780s and was deeply influenced by the English writer's interest in the connection between external stimulus, the internal psychology of human, and how those theories could be used to direct social reform.[51]

The ability to excite and be excited, meanwhile, was only half of the equation in Rush's physiology. Excitement needed to be kept in regular order without fluctuation or imbalance. Again, the connection to political balance is evident. He also emphasized the idea that "excitement" was a fundamental property of all stimuli. This had implications for the roles of different organ systems. In his lectures on animal life, Rush specifically cited Eusebio Valli's (1755–1816) work on "animal electricity" as evidence for a different

---

50 Emphasis added, Samuel Agnew, University of Pennsylvania Kislak Center for Special Collections, Rare Books and Manuscripts Mss Coll 225, Box 4, Item 8, Vol. I, 327.

51 D'Elia, "Benjamin Rush, David Hartley, and the Revolutionary Uses of Psychology"; Hartley, *Observations on Man, His Frame, His Duty, and His Expectations: In Two Parts. Part the First*; Hartley, *Hartley's Theory of the Human Mind, on the Principle of the Association of Ideas*; Priestley, *Hartley's Theory of the Human Mind, on the Principle of the Association of Ideas; with Essays Relating to the Subject of It.*

and weaker view of the nervous system than that of his contemporaries.[52] He argued that the nervous system merely ferried stimuli from the extremities to the brain. Rush, in this manner, broke with some of the dominant trends in British medicine in which physicians and laymen alike were preoccupied with the central nervous system and the possibility of nervous diseases.[53] Rush believed that such focus was misplaced, and that physiology allowed only that the nervous system (which included for him, as for Cullen, the muscular fibers) reacted to external and internal doses of excitement. Nerves opened the gate into the body but did not regulate the passage of excitement. The whole collection of nerves, including muscles and brain, only constituted a twitchy collection of matter that resonated with other systems, which could either abstract or amplify its operation. The one-way street meant that the nerves alone could not account for the circulation of excitement and sympathetic bodily motions.

Famously, Rush renewed medical interest in the circulatory system, both harkening back to and moving beyond his Boerhaavian background. The blood vessels served as the major conduits for excitement throughout the body, for Rush. His use of copious therapeutic bloodletting and purges in cases of yellow fever sealed his reputation as a "heroic" wielder of the lancet. Circulation of the blood meant that excitement could travel in a circular rather than simply linear direction. He also viewed them as the primary movers of the body, going everywhere and able to interact constantly with the environment.[54] When excited, the tension of the arterial wall increased, the heart muscle contracted, and together they propelled the liquid blood throughout the body; its pressure excited other organs. Meanwhile, the mirror system to the blood vessels, the lymphatics and glands, abstracted excitement by absorbing tense blood and connecting the body's internal organs with the skin and outside world. He felt that the best way for a physician to evaluate the state of the body was to pay close attention to the pulse. But this

---

52   Rush, "An Inquiry into the Cause of Animal Life," 450. He probably read about Valli's experiments in a book sent by his former student James Proudfit from Scotland in 1793: Valli, *Experiments on Animal Electricity, with Their Application to Physiology and Some Pathological and Medical Observations.* In other notes and publications Rush also indicated a familiarity with the work of the more famous Italian electrical experimenters physiologists Luigi Galvani and Alessandro Volta.

53   Beatty, *Nervous Disease in Late Eighteenth-Century Britain: The Reality of a Fashionable Disorder,* 12, 22–23, 30.

54   Rush, *Medical Inquiries and Observations: Volume 3,* 10–11.

did not mean that the blood vessels, any more than the nerves, controlled the body alone as "monarch."[55]

The blood vessels meet their equal and opposite match in Rush's lymph vessels and glands. Much of what Rush said about the lymphatic system appears in student lecture notes, Rush's manuscript notes, and vague references in published material. This lack of a systematic, published treatise means that the lymph, like the glands, slips out of the usual Rush narrative. An examination of the manuscript materials, however, tells a very different story, one in which the lymphatics do act as a key system for understanding health and disease. Rush viewed the lymphatic system somewhat idiosyncratically for the period. His idea that the lymphatics were the great abstracters of the body seems novel. British anatomists, on the other hand, emphasized what Rush saw as a very secondary function, the absorption of material from the skin.[56]

Overall, for Rush health depended on an even and regular distribution of excitement and motion, something that the nerves could not accomplish. Blood, as suggested above, could change and impart excitement in its own right as well as react to the reciprocal action of the blood vessels. Nerves and blood vessels connected each of these sites of excitement and thus kept the body in sympathy with itself. No action could go undetected. The blood vessels, meanwhile, delivered excitement from places of high concentration to those of low concentration in an attempt to evenly stimulate the body. Blockages or irregularities *were* disease.

The Nature of Illness

Like others of his generation, Rush viewed disease as a process or state of the body rather than the result of an external and distinct infection. Bleeding and purging draw the attention of modern readers and have become sensational. In part this is the result of mid-nineteenth-century changes in therapeutics

---

55   The metaphor of circulation with respect to commerce and physiology is discussed in Altschuler, "From Blood Vessels to Global Networks of Exchange: The Physiology of Benjamin Rush's Early Republic."

56   Eales, "The History of the Lymphatic System, with Special Reference to the Hunter-Monro Controversy," 280–94; Ambrose, "The Priority Dispute over the Function of the Lymphatic System and Glisson's Ghost (the 18th-Century Hunter-Monro Feud)," 7–15; Monro, *A State of Facts Concerning The First Proposal of Performing the Paracentesis of the Thorax, on Account of Air Effused from the Lungs into the Cavities of the Pleurae; and Concerning the Discovery of the Lymphatic Valvular Absorbent System of Vessels in O.*

that shifted away from the heroic treatments promoted by Rush and his contemporaries. A closer reading of work at this time, however, complicates the story of excessive bleeding and purging. Bloodletting and purging were not thought of as a cure-all nor was it considered appropriate for all diseases or at all times in a disease process. In his 1809 edited edition of *The Works of Thomas Sydenham*, Rush clearly demonstrated his view in a footnote, writing:

> Great judgment is necessary to know when to purge, and when to desist from it in the close of a fever. In general, the state of the pulse as to strength and weakness should be the guide of a physician in the use of this remedy. Purging is likewise more proper in the close of autumnal fevers from the accumulation of bile in the bowels, than in fevers of other seasons.[57]

Once again Rush looked to the pulse as a way of gauging what was happening in the body and how excitement was flowing. That power changed as a disease progressed from initial irritation to crisis to recovery (the longest stage). As discussed by Christopher Hamlin, for example, fevers in the eighteenth century were a diverse set of diseases in this period and they required careful observation and varied care based on their timeline.[58] Rush's observations of the violence of American fevers led him to the conclusion that Americans needed stronger therapeutics early in a fever. American bodies, he suggested, were used to greater stimulation due to their republicanism. This combined with the more violent and varied weather of North America (compared with Northwest Europe) to produce violent and strong fevers for strong constitutions. The logic continued that cures for such diseases required similarly strong therapeutics. The doctor was at war with disease. Copious bloodletting and purging—especially in autumnal fevers—brought the body low and helped remove the irregularity of motion that caused symptoms.

Once the formerly strong body was weak, the physician could regularly and carefully bring it back to full strength. This focus on convalescence tends to be overlooked in fever writing, including that of Rush. Without it, however, the violent therapeutics that Rush is famous for do not make sense. He knew that by bleeding a patient he could bring them close to death (he even faked it as a "cure" for suicidal patients at the Pennsylvania Hospital, as discussed in chapter 7). But he fought a guerrilla war with disease, making the body unable to support the irritations that he believed caused illness. On a larger scale, the fundamental relationship between bodies, excitement, social

---

57   Sydenham and Rush, *The Works*, 23.
58   Hamlin, *More Than Hot: A Short History of Fever*.

interactions, and physical space, had implications for their biological and social relationships. Like Sydenham, Rush believed that geological activity released substances into the air that could encourage putrefaction and disease. In accordance with many colonial counterparts, he argued that maintaining health required adjustments to the local climate in exercise, dress, and diet. Finally, like Montesquieu, Rush believed in a reciprocal relationship between climate, government, and national character. Rush also explicitly linked ideas of environmental distinctiveness to American republicanism. Put together the North American environment and the new government merged to create a unique biosocial space.

In the wake of the Revolution this issue became all the more important. Freedom literally imparted health upon a population by creating "an equilibrium of Irritability & Sensibility." The physiological terms can be traced back to Haller. Rush thought that they could apply to more than muscle twitches and even used them to describe the association between human bodies and political revolution, showing the rational side of medical systems. He went on to provide an example. In 1796, one student recorded in his notebook that Rush followed the physiological comment by saying that such equilibrium "is rapidly taking place in france [*sic*.] . . . Errors are opposed to errors & Truths harmonize with each other."[59] In this reading the physical and political "truth" of freedom would break out across Europe. Like medical therapeutics, the cure could be as violent as the disease. That was certainly the case in the French Revolution, the violence of which shocked many Americans in 1796. Freedom and health, despotism and sickness, the pathophysiology of Benjamin Rush sought to reshape the medical world according to republican principles.[60] Bodies were small republics and eventually would demand that the wider world match biological truth.

The roots of Rush's feelings came from his education. He took the concept of environmentally responsive bodies and nervous physiology from Scottish

---

59 Hare, vol. I (1796). Rush attributed his political radicalization to his time in Edinburgh and London in the mid-1760s, Rush, *The Autobiography of Benjamin Rush: His "Travels Through Life" Together with His Commonplace Book for 1789–1813*. The "correction" Rush referenced with respect to the French Revolution may have been a reference to the establishment of the Directory in 1795 and its new constitution, which looked more like the American system of government than the radial rule during the "Reign of Terror."

60 To hammer the point home all the more, in the case of gout Rush associated monarchy with disease, because gout acted as a monarch and took over the body. Rush, "Observations upon the Nature and Cure of the Gout," 250.

medical training, Enlightenment social theory, and American practice and together concluded that his country was simply different. The unique American climate produced different types and amounts of putrefying effluvia; American bodies performed work under different conditions, and American minds found themselves exercised and challenged by their republican society. American diseases, as a result, were more forceful, came about with a greater degree of excitement and attacked physically stronger bodies. Although general theory could cross oceans, practice could be derived only from local knowledge. In the preface to his 1812 *Inquiries and Observations Upon Diseases of the Mind*, Rush explained his use of older sources by stating "the publication of them, it is hoped, will be excused, when it is perceived, that they are placed under the direction of new principles, and that new inferences of a practical nature are deduced from them."[61] The old could stay, but only in the service of new—and from Rush's perspective more correct—theory.

After Rush's death in 1813, his friend and long-time correspondent John Coakley Lettsom in London wrote a pamphlet reflecting upon the life of his American colleague. The text recounted Rush's youth in a revolutionary country, highlighted key texts, and—most importantly—reflected on Rush's character as a physician. Near the end of the piece, Lettsom compared Rush to the heroes of eighteen-century medicine, writing, "were I to determine the station of our deceased friend, I should place him with Hippocrates and Sydenham, and individually designate him the Sydenham of America."[62] In doing so, Lettsom characterized the foundational role Rush had in nineteenth century medicine. He emphasized Rush's energy as a scholar, the novelty and boldness of American practice (compared with European), and the role of experiment in Rush's practice. Standing outside looking in, Lettsom was positioned in a way to appreciate what made American medicine different and Rush's role in its development.[63]

The following chapters examine the manner in which Rush came to command local information and put it to use.

---

61   Rush, *Medical Inquiries and Observations Upon the Diseases of the Mind*, v.
62   Lettsom, *Recollections of Dr. Rush*, 15.
63   Lettsom, 16.

Chapter Three

Making and Sharing Medical Knowledge

Reflecting on his life in the early nineteenth century, middle-aged Benjamin Rush sat down to sketch out his autobiography. He intended for the text to be read by his children although it is likely he expected others to read it eventually.[1] The book addressed Rush's childhood, education, and political opinions. In it, he also presumed that readers would question the amount of work he completed in his lifetime. Rush assumed that his children would be impressed by his productivity and want to know how he managed to publish so many texts on a variety of subjects.[2] Like his some-time neighbor and political rival Alexander Hamilton, one could argue that Rush wrote like he was "running out of time." The amount of writing he managed to do in his lifetime is simply staggering as was the scope of his projects. Rush wrote frequently for both medical and popular audiences and constantly made connections between different parts of his lived experience. This was aided by his substantial correspondence network that covered the early United States and maintained contacts in the Caribbean, Britain, France, Italy, and parts of Spanish America. Interesting conversations, notes from letters, or thoughts gleaned from reading other texts typically found their way first into his commonplace book and then into lectures, orations, and finally printed texts.

As shown in chapter 2, Rush was socialized in a late-eighteenth-century intellectual culture that valued this kind of collaboration, borrowing, and eclectic approach to knowledge. All characteristics of Scotland and subsequently America's Enlightenment were incorporated. While it doesn't fit

---

1   Jones, "Benjamin Rush, Edinburgh Medicine and the Rise of Physician Autobiography," 97–122.

2   Rush and Biddle, *A Memorial Containing Travels Through Life Or Sundry Incidents in the Life of Dr. Benjamin Rush, Born Dec. 24, 1745 (Old Style) Died April 19, 1813*, 123–25.

with modern ideas about disciplinarity, Rush's writing, thinking, and corresponding created the medical knowledge used to back up his ideas. Tidbits
of information about distant people or places along with personal experience
and case studies mounted up in his notes and commonplace books to support ideas of regularity, the centrality of excitement, and unique variability of the United States. Networked connections with other people were the
most important part of Rush's process. He found inspiration from interactions with others writing, "[i]n acquiring knowledge I did not depend exclusively upon books. I made . . . every person I conversed with contribute to
my improvement. I was visited by many literary strangers, and I kept up
a constant intercourse with several of the most distinguished philosophical characters who resided in, or occasionally visited Philadelphia."[3] Rush's
commonplace books—kept throughout his life—are a treasure-trove of
meetings and musings from which he picked up ideas that wound their way
into lectures and print.[4] In doing so, Rush inserted himself into networks of
knowledge that shaped the intellectual community of the Early Republic. He
also bolstered his empirical credentials, appealing to first- (or second-) hand
information and observation rather than received wisdom from classic texts.

This network-based approach to collecting information was common and
well-suited to the realities of the early United States from the 1780s through
the 1810s.[5] While this form of knowledge production and collection had
European and global counterparts within the self-consciously republican
United States it took on additional significance. Information gleaned from a
variety of sources—in many cases uncredited Black or Indigenous sources—
and filtered through networks of doctors, soldiers, or travelers to reach individuals and institutions at the nation's center. These actions helped build the
nation's sense of self, claim knowledge, and control new territory.[6] Medicine

---

3   Rush and Biddle, 67.
4   Fried, *Rush: Revolution, Madness, and the Visionary Doctor Who Became a
     Founding Father*, 64–68.
5   American scientific networks have been discussed by numerous scholars.
     Examples of this work include: Altschuler, *The Medical Imagination: Literature
     and Health in the Early United States*; Zilberstein, "Inured to Empire:
     Wild Rice and Climate Change," 127–58; Harrison, *Medicine in an Age of
     Commerce and Empire: Britian and Its Tropical Colonies*; Naramore, "'My
     Master and Friend': Social Networks and Professional Identity in American
     Medicine, 1789–1815."
6   Bolton Valencius et al., "Science in Early America: Print Culture and the
     Sciences of Territoriality"; Strang, "Perpetual War and Natural Knowledge

was not different, in great part due to the personal connections Rush maintained with colleagues and students in the United States and beyond.

Rush's system defined health through regularity and motion. Regular stimuli interacted with bodies in a predictable manner and upheld the regular motions of the nerves, blood vessels, lymphatics, and muscular tissue that created healthy life. The world, however, was not always regular. Temperatures changed with seasons and time of day, the chemical composition of the atmosphere shifted based on miasma or geological activity, and political questions and contests stimulated the mind in sudden bursts. In addition to being regular, the republican body needed to be resilient to variation. Looking around the world he inhabited through the lens of his correspondence network, Rush looked for key characteristics of the country that could hold it together. Finding none, he deemed the young nation was unified only in its variation. Between seasons, geography, settlement and "improvement," culture, and weather, the United States between 1780 and 1810 was a country of constant physical and psychological change. This change required vigilance and information from a wide network of correspondents.

While the first two chapters of this book focused closely on Rush himself and his experiences, this chapter zooms out to consider the networks he was connected to and the knowledge they provided. Knowledge production and collection was not a one-way street. Rush made and was made by the exchanges of center and periphery, pupil and preceptor, doctor and patient. This chapter will address each of the interactions to show how the "American system" needed a community of scholars to support it and how Rush gleaned information from a variety of sources. It does so by looking at three forms of interaction: letter-writing, the formation of professional organizations, and one international relationship between Rush and the French travel writer the Comte de Volney.

Networks of Knowledge

Looking out from Fort Pitt in 1780, soldier and Rush correspondent Hugh Martin surveyed the surrounding country with an optimistic eye. In the middle of the American Revolutionary War, the western edge of Pennsylvania was not unknown. It was, however, remote to Anglo-Americans who were not fur traders or land speculators. Martin referred to the region to the north and west of his location as "Indian Country," but implied that the distinction

in the United States, 1775–1860," 387–413; Strang, *Frontiers of Science: Imperialism and Natural Knowledge in the Gulf South Borderlands, 1500–1850*.

would not be meaningful for long. After all, access to "Indian Country" was an important motivation for many revolutionary "patriots" frustrated by the limitations imposed by the Proclamation Line of 1763 and other treaty and trade directives from the British government. Westward migration of white Americans and their demand for land stoked the fires of rebellion in the 1760s and 1770s.[7] Rush certainly took advantage of the changes and invested in western land in the late eighteenth century. Meanwhile, "scientific" details about the climate and situation of Western Pennsylvania and the Ohio Valley remained rare and highly valuable to the intellectual elite (like Rush) and to land speculators (like Rush). Knowledge of land and people constituted one way in which White Americans shaped their identity and laid claim to Indigenous land—doing so using repackaged Indigenous knowledge.

The news that arrived in the 1780s in the crucible of war was even more welcome. Martin admitted that traversing the mountains had been difficult and that spring came later in the west, but he also held that "the Lands on this side of the Mountains are more fertile than any I have ever seen in our Country. These parts abound with the plenteous production of the Animal & Vegetable Kingdoms and as to the mineral we abound in coal, which is our constant fuel."[8] A century later no one could doubt how coal and oil transformed the region around Pittsburgh. Eleven years later, a young James Woodhouse (1770–1809) wrote to Rush from the same region during his military service in Little Turtle's War (Northwest Indian Wars) prior to his appointment as professor of chemistry at the University of Pennsylvania. While serving under General Arthur St. Clair (1737–1818) he described the country, medical practice in the region, and sent botanical samples back to Rush in Philadelphia.[9]

Letters like those of Woodhouse and Martin served as vital tools for the western expansion and economic growth of the United States, often at the expense of other actors in the region. They also provided early information and ideas about how bodies responded to new climates. As noted above,

---

7 For more, see Breen, *American Insurgents, American Patriots: The Revolution of the People*; Choppin Roney, "1776, Viewed from the West," 41; Griffin, *America's Revolution*.

8 Hugh Martin to Benjamin Rush (1780), LCP, Rush Family Papers, Series I, Subseries I, Vol. XXIV.

9 James Woodhouse to Benjamin Rush (1791), LCP, Rush Family Papers, Benjamin Rush Correspondence, Vol. XXVI; Thacher, *American Medical Biography: Or Memoirs of Eminent Physicians Who Have Flourished in America to Which Is Prefixed a Succinct History of the Medical Science in the United States from the First Settlement of the Country, Vol. II*, 220–21.

climate was widely held as a key determinant of health in the eighteenth century. In 1800, one correspondent of Rush from Kentucky wrote "I should as certainly expect to find a difference between the Londoner, fed on luxurious viands and Asian sweetmeats . . . respiring the mephitic air . . . and the Kentukeyan [sic] raised on the Indian Corn and wild beasts of his country, and breathing and atmosphere oxygenated by the luxuriant woods."[10] The chemical terms used indicated both men's knowledge of recent theories—especially Lavoisier's oxygen—and their association with older medical concepts like atmospheric constitutions popularized in the English-speaking world by Sydenham. Conquest of western territory added a new collection of environments for physicians to consider. By the turn of the nineteenth century Rush frequently received mail from patients in Western Pennsylvania, Kentucky, and Ohio seeking advice while also describing their location. Over the course of his career Rush received thousands of letters from students, colleagues, and patients across the continent.[11] This network of information resided in the letters themselves and the published documents they helped support.

Rush's use of correspondence networks to support published arguments was not an exclusive trait. In the introduction to his 1792 volume, *An Historical Account of the Climates and Diseases of the United States of America*, Philadelphia physician, William Currie (1754–1828) explicitly made reference to the necessity of his correspondents for the completion of his work and to provide an accurate picture of the country.[12] Currie was a founding member of the College of Physicians of Philadelphia and had apprenticed under James Kersley in Philadelphia, John Redman's preceptor, and thus connected to Rush through the vital pupil-preceptor relationships of the period. Like Rush, Currie actively participated in the American Revolutionary War. He served in army hospitals and afterwards returned to Philadelphia to have a strong private practice and actively published and contributed to the city's

---

10 Joseph Hamilton Daviass to Benjamin Rush (1800) LCP, Rush Family Papers, Benjamin Rush Correspondence, Vol. 4.

11 Naramore, "'My Master and Friend': Social Networks and Professional Identity in American Medicine, 1789–1815."

12 Rush was one of Currie's correspondents and contributed to the section on Pennsylvania. Transactions of the College of Physicians of Philadelphia (1887), "Currie, William (1754–1828)," in *A Cyclopedia of American Medical Biography, Comprising the Lives of Eminent Deceased Physicians and Surgeons from 1610 to 1910*, 267.

intellectual life.[13] In short, he and Rush were peers who ran in the same professional circles and were familiar with the same medical theories. In the case of his work on the American climate, Currie, like Rush, relied on his professional network. In fact, Rush's ideas and words appear nearly unedited in Currie's discussion of Pennsylvania. After listing the goals of his project Currie wrote, "[w]ith these objects in view, I opened a correspondence with several physicians of talents and experience residing in the several states, and with their assistance, joined to my own personal observations, and such information as I could collect from the few books that contain any thing relative to the subject, have composed the following pages."[14] Without professional contacts scattered throughout the country, synthesizers like Rush and Currie would not have been able to make claims about the country as a whole or presume to represent a national profession. Philadelphia was an intellectual crossroads from which they both benefited. Professional correspondence networks allowed Currie to gain and disseminate knowledge without actual travel beyond eastern Pennsylvania in his book while Rush peppered information in his classes and smaller texts.

Another Philadelphia physician and former Rush student, Benjamin Smith Barton (1766–1815) also actively cultivated correspondents beyond Philadelphia to supplement his own collections and travel experience. Barton's primary interest was in the natural history of the United States despite his medical training. This required a large amount of information and objects from across the country, often obtained from others. Occasionally this took the form of a formal agreement between an employer and employee. In 1807, he hired German-American botanist Frederick Pursh (1774–1820) to collect natural historical information from the Finger Lakes region up through northern New York and into Vermont.[15] In most cases, however, Barton continued in the gentlemanly exchange tradition and used personal and professional contacts to expand his knowledge base.[16] Rush's

---

13   Transactions of the College of Physicians of Philadelphia (1887), 267.

14   Currie, *An Historical Account of the Climates and Diseases of the United States of America and of the Remedies and Methods of Treatment ....*, 1.

15   Between 1807 and 1808 letters arrived for Barton (often asking for money) from Pursh from the Finger Lakes, Milford, Pennsylvania, and Rutland, Vermont. Frederick Pursh to Benjamin Smith Barton (1807–1808), American Philosophical Society, Benjamin Smith Barton Papers, Correspondence, Box 5.

16   For more on the importance of experience in science in the early modern period see Daston, "Baconian Facts, Academic Civility, and the Prehistory of Objectivity," 349; Ponzio, "The Articulation of the Idea of Experience in the

correspondence functioned in a similar way. Case studies and consultations increased both his knowledge and his reputation as a national figure.

Although Rush's interests did not often lead to the swapping of specimens, like Barton, he did engage in the exchange of ideas and publications with colleagues in the United States and Europe. Dozens of letters between Rush and his colleagues referred to enclosed books, pamphlets, or proofs of upcoming work. Glasgow-based physician John Burns (1774–1850), for example, sent Rush early copies of two works on obstetrics, his *Practical observations on the uterine hemorrhage; with remarks on the management of the placenta* (1807) and his *Observations on abortion containing an account of the manner in which it is accomplished, the causes which produced it, and the method of preventing or treating it* (1807).[17] Both volumes included handwritten dedication notes to Rush as well as numerous corrections (mainly printing errors).

Patients also formed a critical part of this exchange and network of ideas. As demonstrated by Convery Bolton Valencius for the antebellum period, physicians, domestic practitioners, and patients generally understood illness the same way.[18] The sick or their relatives wrote to their physicians based on a shared understanding that bodies responded to their immediate

---

16th and 17th Centuries," 193–95; Dear, "The Meanings of Experience," 106–31. For a history of collection, see Findlen, *Possessing Nature: Museums, Collecting, and Scientific Culture in Early Modern Italy*, 1994; Slaughter, *The Natures of John and William Bartram*; Grove, *Green Imperialism: Colonial Expansion, Tropical Island Edens and the Origins of Environmentalism, 1600–1860*; Albritton Jonsson, "Climate Change and the Retreat of the Atlantic: The Cameralist Context of Pehr Kalm's Voyage to North America, 1748–51," 99–126; Judd, *The Untilled Garden: Natural History and the Spirit of Conservation in America, 1740–1840*; Schiebinger et al., *Colonial Botany: Science, Commerce, and Politics in the Early Modern World*; Ratcliff, "The East India Company, the Company's Museum, and the Political Economy of Natural History in the Early Nineteenth Century," 495–517; Phillips, *Acolytes of Nature: Defining Natural Science in Germany*.

17 John Burns to Benjamin Rush (1807), LCP, Rush Family Papers, Benjamin Rush Correspondence, Vol. IIa, Box 6; Burns, *Practical Observations on the Uterine Hemorrhage; with Remarks on the Management of the Placenta*; Burns, *Observations on Abortion Containing an Account of the Manner in Which It Is Accomplished, the Causes Which Prodiced It, and the Method of Preventing or Treating It.*

18 Bolton Valencius, *The Health of the Country: How American Settlers Understood Themselves and Their Land.*

environment. Providing information about the weather, financial situation, occupation, and habits were the equivalent of a medical history. Over the course of decades and thousands of letters from patients, their families, and their doctors, Rush accumulated huge masses of information. It is unsurprising that the experience left him in a position as an expert on American diseases despite the "uniformly variable" climate and his own lack of travel. These exchanges demonstrate the currency of ideas within the medical community as well as the broad influence Rush had in his profession.

Many students and former students also sent Rush essays or published letters on their own practice and a few used Rush as a pathway to formal publication elsewhere. Rush, meanwhile, made a habit of sending out his own publications as gifts to close friends. A much earlier letter from fellow American Edinburgh graduate Samuel Bard (1742–1821) asked for reading suggestions and made some of his own. He wrote, "I have got the <u>Dictionaire de Physic</u> your Recommendation, & am really very much pleased with it—is there anything else new and Excellent, besides Cullen's Lectures which you would recommend to me . . . for I cannot help longing to see what you so much recommend."[19] In later life Rush used students studying abroad to send publications and information, including—on more than one occasion—his son James, who also studied at the University of Edinburgh.

In addition to acting as a node in several correspondence networks, Rush also took advantage of in-person contacts and connections whenever he could. Both Benjamin and Julia Rush frequented private gatherings of intellectuals in Philadelphia and Princeton and occasionally entertained medical students in their home. Rush also tried to invite as many gentlemen visitors in Philadelphia to his home as possible. In essence he started to model himself and his home from those that opened doors when he was a traveler in London, Edinburgh, and Paris. Rush became a bit of an "American Fothergill." Like the Fothergill of his London days, Rush enjoyed meals and regular meetings with strangers to the city. This intellectual sociability was deliberate, as Rush noted in his autobiography.

> In acquiring knowledge, I did not depend exclusively upon books. I made, as far as was in my power, every person I conversed with contribute to my improvement. I was visited by many literary strangers, and I kept up a constant intercourse with several of the most distinguished philosophical characters who resided in, or occasionally visited Philadelphia. As I wished to be correct, in the knowledge I

19   Samuel Bard to Benjamin Rush (1770), LCP, Rush Family Papers, Benjamin Rush Correspondence, Vol. II, Box 3.

acquired by conversation, I made it a practice to record it in a book kept for that purpose after the manner as I supposed of Mr. Boyle. By thus committing it to paper, I was able to use it more confidently in my lectures and publications.[20]

Lecture notes and numerous short publications support the views portrayed in the autobiography. Alongside allusions to texts and personal observations Rush peppered his work with accounts of useful information from international visitors and close friends. Portions of his commonplace books provide examples of how he recorded such conversations. Selections from 1792, for example, include political news gathered on the street, observations of a lion displayed in the city, conversations with Thomas Jefferson on linguistics, observations on slavery by a visiting German physician, multiple discussions of American geography and plant life with French botanist André Michaux, and various other encounters with physicians, clergymen, female friends, and politicians. From this collection of clipped sentences and jumbled anecdotes Rush somehow kept track of the trends and salient examples they set for his medical work. This could take the form of published work, but more often was carried in informal letters and through in-person conversations inaccessible to historians. Reports could be conscious or simply gleaned from the context of a letter. Rush was especially keen to make the most out of truthful reports regardless of the author's original intent. Patients, friends, and physician letters could be used like data sources where a seemingly insignificant note could be read in a larger context. Reliable reporters, including physicians and their patients scattered across the country effectively delivered data about the state of the American environment and its people to the metropolitan centers as part of mundane correspondence. For example, patients wrote to their physicians and described their location, often with details about the weather or geography, due to their shared Hippocratic heritage.

The case of Anthony Jones of Charlotte County, Virginia, in 1801 is a prime example of a patient's self-narrative. Jones was both a patient and a physician, but his descriptions of his own health do not differ substantially from those without a medical education. He wrote to Rush:

> I left Philadelphia, being then in a very bad state of health, with the pulmonary consumption, . . . in 97 I *removed to the County* I am in at present situated on the north side of [the] River, [two miles] above Petersburgh, where it is *very sickly in*

---

20   Rush and Biddle, *A Memorial Containing Travels Through Life Or Sundry Incidents in the Life of Dr. Benjamin Rush, Born Dec. 24, 1745 (Old Style) Died April 19, 1813*, 67.

the fall season, Bilious Remittents & Intermittants prevailing very much, which kept me usually very much employed riding from which I acquired a vigor of constitution that I never before experienced. . . . in the Fall of 1800 I was attacked with a violent Bilious fever which confind [sic] me to bed 9 weeks continued fever, extreme debility & good appetite, & cough as usual, I got upon my feet, but have continued weak & feverish ever since, with a good appetite, I've been forced to bleed very often, during the spring & summer last I was bed ridden & my life much despaired of, *but since the approach of cool weather I've got better* again so that I ride about in my Chair.[21]

Jones described his health in several ways. He noted his personal constitution (consumptive), the general seasonality of disease where he lived, and specific weather conditions of the present year. Furthermore, he included instances where his health improved through riding and relocating. This pattern is common for letters of this type sent to Rush and notes the deep connection between weather, lifestyle, and health. Migration and irregular climates could alter bodies and cause sickness if not handled carefully.

Others wrote about the relationship between situation and chronic ill health. David Campbell wrote to Rush from Abingdon, Virginia, in 1806 claiming that his wife's chronic illness was triggered by dampness and cold.[22] Rush would have understood the weather as causing irregular motions in the body. Joseph Read of Norfolk, Virginia wrote to Rush on behalf of his son in 1802. The son—recently returned from Europe—suffered from ill health, which his father attributed to the climate of Southern Europe and an abundance of salt in the food.[23] Other patients traveled to more salubrious places on the advice of Rush. William Dawson attempted a mineral water cure and traveled to Ball Town Springs (Ballston Spa, New York) in 1807 for an unspecified illness and then claimed to be cured. William Norris of Lewiston, Pennsylvania, made the common trek to Hot Springs, Virginia, in 1812, as did Thomas Perkinson of Amelia County, Virginia. By 1812 Hot Springs and Warm Springs, Virginia were

---

21 Emphasis added, Anthony Jones to Benjamin Rush (1801), LCP, Rush Family Papers, Benjamin Rush Correspondence, Vol. VIII.

22 David Campbell to Benjamin Rush (1806), LCP, Rush Family Papers, Benjamin Rush Correspondence, Vol. III.

23 Js. Read to Benjamin Rush (1802), LCP, Rush Family Papers, Benjamin Rush Correspondence, Vol. XIV.

well-established health spots frequently recommended by Rush and his colleagues after similar reports of success.[24]

The environment also had an effect on professional decision-making. This was especially the case for young men choosing a location in which to practice. In many cases, this meant identifying unhealthy and under-developed areas and those with a high incidence of illness and therefore potential patients. Three medical students—Richard G. Harris in 1796, J. Bullus in 1797 and Edward Anderson in 1809—wrote to their respective preceptors Benjamin Rush and Benjamin Smith Barton, complaining about the health of the towns they had settled in. All three young men initially settled in the mid-Atlantic, Harris in Easton, Pennsylvania, Bullus in Reading, Pennsylvania, and Anderson in Fredericktown, Maryland.[25] None found the success they hoped for as highly educated young medical men. For example, in one letter to Rush, Bullus vented his frustration with the state of the medical profession in Reading and expressed his desire to move to the south. Pennsylvania was both too healthy and had too many medical practitioners—including competition from bleeders and "quacks"—for a young man to make a good living. The south, on the other hand, was considered sickly and feverish and a substantial number of Rush's students who moved for their profession chose a southern route. Physicians in the south (especially South Carolina, Georgia, and by the end of Rush's life the Mississippi Territory) inhabited a growing region with the expansion of plantation slavery in the early nineteenth century. A doctor could attain financial stability by signing on as a contract physician on a planation, caring for wealthy families as well as their enslaved labor force, rather than slugging it out in the established and healthy North.

In addition to migration within North America, American physicians experienced new environments on a global scale through the military and as commercial ship surgeons. The life of Rush student Thomas Horsfield

---

24   William Dawson to Benjamin Rush (1807), LCP, Rush Family Papers, Benjamin Rush Correspondence, Vol. IV; William Norris to Benjamin Rush (1812), LCP, Rush Family Papers, Benjamin Rush Correspondence, Vol. XII; Thomas Perkinson to Benjamin Rush (1812), LCP, Rush Family Papers, Benjamin Rush Correspondence, Vol. XIII.

25   Richard G. Harris to Benjamin Rush (1796), LCP, Rush Family Papers, Benjamin Rush Correspondence, Vol. VII; J. Bullus to Benjamin Rush (1797), LCP, Rush Family Papers, Benjamin Rush Correspondence, Vol. IIa, Box 6; and Edward Anderson (1809), APS, Benjamin Smith Barton Papers, Correspondence, Box 1.

(1773–1859) fits into this category of travel. After completing his MD at the University of Pennsylvania the Bethlehem, Pennsylvania, native started his career at sea on board the Indiaman *China* and eventually settled in Batavia (modern Jakarta), Indonesia. Horsfield stayed in Java for eighteen years, becoming the preeminent scholar of the island's diseases and natural resources.[26] Horsfield wrote back to Rush while recovering from illness in 1803 shortly after his arrival. In the letter he described his research and career plans. Despite his early illness, he had managed to obtain a position at the Dutch East India Company's hospital and promised Rush that he would maintain a rigorous research agenda. The young doctor wrote:

> I have daily opportunities in my observations on the diseases of Batavia of confirming and applying those important truths I acquired by your invaluable instructions. . . . I began some researches into the Natural History and Botany, but especially of the Materia Medica of this Island, I have since continued these investigations under the particular situation. . . . [I have a] view of making such experiments with a number of native medicinal plants as the cases afford—It is in a pleasant and healthy situation; and I have daily opportunities of observing the diseases of Batavia in their different stages and modifications.[27]

Horsfield also planned a trip to the interior of the island to study local languages and "the geology & geography of the same."[28] No further letters from Horsfield to Rush survive, but he did follow through on his scientific endeavors and maintained a research agenda modeled on the observation skill Rush encouraged in the classroom. He continued to collect and study the plant life of the island in particular and took up official duties with the British East India Company after their 1811 takeover of the island. In 1819, Horsfield left Java and settled in England, where he curated the British East India Company's collection and published catalogues of animal life on Java.[29]

---

26 Cowan, "Horsfield, Moore, and the Catalogues of the East India Company Museum," 274; McNair, "Thomas Horsfield -American Naturalist and Explorer," 1–9; Williams, "Discovered in Philadelphia: A Third Set of Thomas Horsfield's Nature Prints of Plants from Java," 169–71.

27 Thomas Horsfield to Benjamin Rush (1803), LCP, Rush Family Papers, Benjamin Rush Papers, Vol. VII.

28 Ibid.

29 McNair, "Thomas Horsfield -American Naturalist and Explorer"; Williams, "Discovered in Philadelphia"; Ratcliff, "The East India Company, the Company's Museum, and the Political Economy of Natural History in the Early Nineteenth Century."

Finally, correspondence networks reveal how physicians constructed reputations outside of formal publication. Few would name Rush as an expert in women's health now; but an overview of his correspondence reveals not only books like Burns' but patients seeking information based his presumed expertise with the female body. This is not the only example of correspondence shedding light on Rush's reputation as a practitioner. Many American colleagues wrote to Rush about both women's health—which Rush hardly wrote about—as well as diseases of the mind decades before his ground-breaking textbook on the subject in 1812. In 1803, for example, a physician who signed his letter E. Daugherty specifically wrote to Rush seeking a cure for goiter—an ailment associated with women—stating, "I beg leave to ask you wether [sic] you have been Discovered any cure for the Goitre a complaint the women are very much troubled with in this country."[30] Rush only dedicated part of one printed essay to diseases of the thyroid, however, questions about goiter followed him for years as discussed in chapter 6. Correspondence, networks, and reputation spread information differently than the limited world of publication. Publications, however, also have their place in this history, which was deeply connected to those preexisting correspondence networks.

Medical Journals and Associations

In addition to personal correspondence, professional associations and journals helped knit the American profession together and contributed to the expansion and exchange of medical knowledge. As should be evident at this point, the construction of scientific knowledge at the turn of the nineteenth century was decidedly social rather than solitary or strictly institutional. Therefore, the early institutions that did promote and encourage scientific development copied existing social networks and practices. Philadelphia's College of Physicians, established in 1787, is the most notable example of the early medical organizations and counted Rush, Currie, Redman, and Shippen among its founding members. It was not, however, a lone project, but rather emblematic of a wider impulse throughout the country.

Physicians wanted to organize to share information and build a sense of professional community. They also worked to distinguish themselves from other kinds of healers, including midwives, apothecaries, bleeders, and bonesetters. In 1788, the College of Physicians of Philadelphia received a

---

30 E. Daugherty to Benjamin Rush (1803), LCP, Rush Family Papers, Benjamin Rush Correspondence, Vol. IV.

letter from the Medical Society of New-Haven County, Connecticut, which requested it "to honour them with the annual communications of your learned society. [and that] They [the Medical Society of New-Haven County] would have been happy in rendering their publications more deserving the notice & attentions of your very respectable institution."[31] Physicians in Delaware and Massachusetts formed medical societies in 1789. In New-York, a hierarchical state-wide medical society with representatives from each county facilitated the flow of information and was empowered by the state to grant medical licenses, merging both the old corporate power of medical organizations and the newer impulse of exploration. By the early nineteenth century new western states and cities copied the impulse as well and formed organizations in Kentucky and Ohio.

Not all physicians, however, had ready access to medical associations. Most practitioners worked in rural areas where they could feel isolated. Without community these men struggled to find community. Other options were required for these men to reinforce their own identities. Some was likely in person notes and casebooks like those of later-nineteenth-century American physicians, but public writing also played a critical role.[32] Virtual connections fostered by correspondence and formal magazines and journals stepped in to fill the gap. Medical journals first appeared in substantial numbers in the United States at the turn of the nineteenth century and solicited material well beyond their metropolitan publishing locations in Philadelphia and New York. Like the societies which privileged transactions, journals replicated the conventions of professional sociability present in professional organizations and correspondence. They also encouraged the sharing of weather data in a public forum. Regular weather reports appeared in medical journals alongside articles, book reviews, and published correspondence. New York's *American Medical and Philosophical Register* (1811–1814) included temperature, rainfall, and disease data for the City of New York in each issue. Although journals lacked the professional power of some medical societies— a journal could not grant a medical license, for example—they did collect and disseminate information in a similar way and warrant consideration here. Furthermore, both American and British medical journals acted as sources of

---

31   Medical Society of New-Haven County to the College of Physicians of Philadelphia (November 29, 1788), CPP, Manuscript Archives of the College of Physicians of Philadelphia, 1781–1847.

32   Thompson, "Beyond Imperturbability: The Nineteenth-Century Medical Casebook as Affective Genre," 188–190.

information for Rush, his colleagues, and his students. Numerous citations to journal articles appear in Rush's commonplace books and medical notes, outnumbering those referring the reader to medical books. On May 15, 1810, for example, Rush wrote that he had read from two American medical journals finishing "'Pathological Remarks upon Certain Diseases of the Liver' for Dr. Coxe's *Museum* and 'An Inquiry into the Use of the Thymus Gland for Dr. Miller's *New York Repository.*"[33] In teaching, he encouraged students to follow his example. Rush argued that journals did not possess the same pitfalls he believed existed in medical books. They largely contained short factual accounts that the reader could interpret for himself (allowing him to apply a different theory than that subscribed to by the author), and frequent publication prevented knowledge from becoming stale.[34] In this sense, medical journalism was journalism in the sense that it privileged the recording and transmitting of news in the form of personal observations and records.

Each of the early journals took on their own characters and forms of published material covering a slightly difference selection of medical science. Benjamin Smith Barton's *Philadelphia Medical Museum* (1805–1811), for example, included large sections of Barton's own observations or reprinted his personal medical correspondence. It was, in some respects, like a peek into his mailbox. Other journals reprinted medical material from foreign journals or focused on medical book reviews. Even their definition of "medical" varied, with Barton's publication often leaning toward natural history and away from medical practice. Few of the American publications of Rush's time lasted long. The first journal, New York's *The Medical Repository and Review of American Publications* (1797–1824) had the longest print run. Nevertheless, they had support from the American medical establishment and were praised by Rush as a good alternative to medical books for information. He did not, however, submit much of his own work, preferring pamphlets and popular magazines to medical journals in order to get his ideas into the public square. Nevertheless, Rush understood journals and transactions, both American and European, as sources for trustworthy descriptions of illness. Both his commonplace books and lecture notes include references

---

33 Rush, *The Autobiography of Benjamin Rush: His "Travels Through Life" Together with His Commonplace Book for 1789–1813*, 290.

34 Notes of Henry Powell (1809), KCRBM, Mss. Coll. 225, Box 3, Item 7, Vol. I, 3–5.

to journal articles, with the *Edinburgh Medical and Surgical* journal as the most common. But American journals also appeared frequently.[35]

Each journal, like each medical society or personal correspondence network possessed also a slightly different geographic footprint. New York and Philadelphia represented two publication hubs, each with multiple medical journals. Boston produced one journal during this period, *The New England Journal of Medicine and Surgery*, beginning in 1812. Beyond cities of publication, the various journals drew information from throughout the United States, often along lines that related to professional associations and personal connection.

By the end of the 1810s, American medical journals had printed information from both eastern cities like Philadelphia, New York, and Boston, and western outposts on the frontier, marking the expansion of the profession with the migration of Americans more generally. This geographic distribution indicated the existence of some form of professional unity rather than sectionalism, however fragmented it might have been otherwise. It also connected rural and Western physicians to ideas and people in urban centers while providing those in the metropole like Rush with direct insight onto the edge of the American empire.

Volney and Rush—An Example of Transatlantic Networks

At the end of the day, networks of knowledge exchange and production were simply an aggregate of real human relationships. Individuals built trust with each other, and that trust and camaraderie (in theory) echoed down the lines of exchange. Being part of the "Republic of Letters" gave correspondents a standing among their peers and allowed for their work to be taken seriously. This chapter concludes with a discussion of just one of those friendships and highlights the way international as well as national exchanged shaped American medicine, that between Benjamin Rush and the Comte de Volney (1757–1820). Rush developed a personal connection with Volney, who visited the United States between 1795 and 1798. Like many visitors to Philadelphia, he spent time in the Rush home and in deep conversation with its owner. The two men seemed to appreciate each other's company and discussed the future of the United States over various refreshments (Rush, like Fothergill, enjoyed company for breakfast), which gave Rush an opportunity to practice his French.

---

35   Rush, *The Autobiography*.

By the late 1790s, Volney was already a well-known author of travel literature in France and the United States after the success of his *Travels in Syria and Egypt*. The text was in the popular nonfiction genre of travel literature and history with a sprinkling of medical topography.[36] Rush and other Americans had access to French editions soon after the book's publication. Both Rush and Noah Webster used Volney's descriptions of the Mediterranean plague in their own observations about epidemic diseases published in the wake of the first yellow fever outbreaks in New York and Philadelphia, between 1792 and 1793. American-printed English translations were available by the end of the decade.[37] In his work on the United States, Volney self-consciously pushed the borders of "travel literature" to create something closer to a natural history of North American people and spaces. He noted that compared to the work on Egypt and Syria his new work was "more grave and scientific" than its predecessor.[38] While he still wrote about the culture of the United States and his own experience, the book also includes lengthy scientific passages and comparison of weather data between the United States and Europe. This hybridization brought him into the social and professional spheres of physicians in Philadelphia, Charleston, and New York. These were the same circles within which Rush exchanged information and crafted theories. Volney and Rush directly exchanged ideas and information both in writing and in conversations at Rush's home. In short, Volney became part of the American medical and scientific professional network for the duration of his stay while maintaining an outsider's perspective.

The connection between the two men certainly made sense. Like Rush, Volney was interested in the politics of the new nation as well as its geography and natural history and wondered how they interacted. It is easy to imagine the two men sitting in Rush's parlor bouncing from political discussions to the weather to the geography of the Near West. Of course, their motivations differed. Rush was interested in the perfection and improvement of his own country while Volney (like other French visitors to the United States) looked for examples of a functional republic that could be instructive

---

36 Volney, *Travels Through Egypt and Syria, in the Years 1783, 1784 & 1785: Containing the Present Natural and Political State of Those Countries; Their Productions, Arts, Manufactures & Commerce; with Observations on the Manners, Customs and Government of the Turks.*

37 Volney; Webster, *Noah Webster: Letters on Yellow Fever Addressed to Dr. William Currie*, 28.

38 Volney, *View of the Climate and Soil of the United States of America: To Which Are Annexed Some Accounts of Florida, the French Colony on the Scioto, Certain Canadian Colonies, and the Savages or Natives*, xxi.

to the rest of the world. In the preface to the 1804 English edition of his *View of the Climate and Soil of the United States of America*, Volney described his state of mind as he "embarked at [Le Havre] with that disgust and indifference, which the sight and experience of injustice and persecution impart . . . to try whether a sincere friend of that Liberty, whose name had been so profaned, could find for his declining years a peaceful asylum, of which Europe no longer afforded him any hope."[39] Volney left France disappointed in his country's revolution (and after imprisonment during the terror in 1794–1795) and hoped to find a moderate republican refuge and country at peace in the United States. Ultimately, he was disappointed in the Federalist leadership of the young nation and returned to France due to surging fracophobia during the Quasi-War of the Adams administration.[40] That disappointment echoes throughout the text and certainly tainted his general impression of the United States.

Nevertheless, Volney produced a comprehensive account of his experience and considerable travel while in the United States. With respect to natural history Rush's influence is evident. On the American climate, Volney, like Rush, characterized the country by its extreme variability and assumed a connection between what he considered physical and political bodies and the nation and body politic. Wary of the country's size and diverse climates he predicted that disunion was inevitable, especially in the West.[41] He also compared various regions to analogous spots in Europe, Africa, and Asia, like Rush. Volney's relationship with Rush led him to defer to the American's observations on the local climate and geography. In addition to using Rush's weather data, he credited the American for correctly noting the similarity of Pennsylvania's climate with that of Northeastern China and Tartary. This was despite the fact that neither man had actually traveled to Central or East Asia.[42] From his own experiences, Volney claimed to have experienced many of the same conditions he attributed to the hot countries of the Eastern Mediterranean discussed in his first book.

Of course, the United States was not uniform. Volney saw much of the nation firsthand, even traveling as far West as the Wabash River and certainly encountered very different climates. To account for variation in his narrative, Volney organized the country into four clear divisions: (1) the cold New England climate; (2) the variable middle climate of southern New York,

39   Volney, *View*, iv.
40   Volney, *View*, iv–v.
41   Volney, *View*, 4–5.
42   Volney, *View*, 33, 130, 239.

Pennsylvania, and Maryland; (3) the hot climate of Virginia, the Carolinas, and Georgia; and (4) the western climate of Tennessee, Kentucky, and the Northwest Territories. He argued that these divisions reflected elevation as much or more than latitude in an attempt to account for the perennial American climate problem.[43] For over a century the continental climate of North America (especially its relatively extreme seasons compared to Northwestern Europe) baffled Europeans who expected regions with the same latitude to have the same weather. American locations from Virginia to Canada confounded these expectations.[44] Within specific locations he complained about the dangerous variability of weather and its ill effects on his own health, especially in fickle Philadelphia, which existed in a variable climate zone and suffered from urban epidemics.[45]

Unlike Rush or other Americans who took variation in stride, Volney was deeply concerned with the dangers associated with variable weather and the nation's recent experience with epidemic disease writing, "all Europeans agree in condemning the extreme variableness of the weather from cold to hot, and from hot to cold: but the Americans . . . defend their climate as their property, and have three powerful motives of partiality to it . . . individual self-love . . . national vanity . . . and a pecuniary interest as dear to the state as to individual, that of selling land, and attracting foreign purchasers and foreign capitals."[46] While pride and profit certainly effected American attitudes, living with variation and thriving with problematic weather became part of the American identity. Native-born Anglo-Americans were suited to their climate—in their own minds—because it was what constantly surrounded them. Living with variation was fundamentally different from "seasoning" in a new setting and required a different medical approach.

Volney described how he was overwhelmed by the country's wildness and diffuse population when compared with that of France. He wrote that "[t]o a European traveler . . . the prominent feature of the American soil is a wild appearance of almost uninterrupted forest, which displays itself on the shores of the sea, and continues growing thicker and thicker as you proceed into

---

43 Volney, *View*, 5–6.

44 Kupperman, "Fear of Hot Climates in the Anglo-American Colonial Experience.," 213–40; White, "Unpuzzling American Climate: New World Experience and the Foundations of a New Science," 544–66; Kupperman, "The Puzzle of the American Climate in the Early Colonial Period," 1262–89.

45 Golinski, "Debating the Atmospheric Constitution: Yellow Fever and the American Climate," 157.

46 Volney, *View*, 328–29.

the interior of the country."[47] This description was not without evidence. Volney did travel extensively in the United States including to its western border: the Mississippi River. His travel in 1796 took him through all four of the climatic zones he proposed and levels of Euro-American settlement and "improvement" of the land. Concern about the forest recapitulated a common worry in eighteenth-century natural history. In northern climates, too much forest cooled the area and marked a lack of agricultural production.[48] In warmer regions open space was thought to aid in cultivating cooling breezes.[49] Rush worried that a lack of barriers between settlements and wetlands could lead to disease-producing miasma or gasses that could cause illness. Based on his travels, Volney attributed increased drought and larger rivers to forest clearing in Tennessee and Kentucky, indicating poor management of new farmland.[50] These complaints about the American farmer highlighted the presumed reciprocal nature of humans and their environment. Poor climates encouraged poor farming, which worsened the climate. Following a statement about the irregularity and unkemptness of American farms he wrote:

> Add to this a fickle and variable sky, an atmosphere alternately very moist and very dry, very misty and very clear, very hot and very cold, and a temperature so changeable, that in the same day you will have spring, summer, autumn, and winter, Norwegian frost and an African sun. Figure to yourself these, and you will have a concise physical sketch of the United States.[51]

---

47 Volney, *View*, 7.

48 Glacken, *Traces on the Rhodian Shore: Nature and Culture in Western Thought from Ancient Times to the End of the Eighteenth Century*; Judd, *The Untilled Garden: Natural History and the Spirit of Conservation in America, 1740–1840*; Rockman, "New World with a New Sky : Climatic Variability , Environmental Expectations , and the Historical Period Colonization of Eastern North America," 16; White, "Unpuzzling American Climate: New World Experience and the Foundations of a New Science," 560–61; Vogel, "The Letter from Dublin: Climate Change, Colonialism, and the Royal Society in the Seventeenth Century," 111–28.

49 Kupperman, "Fear of Hot Climates in the Anglo-American Colonial Experience," 234.

50 Volney, *View*, 25.

51 Volney, *View*, 12.

While he did not agree with American optimism about the climate, Volney did value American information and Rush valued his experience. While in Philadelphia, the Frenchman obtained climate data from Rush in an informal manner. The data on Pennsylvania's climate comes almost entirely from Rush's notes. Rush's commonplace book indicates that much of his contact with visiting scientists, politicians, and public figures occurred during such private calls. Volney met colleagues throughout his travels for breakfast, supper, and in groups at Philadelphia's salons and societies. It was not uncommon for him to collect and quote physicians, naturalists, and other intellectuals in the text. He used Jeremy Belkap's *History of New Hampshire,* visited Thomas Jefferson at Monticello, gathered information on minerology from an organization of New York doctors, and Native American linguistics from Benjamin Smith Barton.[52] On February 9, 1798, Rush met Volney to discuss a variety of topics, including the climate of the southern states as well as whether "the bones of an Italian, and Spaniard [were] heavier than the bones of a German, Hollander, and Frenchman" and whether or not suicide resulted from mental derangement.[53] The wide-ranging topics are common for Rush's conversations among colleagues who were as interested in philosophy as in empirical science. It is likely that Rush shared his ideas about the American climate as well as his meteorological data with Volney in such a meeting. By the late 1790s, Rush acknowledged the dangers of the local climate and, in the wake of several yellow fever outbreaks in American cities, was well versed in the dangers of artificial heat and city filth.

Of the data Rush provided, rainfall was perhaps the most important for Volney in constructing a generalization of the American climate. Based on Volney's tables, at 30 inches per year, Philadelphia received significantly more rain than Paris (21¾ inches) or other European cities, but did not differ substantially from American towns. These tables put numbers on the long-held assumptions that the coastal United States was wetter than comparable regions in Europe. The dampness of the country proved an explanation for illness, especially remittent and intermittent fevers associated with swampy areas. Volney summarized by stating, "that in Europe, at a medium, one third less rain falls than in North America" and "that in America it falls in heavier storms, in Europe in gentler showers; and we have seen, that facts accord

---

52 Volney, *View,* 33, 48–49, 51.
53 Benjamin Rush, Commonplace Book (1792–1813), APS, MssB.R89c, 172.

with this reasoning."[54] Dampness, especially in the presence of heat, was associated with putrefaction as a major source of disease. This placed temperate North America in a similar position as the tropics. Like White Americans themselves who were from both European and other nations, the climate they lived in was both familiar and foreign. This position, while unsettling to Volney, would prove useful for Americans like Rush when declaring their uniqueness.

Ultimately, North America's relationship with weather confused Volney in the same way it had confused newcomers for centuries. The east coast's relationship with rain serves as an example of this confusion. It had fewer rainy days, but more rainfall, and the rain evaporated more quickly than in Europe.[55] Philadelphia could experience rapid freezing in the winter and tropical storms and heat in the summer. Between his political disappointments and concerns about the nation's health, Volney's account would not serve to boost American settlement or promote the national interest. Surprisingly, Rush did not censure Volney nearly as much for his negative views on the United States as he did Pehr Kalm or Buffon. Perhaps their personal connection softened Rush's view, or, as with the American editions discussed further on, he valued the factual content of the book even if he reinterpreted the data to suit his own experience. Perhaps he simply respected the French traveler's commitment to observing the country he visited. After all, Volney saw more of the United State in the few years of his residency that Rush did in his entire life. Volney's work appears in seven notebooks of Rush's students, including all four volumes written by Samuel Agnew in 1801. Volney had a lasting influence on Rush. The French traveler provided Rush with information about the United States from regions Rush never saw firsthand. When making claims about American uniqueness, Rush needed to rely on external sources, including the careful observations of Volney.

Although Rush never completed a major work on the American climate, he regularly used weather data, geographic descriptions, and theories of improvement to diagnose cases and make suggestions for the improvement of health. Throughout his career Rush fostered relationships with naturalists and physicians who could furnish him with additional information about geography and health. Among his most frequent correspondents were his own patients and students, scattered in communities throughout the United

---

54 Volney, *View*, 239–40.
55 Volney, *View*, 240.

States. Over the course of his career Rush received thousands of letters from physicians, patients, and friends from all parts of the United States and many places beyond. By collecting, comparing, and contrasting information Rush started to claim American knowledge as his own by the turn of the nineteenth century. The next chapter will return to Rush, his medical practice, and the information provided by bodies to round out his physiology.

Chapter Four

Learning from Bodies

William Baker—a physician in Elkridge, Maryland—wrote to Benjamin Rush in 1770. The letter described a series of medical experiments he conducted as part of his practice. The form of the letter suggested that Baker looked up to Rush as a preceptor-figure despite the fact that the men must have been around the same age—in their mid-twenties. Opportunities for experimentation were rare in the American colonies and were often shared when they occurred. Physicians usually lacked control over the sick and hardly ever had access to enough bodies to make comparisons or broad claims at the same time. The few exceptions occurred in the military, during epidemics, and on plantations with large numbers of enslaved people. Baker's experience fell into the final category. Despite Rush's early antislavery writing and feeling, he willingly used and referenced the work of plantation physicians from published sources from the Caribbean to correspondence, like that of Baker.

Charles Carroll contracted Baker (and the senior physician he studied under, Dr. Howard) to inoculate 110 enslaved people against smallpox.[1] The action certainly saved lives, but Carroll was likely making a financial calculation rather than a moral decision. Smallpox was deadly in the eighteenth century with mortality rates hovering around 10 percent. An outbreak on a plantation with crowded and insufficient housing could be biologically and financially catastrophic. Meanwhile, the immune status granted by either "natural" or inoculated experience with the disease appears in advertisements for enslaved Africans and African-descended people, suggesting their increased value in slave markets.[2] Whatever the reason, Carroll's decision

---

1   William Baker to Benjamin Rush (1770) LCP, Rush Family Papers, Benjamin Rush Correspondence, Vol. II, Box 1, Folder 6.

2   Schiebinger, "Medical Experimentation and Race in the Eighteenth-Century Atlantic World," 378.

allowed the physicians to have a steady source of work for a few weeks and the control over sick bodies to test out new ideas about therapeutics.

Baker's letter described the circumstances of the inoculations and the follow-up treatment he provided. At the time, doctors debated the best time to inoculate and how to care for patients before and after the procedure.[3] The treatment was introduced to the American colonies in 1716 by an African man known to us as Onesimus. When asked by his enslaver, theologian Cotton Mather of Boston, if he had ever contracted smallpox, Onesimus essentially replied "yes and no" and described the procedure of introducing smallpox to the system on purpose. Mather later promoted the idea during an outbreak in Boston.[4] Inoculation (unlike vaccination) induced weak but active and contagious disease in patients that could spread to the uninfected, creating "natural" disease. Therefore, many communities required inoculated patients to be isolated from others during their recovery. Many only felt comfortable allowing inoculation during an active epidemic anyway, or as in the case of the Carroll plantation, inoculated as a large group.

Physicians and patients both viewed preparation and recovery as essential for a successful inoculation even as the procedure became routine in the mid-Atlantic colonies by the 1760s.[5] Baker's experiment was aimed to disprove the utility of mercury—an old Boerhaavian practice—in patients with smallpox. He wrote, "I had a fair opportunity to confirm That Theory which you deliver'd with so much accuracy to your pupils i.e. exploding the use of Mercury . . . and introducing the more diligent observance of the Cool Regimen—Truly Sensible of the ingenuity & Propriety of the Doctrine and the experiments which had been made so much in favour of it I was determined to try it."[6] In other words, the 110 enslaved and inoculated people under Baker's control did not receive the more common care, but a newer and experimental procedure promoted by Benjamin Rush to his students. Baker claimed that the experiment was successful, supporting Rush's new ideas over the aging theories of Boerhaave.

---

3   Block, *Colonial Complexions: Race and Bodies in Eighteenth-Century America*, 52–53.

4   Fenn, *Pox Americana: The Great Smallpox Epidemic of 1775–82*, 32–33.

5   Stidstone Gronim, "Imagining Inoculation: Smallpox, the Body, and Social Relations of Healing in the Eighteenth Century.," 247–68.

6   William Baker to Benjamin Rush (1770) LCP, Rush Family Papers, Benjamin Rush Correspondence, Vol. II, Box 1, Folder 6.

Baker's letter draws attention to the manner in which experimentation and clinical practice intersected with power, race, and unfree status in the American colonies. Authority needed to be tested and patient bodies were the places that testing occurred. Rush's response to Baker does not survive. His feelings, if he had any, about the ethics of this experiment are lost. He may not have thought about those aspects of the scenario much at all. Baker was not the only correspondent to write to Rush about experiments on Black bodies, military bodies, or (slightly later) poor hospitalized bodies. Rush himself collected information from patients in the Pennsylvania Hospital and the outpatient Philadelphia Dispensary (both of which catered to the city's poor in tacit exchange for providing experience and experimental material for doctors and medical students) by testing new treatments and dissecting the bodies of the deceased, searching for information about pathological processes.[7] The knowledge garnered from such interactions seemed to outweigh concerns about patient feelings or consent. Despite an acute awareness of how a doctor-patient relationship was negotiated during house calls, Rush pulled information from bodies and put it in aggregate when possible, hiding that collaboration. His notes predate the widespread use of modern statistics in medicine. As a result, Rush's arguments are more impressionistic than data driven. He kept tabs on things that interested him and jotted down thoughts on old age, dissections of children with hydrocephalus, and prevailing illnesses in conjunction with weather patterns (following the lead of physicians from Hippocrates to Sydenham).[8] These all represent typical behaviors for someone of Rush's background. Evidence from encounters like Baker's were useful for him. So too were his daily actions as a physician and medical educator. Physicians had to learn from the bodies they encountered.

Previous chapters have outlined Rush's education, identified his American system, and highlighted the way American doctors built a system of shared information. The daily work of medicine, however, is interaction with specific bodies. In addition to an avid reader, educator, and medical theorist, Rush was also a physician. He spent hours each day in the presence of bodies and minds that appeared diseased. He also spent hours each day with the healthy bodies of friends, family, and students, all of whom came under his clinical gaze. Determining health and illness required careful observation of both. This chapter narrows our lens of analysis to focus on Rush's encounters with patient bodies and the use of bodies as raw data for his work. This

---

7   Rush, *Medical Inquiries and Observations Upon the Diseases of the Mind*, 13, 316.
8   Benjamin Rush "Medical Notes, 1789–1809" LCP, Rush Family Papers, Benjamin Rush Papers, Subserives V. Medical Research and Notes, Vols. 85–87.

includes the incorporation of information from "trusted" sources like Baker. Over the course of his career Rush treated hundreds of individuals in person and consulted on cases around the country. It also pays special attention to Rush's understanding of American bodies that did not quite fit into the body politic. Articulating the "otherness" and differences introduced by gender and race was part of his system. The following pages present the source material for Rush's "American System": the patients and patient interactions that shaped his worldview. This is especially evident in his response and discussion of sex and race in student lectures and published documents.

Rush in the Clinic and the Lecture Hall

Despite what he considered a rough start in the early 1770s, Rush headed a successful medical business. In 1776, he finally found himself in a position to marry, and the ideal candidate to be his wife was Julia Stockton. Although separated at times by war, as noted in the previous chapter, the family grew quickly. By the late 1780s, Rush was part of a growing household that included himself, Julia, a growing number of children, a handful of servants, at least one enslaved man named William Grubber (later manumitted), and at times one of his sisters to help keep house. The busy home also included anywhere between three and five private pupils who paid for their education, room, and board as Rush had done with Redman two decades earlier. Home and work were blended in the eighteenth century for most families, and doctors were not an exception. Throughout his career Rush sold medications from his home and occasionally saw patients who dropped in for advice. It was also a classroom. While formal lectures were outside the home and given only in the winter, the informal teaching of private pupils could occur at any time during the day when an instructional moment arose.

Based on letters, Rush's autobiography, and case notes, he could expect to have a call or two from patients most days. Students often accompanied him, preparing for a time in which they would visit the sick on their own when Rush was too busy to attend himself. Philadelphia's population continued to grow throughout the early nineteenth century. However, its physical footprint remained walkable. This put people of all classes and backgrounds in close proximity to one another and the docks on the Delaware River, which served as the economic lifeblood of the city. In his daily rounds, Rush *saw* the American republic as a combination of people of different ages, classes, genders, races, and faith traditions, each contributing to a new society. Inside homes, the republican analogies continued on a smaller scale between family members. Physicians entered the most private parts of a home to intimately engage with sick bodies and minds. They relied not only upon their expert observations, but the narrative the sick person and their family members could give of their own illness and accounts from family members. The experience could be long or short but was always intimate.

In medical lectures, Rush addressed the importance of conduct in the sickroom. He told his students that good relationships with "ladies" were essential for a practicing physician. In some ways the doctor entered an otherwise feminine domain by interacting with the sick. In eighteenth-century Philadelphia women typically called physicians, introduced them to patients, and managed the nursing care of family members after the doctor left. Midwives and other women healers also acted as important intermediaries between physicians and possible patients. As discussed above, Rush specifically noted his indebtedness to a Philadelphia midwife—known only as Mrs. Patten—for helping him find clients in his autobiography. He also worked with more general women healers and apothecaries who conducted business within the city or ladies interested in medical science who volunteered their skills.[9] In this respect, communication and collaboration with women were both vital for a physician's reputation and livelihood. In his fourth lecture of the year in 1802, Rush specifically addressed decorum in the home of a patient and the typical steps taken in a house call.

> Observe a due respect and the rules of good breeding toward every part of the family in your visits to see a patient. If a lady conduct[s] you up stairs [sic] to see the patient, always walk up before her, but let her enter the sick room first: and in returning downstairs walk behind her . . . Always let the patient know of your arrival before you enter the room; this you may apprise him of by your walk, or by speaking. The consulting physician should avoid visiting the patient alone; as questions may be asked, or he may make use of expressions, which will produce embarrassment afterwards. Let the attending physician speak to the patient first; and make the first enquiries. Do not feel for the pulse immediately on entering the room of a sick person. Sit down on a chair, or trunk, or some convenient place (but the pulse should be felt before the patient describes the disease, as speaking accelerates the pulse) and converse with the patient on some unimportant subject; but never introduce foreign subjects nor speak of them, unless introduced by the patient—when the patient becomes perfectly at his ease introduce the subject of his complaint . . . let him tell you all he knows respecting it before you ask any questions; for the sick can generally give the best description of their situation, if not interrupted by interrogatories; though they seldom give a correct account of the causes.[10]

---

9   Brandt, *Women Healers: Gender, Authority, and Medicine in Early Philadelphia*.

10   Amos A. Evans, "Notes Taken From Dr. Rush's Lectures upon the Institutes and Practice of Medicine and on Clinical Cases, Vol. I" (USS Constituion

The interaction described here is one of consultation. It is, of course, idealized and makes key assumptions about the nature of the home in question. The patient has a family, is able to give some description of their disease, and is free to listen to or ignore the doctor. This agency so central to the free person's house call and construed as normal was complicated by slavery and by hospitalization as discussed below. The account provided in the lecture notes highlights important aspects of the relationship between a physician and his patient, his colleagues, and the patient's family. Patients and their families were the first experts on illness and their narratives acted as important data points for a physician. Furthermore, the text notes the importance of behaving in a sociable as well as professional manner. Barging into a room and immediately asking about illness or reaching out for a pulse was not only rude but could affect the body of the patient and provide false information (an eighteenth-century white-coat syndrome). Finally, unlike a hospital, military encampment, or plantation, the physician in the home of free people (especially those of equal or higher class status) had to share his power.

In some respects, physicians around the turn of the nineteenth century were detectives. The purpose of a doctor was to explain, predict, and ease a patient's course through illness. Doing so required a considerable amount of information about the history of the patient and his or her physical circumstances. This is worth reflecting on because it is fundamentally different from the medical exchanges of the twenty-first century. Modern diagnosis as a result of standardized signs and symptoms did not make sense in the fluid- and system-driven world of Rush. Disease was a process to be overcome not an event to be eliminated with a quick round of antibiotics. When Rush recommended bloodletting, for example, it was not in some hope that releasing blood would cure the disease but that it would alter the body and make it able to undo the damage wrought by irregularity. Afterward the patient would need to maintain a strict diet and exercise regimen to build strength back in a regular manner. Convalescence was serious business. For any two-week fever a patient might reasonably assume about a month of careful recovery. This meant that doctors had a different relationship with patient bodies. The narrative of illness remained key as well as the specific alterations between diseased state and health for each body.[11] It also meant that each illness contributed to a physician's collective experience with different diseases and constitutions.

Museum, access via Internet Archive, 1802), 23–25, http://www.archive.org/details/notestakenfromdr00evan.

11 Hamlin, *More Than Hot: A Short History of Fever*.

Some doctors found the negotiation of the sick room to be grating and preferred to exert control over sick bodies without argument. James Woodhouse, a young correspondent of Rush's in the 1790s, spoke excitedly of the increased control he had over military patients housed in a hospital boat compared to civilian patients.[12] Unlike the home visit, hospitals and dispensaries provided a chance for doctors to see multiple patients at once and (at least attempt to) exert more control over those patients. The Pennsylvania Hospital offered additional opportunities for Rush to observe human bodies, both alive and deceased. In his 1802 lectures Amos Evans reported Rush's descriptions of how bodies should be arranged with separate wards for patients with fevers and a significant distance between patients and the surgical amphitheater. Rush also noted the ideal institution would have a space reserved for the examination of dead bodies.[13] While the lecture notes do not clearly state the purpose of such examinations, other Rush writings suggest that he actively searched for physical alterations in organs that could shed light on the fatal disease. Similar searches for lesions or other structural changes among French physicians have been described by historians as part of the revolutionary turn toward clinical medicine.[14]

Rush used bodies differently. There is little evidence that Rush cared about Parisian clinical medicine even if he had been aware of the work of contemporaries like Xavier Bichat (1771–1802) or François-Joseph-Victor Broussais (1772–1838). He may have received some information about their work through correspondents in France, although most of his connections were with the Montpellier vitalists.[15] Rush looked to structural changes to support not supplant an idea of disease as an individualized process and state

---

12   James Woodhouse to Benjamin Rush (1791), LCP, Rush Family Papers, Benjamin Rush Correspondence, Vol. XXVI.

13   Evans, "Notes Taken From Dr. Rush's Lectures upon the Institutes and Practice of Medicine and on Clinical Cases, Vol. I," 5.

14   Weiner and Sauter, "The City of Paris and the Rise of Clinical Medicine," 23–42; Williams, "Neuroses of the Stomach: Eating, Gender, and Psychopathology in French Medicine, 1800–1870," 54–79; Jean Nicolas (baron) Corvisart des Marets, C.E. Horeau, and Jacob Gates, *An Essay on the Organic Diseases and Lesions of the Heart and Great Vessels From the Clinical Lectures of J.N. Corvisart*; Miller, *A Modern History of the Stomach: Gastric Illness, Medicine and British Society, 1800–1950.*

15   For more on the theories present in Montpellier, see Cimino et al., *Vitalisms: From Haller to the Cell Theory*; King, *The Medical World of the Eighteenth Century*; Sykes, "The Art of Listening: Perceiving Pulse in Eighteenth-Century

of bodily disfunction. Observing the brains of children who died of encephalitis and adults who perished in the Pennsylvania Hospital's wards for "diseases of the mind," he looked for the scars of physiological actions. Damaged tissues indicated the presence of poorly managed "excitement" and the flow of that excitement in bodies. In this way Rush's morbid anatomy was not so different from earlier anatomical work that hoped to explain the mechanisms behind healthy function.

Together these ordinary events of viewing patients in their homes or in the hospital formed the raw material of medical theorizing. Rush encountered bodies in the narrative context of disease. The medical encounter represented only one part of a body's journey from health through illness to recovery or death. Healthy bodies possessed variation that doctors needed to understand as well. Weather, cultural, and political situations could alter health as noted in the previous chapter. Other differences, however, appeared more essential in Rush's work. Sex difference in particular looms large as a rare instance where he clearly put bodies into unchanging groups. He treated male and female bodies as fundamentally and irrevocably different.

Sex and Gender in the American System

For the most part, all bodies were created equal in Rush's medicine. Time, place, age, inherited peculiarities, and climate physically altered them, creating individuality, but the underlying systems functioned the same way. Those alterations also changed the body's relationship to physiological excitement and altered the balance of healthy systems. Rush's peculiar interest in excitement aside, his general views recapitulated the theories of numerous physicians and naturalists of his day. Frequently, this resulted in a clear pronouncement followed by numerous alterations in his published work or medical lectures. This occurred in 1802 when he considered the normal function of the pulse. After clearly noting the expected heart rate for healthy people based on age (66 strokes per minute for an adult, 140 from birth to age three, and between 80 and 108 for children between three and seven), he introduced the role of variation while clearly relying on the work of others writing "[t]he pulse is influenced by the sex—quicker in females as well as more frequent—Seldom & slow among Savages—quicker in large cities— In short people—Climate & Season influence the pulse—heat accelerates

France,"; Williams, *A Cultural History of Medical Vitalism in Enlightenment Montpellier.*

it—Slow in cold climates—seldom above 40 strokes in a minute in a green-lander [sic]."[16] Knowing how the pulse changed would have been critical for a physician lest he treat a healthy child for fever because her pulse was greater than an adult man's. Climate, sex, and level of "civilization" all played a role in shaping this most important physiological marker in Rush's therapeutics.

Rush thought that the combination of these circumstances resulted in the differential health between individuals as well as the shared general health, characteristics, or illness of groups. This explained the differences between cultures and accounted for both individual and epidemic diseases. Major changes to the chemical makeup of the atmosphere, for example, could trigger epidemics. Meanwhile, variations in height, skin color, or general health could be the result of cultural practices, time outdoors, or diet, as discussed at the end of this chapter. Only two categories appear across cultures in Rush's writings as unchanging differences: age and sex. The former, as noted in the case of the pulse, created a framework to understand change over time in individual bodies. Both childhood and old age held special significance in Rush's writings. Knowledge of children's bodies and minds informed his view of childrearing and education discussed in chapter 8. Meanwhile, Rush had an unpolished curiosity about the particularities of old age. He published little on the subject but kept a notebook containing the medical histories of his oldest patients without analysis.[17] Sex, however, was the primary division—perhaps *the* essential division—that Rush explored in healthy bodies. In this section the terms *sex*, *male*, and *female* are used to describe the presumed physical sex of bodies. *Gender*, *man*, and *woman* are used when discussing how Rush blended ideas about physical bodies with socially prescribed attributes attached to those assumed to be men or women. For Rush sex, gender, and gender roles were synonymous rather than separate biological and social categories, respectively.

After 1789 Rush took over the role once held by John Morgan in teaching theory and practice of medicine. These courses are critical for understanding Rush's evolution as a medical system builder and cornerstone of the American profession, ushering thousands of men into their vocation. Each year he presented students with guidance on the general treatment of healthy and sick bodies, the role of a physician, and how medical knowledge was

16 Evans, "Notes Taken From Dr. Rush's Lectures upon the Institutes and Practice of Medicine and on Clinical Cases, Vol. I," 35.

17 Rush, "Histories of the Manner of Life of Sundry Men and Women Above 80 Years of Life, 1798," LCP, Rush Family Papers, Series I Benjamin Rush Papers, Subseries V Medical Research and Notes, Vol. 88.

produced. This included long discussions of the differences between the bodies, minds, and treatment of men and women.

Rush's published and manuscript lectures on physiology implicitly emphasized sexual difference as essential knowledge for medical men by literally foregrounding the uniqueness of female bodies in the lecture order. In addressing sex, Rush focused mainly on the distinctness of women to his male audience. He not only argued that women were physically distinct from men, but that their physiology determined their appropriate role in society. This applied to men as well, but women's bodies were presented as more transparent, and more essentialized. Women, in Rush's opinion, had physiological requirements that were the opposite of those needed by men. As a result, their interactions with the world, their own bodies, and disease did not follow the same patterns as those of men. Female bodies needed to throw off excess excitement and demonstrated their illness or malfunction through alterations in regularly observable events like menstruation, pregnancy, and childbirth.

Rush specifically noted that it likely took about a month for a female body to collect excess excitement and fluid and then discharge it in the form of a menstrual period or other forms when menses were blocked.[18] Diseases associated with reproduction formed a foundation for the discussion of women, their roles in society, and the utility of Rush's system. This anticipated a view of women's bodies common in the nineteenth century when medicine reinforced concepts of female weakness and domesticity.[19] Rush did not explicitly argue that women were "weak" but did describe female bodies as inherently suited to a Western cultural view of domesticity and that deviation from such roles led to disease through excessive excitement bombarding their bodies, especially if it came from physical labor. As discussed below, women who did experience excessive excitement were pathological and perhaps unsexed. Rush worried that too much labor resulted in lower fertility rates, delayed menstruation, and disease, especially among Indigenous and African-descended enslaved women.[20]

As Rush put it, gender came from "an original difference in the bodies & minds of men & women, stamped upon both in the womb, by the hand

---

18 Rush Lecture Notes on Physiology, LCP, Rush Family Papers, Series I Benjamin Rush Papers, Vol. 180, 732.

19 Smith-Rosenberg and Rosenberg, "The Female Animal: Medical and Biological Views of Woman and Her Role in Nineteenth- Century America," 332–56.

20 Rush Lecture Notes on Physiology, LCP, Rush Family Papers, Series I Benjamin Rush Papers, Vol. 180.

of nature."[21] This is a strong endorsement of a "two-sex" model of anatomy and physiology described by Thomas Laqueur. Essentially, those who supported this model argued that male and female bodies were not variations on one another but different machines entirely that required a different set of guidelines to keep them healthy.[22] Rush—and many of his contemporaries—believed that women in different societies suffered from and had to compensate for their "unhealthy" lifestyles because they naturally required a sedentary and domestic life. Enlightenment concepts like stadial theory—a means of understanding social "progress"—also relied on assessments of the social and physical state of women. According to many Scottish theorists advances in "civilization" improved women's social standing and women's health when compared with "savage" societies. Rush would take this further and suggest that the American republic would specifically create a society to provide the best and healthiest opportunities for women as well as men, at least by process of elimination in his lectures.[23]

Rush found markers of sex throughout human bodies.[24] As discussed in chapter 2, his physiology assumed that bodies needed a balanced and regular flow of excitement. In terms of that balance, men and women were opposites and in turn had opposite management styles. Using Rush's physiological terms, male bodies absorbed, and female bodies abstracted stimulus or "excitement." In Rush's reasoning, this fundamental difference written throughout bodies and not just in the organs of generation dictated the social roles suitable to each gender. In this manner, sex acted as a category that dictated all parts of a person's life. Recall that in Rush's physiology, all human actions contributed to the careful balance of excitement required for healthy function. If men and women needed and reacted to excitement in fundamentally different ways, then they needed to live fundamentally different lives. Each year in his medical lectures Rush discussed the physiological differences between male and female bodies. Beginning with women (the presumed "other") and a room full of men he discussed the general differences between the sexes, differences deemed obvious to the casual observer. Anyone could point to a woman's stature or lack of beard to identify her as

---

21 Rush Lecture Notes on Physiology, LCP, Rush Family Papers, Series I Benjamin Rush Papers, Vol. 166.

22 Schiebinger, *Nature's Body: Gender in the Making of Modern Science*; Laqueur, *Making Sex: Body and Gender from the Greeks to Freud.*

23 Rush, Lecture Notes, LCP, Vol. 165.

24 Laqueur, "Orgasm, Generation, and the Politics of Reproductive Biology," 1–41; Laqueur, *Making Sex: Body and Gender from the Greeks to Freud.*

female as easily as clothing. Beyond obvious structural differences, however, lymph, glands, and the system of abstraction they belonged to, helped create that distinction under the skin.

Focusing on women and female bodies provides a fuller picture of Rush's ideas surrounding physiology. In much of the secondary literature, Rush's medical system is best known for therapeutics that caused sudden abstraction of excitement by targeting the organs that transmitted that excitement to the body via the blood vessels. Bleeding pulled excitement out of the vessels by reducing the physical pressure of the blood on the vessels themselves. Likewise, purges and emetics loosened the body and released dangerous tensions caused by fevers. A simple reading might suggest that Rush viewed illness as an excess of excitement. Rush's physiology, however, was more nuanced, emphasizing regularity of motion rather than amount of excitement. In his lecture notes on the subject, he wrote that the body "in a morbid State . . . is in a State in which its functions are performed with difficulty, & irregularity" and that a weakness could predispose a body to fall ill. Bringing the body to a state of low excitement allowed for a safe "reboot" of the system to remove the predisposing debility.[25] Women's bodies provided a blueprint for understanding the natural processes of absorption and abstraction.

To understand natural abstraction, we need to shift our attention from the flashy therapeutics and focus on the fundamentals of Rush's female physiology. Numerous physicians pointed to the definitionally female processes of menstruation, gestation, and lactation to explain the less energetic or less tense female body.[26] By releasing fluids they were viewed as releasing tension, stimulus, or energy. This was especially the case in warm climates where both women and effeminate men were considered to be more resistant to fevers that claimed the lives of more masculine men with tenser fibers. Rush, however, went beyond these actions. He looked for a means of explaining sexual differences at all points in men and women's lives, not only those associated with reproduction. After all, young girls and elderly matrons were still female even if they did not menstruate. The masculine blood vessels needed an equal and opposite system in the body. That system of abstraction, Rush presumed, could be found in another set of vessels and organs: the lymphatic vessels and glands.

---

25   Rush, "Notes on Materia Medica" (c. 1799), LCP, Rush Family Papers, Benjamin Rush, Box 2, Vol. 133.

26   Seth, *Difference and Disease: Medicine, Race, and the Eighteenth-Century British Empire.*

In Rush's theory, glands like the thyroid (which he thought absorbed excitement by redirecting blood away from the brain) and the lymphatic vessels protected bodies by moving excitement out of the body and disbursing it on the skin. This was essential for female bodies that lived in a world full of excessive excitement. It is not completely clear what Rush was referring to when he wrote about the lymphatic vessels, which were still somewhat mysterious in the late eighteenth century. They clearly included vascular structures found throughout the body, which did not carry blood. Occasionally, he lumped lymphatics together with the lacteals (vessels found in the abdominal cavity) or assigned similar functions to the two sets of vessels: the movement of excitement from inside the body to the skin's surface.

Rush's first exposure to the lymphatics as important structures probably came from Boerhaave. In a volume of Boerhaave's lectures owned by Rush, the Dutch physician described the lymph fluid as a rarefied form of blood (lacking red globules or red blood cells) and the lymphatic vessels as a small continuation of the circulatory system.[27] Rush did not follow Boerhaave's anatomical assertion, however, his association of lymphatic vessels with the larger circulation does resemble Boerhaave. He benefited from the experiments of Alexander Monro and Willian Hunter on the structure of the vessels. In a letter discussing his dispute with Hunter and Hewson, Monro recounted his experiments on the lymphatic systems of animals, which he carried out in the late 1750s and early 1760s. By summer 1759, he was convinced that the lymphatics were a separate system from the circulatory system and responsible for the absorption of substance from the skin into the body. He taught this viewpoint in his classes throughout the 1760s, including those attended by Rush.[28] Although Rush used the structures promoted by Monro, Hunter, Hewson, and others, he moved the focus away from

---

27 Boerhaave, *Dr. Boerhaave's Academical Lectures on the Theory of Physic Being A Genuine Translation of His Institutes and Explanatory Comments, Collated and Adjusted to Each Other, as They Were Dictated to His STUDENTS at the University of Leyden, Vol. II.*, 227.

28 Monro, *A State of Facts Concerning The First Proposal of Performing the Paracentesis of the Thorax, on Account of Air Effused from the Lungs into the Cavities of the Pleurae; and Concerning The Discovery of the Lymphatic Valvular Absorbent System of Vessels in O.* Eales, "The History of the Lymphatic System, with Special Reference to the Hunter-Monro Controversy"; Ambrose, "The Priority Dispute over the Function of the Lymphatic System and Glisson's Ghost (the 18th-Century Hunter-Monro Feud)."

absorption of material and toward the abstraction of excitement. In doing so, they became gendered organs.

Contemporaries' writing on the glands also contributed to Rush's construction of a system of abstraction. By the early nineteenth century, it was common knowledge in medical circles that women had proportionally larger thyroids than their male counterparts. From Rush's perspective, this difference made perfect sense and reinforced his ideas regarding thyroid function. In his 1801 lecture notes, Rush student Russel Clark noted that the larger thyroids of women led Rush to believe that the organ was associated with the protection of the sensitive female brain.[29] Going the other direction, during a paroxysm of mania or hysteria the thyroid could swell and take in blood from the head in a condition called *globus hystericus*. Later, in his psychiatry textbook, *Diseases of the Mind* (1812), Rush listed *globus hystericus* as one effect of fear. The strong passion, he argued, could trigger many physiological effects, including the rush of blood and subsequent swelling of the thyroid.[30]

Between the existence of a mirror system to the exciting and masculine circulation and larger female glands, Rush had the blueprint for a feminized body, which needed to throw off excitement rather than circulate and accumulate the substance. Women, according to Rush, possessed a higher sensitivity to environmental stimulus. This ability allowed them to live the sedentary domestic lives he believed they were designed for; however, it also left them in greater danger of disease. The larger thyroid enabled women to abstract excess excitement that might take their systems by surprise. Rush explained that the larger thyroids were "necessary to guard the female system from the influence of the more numerous causes of irritation and vexation of mind, and the more acute bodily disease, to which they are exposed than the male sex."[31]

The lymphatics even managed to take on an additional subsidiary role in women with respect to reproduction. In lectures and his own notes, Rush suggested that semen entered the lymphatic vessels after being absorbed by the walls of the vagina.[32] Rush rejected the notion that sperm and egg met in either the fallopian tubes or uterus. His reasons were mechanical. Firstly, penis size or location of ejaculation in the vagina did not appear to alter a

---

29   Russel Clark, Lecture Notes (1801), KCRBM, ms. Coll 225, Item 11, Vol. I.

30   Rush, *Medical Inquiries and Observations Upon the Diseases of the Mind*, 323.

31   Rush, "An Inquiry into the Functions of the Spleen, Liver, Pancreas, and Thyroid Gland," 28.

32   Benjamin Rush, Lectures on Physiology, Library Company of Philadelphia, Rush Family Papers, Volume 181, Yi2 7397 F.L8.

person's chance of becoming pregnant. Rush's version of his lectures included a footnote stating, "I knew a student of Physic in Edinburgh who was called upon to marry a girl to whom he was engaged, in consequence of her having become suddenly pregnant, who assured me that he had never had such a connection with her as had injured her badge of virginity." In addition to several cases of pregnancy in young women who appeared "intact," related by man-midwives, Rush concluded that semen did not need a deep entry into the female system to fertilize the ovum.[33]

The second reason Rush rejected the concept of fertilization within the uterus had to do with ectopic pregnancy. If sperm traveled through the vagina and uterus, then how did it then manage to exit the female reproductive tract altogether and help create an embryo in the abdominal cavity? At the time, Rush considered this route for fertilization other American physicians were taking a public interest in the phenomena, many of whom were likely former students. At the end of the eighteenth century, the first American medical journals published several cases of the disorder.[34] Each of these accounts show an interest in the immediate cure of an extrauterine event. They are, essentially, surgical studies. Although physicians typically considered extrauterine pregnancy a death sentence, William Bayham claimed success in treatment, reporting two cases in which he removed fetuses surgically from the abdominal cavity of women who survived.[35] Rush's interest brings the narrative back to the lymphatics and the female body as a whole. If extrauterine events occurred, which based on the articles might have *seemed* surprisingly frequent in the early nineteenth century, then semen needed a way out of the female reproductive structures that still brought it into contact with the ovum.

Rush also suggested that peak health of the lymphatics could improve fertility, further imbedding them in his definition of the female body. Following his arguments on unwanted conceptions Rush wrote of the importance of

---

33 Ibid.

34 William Bayham to College of Physicians of Philadelphia, "Case of an extrauterine Conception" May 12, 1796, College of Physicians of Philadelphia Manuscript Archives; Baynham, "An Account of Two Cases of Extra-Uterine Conception; in Each of Which the Foetus Was Extracted by an Operation with Success," 161–70; Smith, "A Case of Extra-Uterine Conception, in Which an Operation Was Performed," 54–57; Ramsay, "A Case of Extra-Uterine Foetus, with Some Observations on the Subject Generally," 221–28; Clark, "Case of Extra-Uterine Gestation," 292–95.

35 Baynham, "An Account of Two Cases of Extra-Uterine Conception; in Each of Which the Foetus Was Extracted by an Operation with Success."

strong lymphatic movement to absorb and circulate the semen as a matter of the system as a whole. To encourage pregnancy, he had the following advice:

> The two last [power of lymphatic vessels and state of ovaria] are greatly influenced by a peculiar *state of excitability in the female system*—hence we find conception to be most certain, immediately <u>before</u> or <u>after</u> menstruation—after a fit of sickness particularly a malignant fever, after a long bdomen [sic]—After the action of fresh steam upon the system by a woman's <u>visiting a foreign country</u> and after using the warm Bath.[36]

Each of the above-mentioned instances would have increased the general excitement of the female body in a healthy manner making it ready to bear children. Following the logic of Rush's system, this increased excitement would have stimulated the lymphatics into action, circulating and disposing of excitement, but also of sperm, as needed. These preactivated lymphatics (and in this particular case ovaries as well) were in an ideal position to efficiently circulate semen and deposit it in the correct location.

The idea that the lymphatics played a role in reproduction is an example of Rush's firm belief that men and women possessed different physiologies suited to different social and biological tasks. Even in children, sex made its mark. In 1796, one student, surname Hare, noted that even in very small children who still dressed alike respiration could give away their sex to the careful on-looker. Very young children all wore simple dresses in this period and wore similar hair styles regardless of sex. Nevertheless, Rush believed that gender was so essential that bodies could not be confused. He wrote, "[r]espiration is performed differently in the male and female. A Girl moves her breast more and her bdomenn [sic] less than a boy. This is wisely intended to favor gestation."[37] Based on this assumption, Rush claimed he could determine sex gender even in infants. The exact manner in which breathing favored gestation is not discussed, but likely these hint at a mechanical explanation. If women moved their abdomens while breathing it would either disturb a fetus or inhibit the breathing of a pregnant woman. By taking shallower breaths from the chest, Rush's reasoning went, the growth of a fetus would not take up space usually used by the lungs for respiration. Either way, this example, like that of the lymphatics or thyroid, shows how healthy

---

36   Benjamin Rush, Lectures on Physiology, Library Company of Philadelphia, Rush Family Papers, Volume 181, Yi2 7397 F.L8.

37   Hare, Lecture Notes 1796, UPenn Kislak, Ms. Coll. 225, Item 9, Vol. I; M. Wallant, Lecture Notes 1798, UPenn Kislak, Ms. Coll. 225, Item 10; Samuel Agnew, Lecture Notes 1801, UPenn Kislak, Ms. Coll. 225, Item 8, Vol. I.

male and healthy female bodies possessed fundamentally different forms that hinted at their preordained social and biological functions.

The process of maturation acted as a key point of inquiry regarding the specific influences of the environment of human bodies, cultures, and practices. Physicians at the time thought that age at first and last menstrual period was closely connected to environment and culture. Some physicians claimed that nonwhite women matured faster than their European counterparts. In Jamaica, British physician Hans Sloane (1660–1753) argued that after moving to the island English and Scottish women experienced shorter cycles in the heat (a century later Rush believed the opposite).[38] At the turn of the nineteenth century, Rush argued that warm climates brought earlier and longer periods and aged women more quickly. Meanwhile, the cold weather of northern New England might delay a girl's first period until she was nearly eighteen years old. Loss of blood in cold weather could trigger an imbalance of excitement and lower the base level of excitement in the female body too much. Menstrual blood both released excess excitement, plethora, and signified a healthy female body possessed of requisite excitement for procreation. The reduction of excitement came from the loss of blood pressure during menstruation akin to bloodletting. The fact that there was sufficient excitement to lose blood, meanwhile, indicated that excitement was cycling, and could both deliver sperm to egg and support the needs of a growing fetus.

If women differed fundamentally from men, could their bodies reveal different information based in new mental and physical environments? Rush's answer was an unequivocal "yes." His observations of women lent support to the idea that they were physically determined to live sedentary lives, raise children, and govern morality as discussed in chapter 5. Republican wives and mothers would raise children in a moral population prepared for democratic governance, which in turn would literally produce a healthier country. In the west, life looked less certain. Rush, like many supporters of environmental "improvement" of his day, looked forward to a time in which the settled and agrarian lifestyle idealized in American culture expanded seamlessly beyond the Appalachian Mountains. Cultivation and a widespread population would limit disease and encourage the democratic ideals that filled Thomas Jefferson's dreams. Reaching this goal, however, proved less straightforward. The experiences of colonization, epidemic disease, and western

---

38   Bullough and Voght, "Women, Menstruation, and Nineteenth-Century Medicine," 66–82; Seth, "Materialism, Slavery, and The History of Jamaica," 767; Churchill, "Bodily Differences?: Gender, Race, and Class in Hans Sloane's Jamican Medical Practice, 1678–1688," 417–22.

revolts showed Americans that optimistic improvement schemes were not as simple as they sounded.[39]

Making Race in Rush's World

If sex is a rare example of how bodies could be clearly grouped in Rush's physiology, then race demonstrates the far more common kind of grouping in Rush's view: a variable and unstable category. Besides sex and small individual differences between different bodies, he believed that human beings were essentially the same. However, by the turn of the nineteenth century European-descended Americans recognized three different groups of North American inhabitants: white, Black, and Indian. As discussed by Sharon Block, this shift to a racialized understanding of bodies went beyond merely skin color, to include facial features, personality traits, employment, and cultural practices.[40] It developed over time to flatten out distinctions between individuals, communities, and nations and serve as a shorthand for social dichotomies including free or enslaved, citizen or noncitizen, "civilized" or "savage." Those who believed in a single origin for all humans (monogenesis) like Rush argued that cultural practices and climate worked together to create racial difference over time. In the late eighteenth century, this group made up the majority of American men of science. Race in this sense was fluid. That did not mean, however, that it wasn't a social reality that became entangled with medical theorizing. Nor did it mean that Rush was immune from notions of racial and especially cultural hierarchy, the foundation for racist and xenophobic ideas. It did mean that by the late eighteenth century, Rush was at some pains to try and explain how, after over a century of European settlement in North America, three "races" inhabited the same space without starting to resemble one another.

Sitting between European and non-European cultures in the midst of revolution, white Americans found themselves in an unstable racial space. As a young doctor in 1774, Benjamin Rush delivered an oration on comparative medicine and ethnography to the American Philosophical Society that addressed this instability. Although the American speech took place early in his career, only five years after his return from Britain and two years before

---

39   Golinski, "Debating the Atmospheric Constitution: Yellow Fever and the American Climate"; Hedges, "Benjamin Rush, Charles Brockden Brown, and the American Plague Year," 295–311; Onuf, "Liberty, Development, and Union : Visions of the West in the 1780s," 179–213.

40   Block, *Colonial Complexions: Race and Bodies in Eighteenth-Century America.*

the American colonists declared independence, it demonstrated principles that informed his work for decades. Rush included it in his anthologized medical text, *Medical Inquiries and Observations,* as late as 1805, indicating his continued interest in the topic and some consistency in his theory.

This theory effectively made race a product of culture, but that did not take away from the fact that Rush gave "race" a biological reality. As demonstrated below, difference in disease expression became a key marker of culturally determined biological difference in Rush's view. The result is as disturbing as any assertion of scientific racism or arguments of racial superiority. More than skin color or any other physical feature, this difference—the presence or absence of disease and expressions of culture—clearly marked one race from another and suggested that they had little to learn from each other. Little mention was made of medicinal knowledge that had entered Euro-American practice from African and American societies, from cinchona bark to smallpox inoculation. In Rush's mind a body, for example, exposed to a variable climate was so different from and equivalent to a body in the same location but shielded from the elements that they were medically incompatible. Rush defined racial boundaries in this essay by essentially saying, "we don't have the same diseases as you."

That idea carried on as a core means of noting difference between groups based on culture and climate. Even within groups considered to be of the same "race" there existed considerable variation based on location, class, and travel, all of which had consequences for medical treatment. When instructing students to interact with patients Rush noted this explicitly, stating:

> Inquire the native place of the patient. For the disease of foreigners are often influenced by those of their own country. At the time when the fever prevailed at barbadoes [sic] which was accompanied with, or succeeded by swelled legs those natives who came to this country, and merely had our common intermittents, have obstinate swellings of those parts. People from warm climates bear bleeding less when they settle in more northern than the natives of those climates and those from cold countries will bear greater bleedings when they go southward, than those among whom they go.[41]

Living in an Atlantic trade hub, Rush had plenty of opportunities to treat and converse with long-distance travelers or migrants to and from the mid-Atlantic. The differences encountered between European-descended and Native American bodies, meanwhile, appeared all the more extreme in his essay.

---

41 Evans, "Notes Taken From Dr. Rush's Lectures upon the Institutes and Practice of Medicine and on Clinical Cases, Vol. I," 27–28.

In the 1774 essay, Rush attempted to use comparative ethnography of Native Americans and to a lesser extent elite Britons to argue for a unique Euro-American culture, neither British nor Indigenous. This new culture, he felt, had the potential to be healthier than either of the others and be the best suited (biologically speaking) to live in and "improve" North America. The two cultures he compared stood at opposite ends of an Enlightenment-era spectrum of "civility." Rush specifically defined the different states of "civilization" by how they obtained food: "the savage lives by fishing and hunting; the barbarous, by pasturage or cattle; and the civilized, by agriculture."[42] American Indians remained largely in what he considered a "savage" state, whereas the British (especially the well-to-do of London, Edinburgh, and Bath) sat at the pinnacle of refined and sensible society, perhaps even over-civilized.[43] It was too refined a society by his measure. Americans of European descent had not, in Rush's view, firmly settled into a pattern and had the ability to plan their institutions around the knowledge presented. During the American Revolution, Rush used the oration to make a statement about what type of people Anglo-Americans could be if they applied themselves. They were neither Native nor British and had the ability to maintain healthy, informed, balance.

---

42 Irving-Stonebraker, "Nature, Knowledge, and Civilization. Connecting the Atlantic and Pacific Worlds in the Enlightenment," 93–107; McCosh, *The Scottish Philosophy, Biographical, Expository, Critical, From Hutcheson to Hamilton*, 263; Wolloch, "The Civilizing Process, Nature, and Stadial Theory," 245–59; Moran, "Between the Savage and the Civil: Dr John Gregory's Natural History of Femininity"; Haakonssen, *Medicine and Morals in the Enlightenment: John Gregory, Thomas Percival, and Benjamin Rush*; McCullough, "Hume's Influence on John Gregory and the History of Medical Ethics," 376–95; Gregory, *Observations on the Duties and Offices of a Physician and on the Method of Prosecuting Enquiries in Philosophy*; Gregory, *A Father's Legacy to His Daughters*; Moseley, *Medical Tracts*; Cadogan, *Dissertation on the Gout, and All Chronic Diseases, Jointly Considered, As Proceeding from the Same Causes; What Those Causes Are; and A Rational and Natural Method of Cure Proposed*; Hume, "Essay XXIV: Of National Charactes,"; Montesquieu et al., *The Spirit of Laws, Vol. I*; Beattie, *Elements of Moral Science*; Reid, *Essays on the Powers of the Human Mind*.

43 Rush, "An Inquiry into the Natural History of Medicine among the Indians of North-America; and a Comparative View of Their Diseases and Remedies with Those of Civilized Nations," 5.

Rush highlighted the comparative nature of his work in the paper's title "An Inquiry into the Natural History of Medicine among the Indians of North-America; and a Comparative View of Their Diseases and Remedies with Those of Civilized Nations." As noted previously, disease, cure, and culture could not be separated in Rush's view of physiology. How someone lived altered the manner in which they exposed themselves to and managed their excitement. Therefore, right living and the prevention of illness in the first place was the best cure. A poorly planned city, miasma-ridden home, or improper labor for women could lead to pathological excitement and disease. Society functioned analogously. If a group of people engaged in culturally mandated unhealthy or healthy behavior it would show in their bodies. A key example of this is found in a slightly later ethnographic work on Pennsylvania's German population, *An Account of the Manners of the German Inhabitants of Pennsylvania* (1789). Germans, Rush argued, maintained their characteristic robust health though the consumption of vegetables all year by using sauerkraut in the winter. German-American health stood in stark contrast to the illness of fashionable Anglo-Americans and their meat-heavy diet.[44]

As with his German neighbors, Rush relied on first-hand knowledge from his time as a student in Edinburgh and London to address British health. He also had access to numerous texts on the diseases of the British elite, most famously George Cheyne's *The English Malady*.[45] Worry about nervous diseases only grew over the course of the century aided by the nerve-centric physiology promoted at the University of Edinburgh. During Rush's student days, the diseases were closely associated with the British gentry and middling sorts. By the turn of the nineteenth century, it was considered a danger to all people as nervous fevers attacked the poor as well as the rich.[46]

In the case of people of African descent, Rush relied on his daily practice as well as gleaning information from correspondents and printed texts (albeit

---

44   Rush, *An Account of the Manners of the German Inhabitants of Pennsylvania*, 18–19.

45   For a discussion of the Cheyne's life and work, see Guerrini, *Obesity and Depression in the Enlightenment: The Life and Times of George Cheyne*.

46   Bynum, "The Nervous Patient in Eighteenth- and Nineteenth-Century Britain: The Psychiatric Origins of British Neurology," 89–102; Beatty, *Nervous Disease in Late Eighteenth-Century Britain: The Reality of a Fashionable Disorder*; Hare, "The History of 'Nervous Disorders' from 1600 to 1840, and a Comparison with Modern Views," 37–45; Wild, *Medicine-by-Post: The Changing Voice of Illness in Eighteenth-Century British Consultation Letters and Literature*, 116–20; Berrios, "'Febrile Anxiety', by Robert James (1745)," 114.

ones with unreliable narrators, like Baker at the beginning of this chapter). Rush's practice notes included multiple references to "negros" he treated, and he also had close ties with leaders in the African American community, especially A.M.E. ministers Richard Allen and Absalom Jones.[47]

Rush's interactions with Indigenous people, however, were far more limited. Although Native people would not have been strangers to eighteenth-century Philadelphia, it is not clear if any appeared in Rush's patient lists. His commonplace book claims that he did meet Little Turtle in Philadelphia in 1798, describing him as "the Chief of the Miami Tribe, who commanded in the defeat of General St. Clair and whom I had inoculated."[48] However, in 1774 Rush's knowledge of Native Americans came from a combination of written sources, stereotypes, and conversations with western travelers with varying degrees of reliability. Although he certainly would have seen American Indians in eighteenth-century Philadelphia on occasion, the ethnographic work addresses a world far beyond the Schuylkill. Rush specifically cited written histories of Canada and the verbal testimony of physician and Revolutionary War general, Edward Hand (1744–1802).[49] From these sources he generalized about Indigenous traditions and made no attempt to differentiate by region, tribal nation, or language group.

Within his comparative ethnography Rush described the actions of both American Indians and wealthy Britons in sickness and in health. Although he dedicated more space to Indian bodies, both received critique and analysis. Rush's complaints about British habits and the pathological nature of their society from the perspective of a colonial subject (and in 1774) may have figured into the advice by London booksellers Edward and Charles Dilly against his publishing in England.[50] This oration is an early attempt by Rush to document the specific alterations that culture and climate made on individual bodies. In the case of his Anglo-American audience, they found themselves in a sort of limbo—not fully British due to their climate, and not

---

47 Rush Practice Notes (1789–1813), LCP, Rush Family Papers, Benjamin Rush Papers, Subseries V Medical Research and Notes, Vol. 85–87.

48 Rush and Biddle, *A Memorial Containing Travels Through Life Or Sundry Incidents in the Life of Dr. Benjamin Rush, Born Dec. 24, 1745 (Old Style) Died April 19, 1813*, 156.

49 Presumably Hand obtained information prior to the war; however, Rush notes that his information from Hand came via conversation and tracking down its source is impossible. Rush, "An Inquiry," 6, 7.

50 Edward Dilly and Charles Dilly (1774), LCP, Rush Family Papers, Benjamin Rush Correspondence, Vol. XXXI.

Indian because of their culture. During the American Revolution, however, Anglo-Americans self-consciously tried to recreate the world. Knowledge gleaned from around the globe, from physiology, travel literature, and philosophy could explain physical human difference and provide the rules with which a new republican society could flourish. Choices helped construct the perceived differences between white and Indian bodies. Rush therefore attributed any "inferiority" on the part of Indigenous people to their "savage" state rather than to heredity. To the eyes of an observer like himself, the two groups, the British and the Native American, possessed obvious physical differences. The most striking seemed to be the diseases the groups were susceptible to and the best means of cure. Those physical differences, however, were not as "natural" as they first appeared.

In his lecture to the American Philosophical Society Rush took an ethnographic approach and used both his own observations and those of others to generalize about the lifestyle of his two study groups. In both cases, he followed the same mode of inquiry:

> First, Mention a few facts which relate to the birth and treatment of their children.
>
> Secondly, I shall speak of their diet.
>
> Thirdly, Of the customs which are peculiar to the sexes, and,
>
> Fourthly, Of those customs which are common to them both.[51]

The first step stands out as quintessentially Rush. In his general physiology lectures, he presumed an infant's early care substantially affected its future health and well-being. In medical lectures the treatment of newborns and mistakes of midwives are found early on and in multiple student notebooks. Following the lead of British writers like Gregory and Cadogan, Rush worried that early shocks to the system could turn into permanent alterations to the constitution and leave a child susceptible to disease throughout his or her whole life. For example, he blamed midwives for tight swaddling in infancy leading to later pulmonary problems.[52] Meanwhile, British émigré and physician, Benjamin Vaughan (1751–1835), lamented in an 1807 letter to Rush that poor infant care in Maine led to disease. He encouraged Rush to address the subject:

---

51 Rush, "An Inquiry," 6.

52 William Simontown, KCRBM, ms. Coll 255, Item 5, Vol. I.; Christopher Heydrick (1790), KCRBM, ms. Coll. 225, Item 20, Vol. I.

Permit me to suggest that the subject in this country [Maine] solicits your best attention, because the sickness & the mortality of children is beyond its proportion, compared with that of adults; notwithstanding a mother's milk & a country air are so generally their lot here.— I cannot but observe in these parts a want of cleanliness, & thin clothing, and coarse addition to their diet, as among the probable causes of a part of their misfortunes; & that multitudes of children pine till they come to the ages when these are circumstances do them less mischief.[53]

Vaughan's account assumes a shared concern between the two men about the health of children and cultural practices. Poor clothing and exposure to the excitement of the outside environment cause sickness in infants despite the otherwise healthy influences of fresh air and breast milk. In addition to physical transformation, Rush believed the influence of culture at this stage was at its strongest.[54] All bodies were fundamentally shaped by their environment, but in infants the clay was at its softest, easily molded by the hands of nature and of parents. In infant care, Rush agreed with Vaughan's concerns and suggested that in many ways American Indian parent served their children better than their white counterparts.

In the case of Native Americans, Rush argued that the actions of parents on their children consistently reinforced a "hereditary firmness of constitution."[55] The theme of Indian "firmness" appears frequently in this essay and fits general stereotypes perpetuated by European settlers.[56] The concept of a strong "noble savage" living close to nature permeates the essay. As such Rush claimed that all Indian babies were purposefully "hardened" in cold water, shaped on cradleboards, and given strong nourishment as a result of prolonged breastfeeding.[57] The low temperature of the water caused the body to tense and, over time, hold that shape. Similarly, the cradleboard, he claimed, encouraged the growth of straight and strong limbs, accounting

---

53   Benjamin Vaughan (1807), LCP, Rush Family Papers, Benjamin Rush Correspondence, Vol. XVIII.

54   Rush, "Thoughts upon Female Education, Accomodated to the Present State of Society, Manners, and Government, in the United States of America. Addressed to the Visitors of the Young Ladies' Academy in Philadelphia, 28th July, 1787, at the Close of the Quarterly E," 82–83.

55   Rush, "An Inquiry," 7.

56   Block, *Colonial Complexions: Race and Bodies in Eighteenth-Century America*, 46; Chaplin, *Subject Matter: Technology, the Body, and Science on the Anglo-American Frontier, 1500–1676*, 100.

57   Rush, "An Inquiry," 7; Norton, *Liberty's Daughters: The Revolutionary Experience of American Women, 1750–1800*.

for adult physical strength. Suitable nutrition, in turn, aided both of the previous practices. Rush wrote that babies needed only the simple nourishment from milk and encouraged Anglo-American mothers to breast-feed for a minimum of twelve months. Indian mothers, he argued might breast feed for twice as long. He claimed that in "civilized" societies parents gave children solid food, especially meat, before their bodies could properly digest flesh. As a result, he claimed Indian children grew up to be vigorous and develop societies that lacked debility or "deformity."[58]

Despite the general health of the food itself, Rush fell back on stereotypes of laziness and stoicism with respect to Indian reliance on hunting and fishing. This idea was one of the older European complaints about Native American cultures and a fundamental misunderstanding of gender roles in many tribal nations. Early modern Europeans considered hunting and fishing to be leisure activities and not part of subsistence. As such they stubbornly continued to think of Native men engaged in hunting and fishing as relaxing while all "real"—that is agricultural work—was completed by women.[59] Rush also expressed surprise at the absence of salt in Indian diets or as a means of preserving meat despite the fact that "the interior parts of our continent abound with salt springs."[60]

Ultimately, Rush presumed a certain "naturalness" to the Indian lifestyle. Recall, that "natural" was not a positive term from Rush's perspective. He strongly rejected the "natural" approaches to medicine and letting "nature take its course." Nature was imperfect and thus following nature alone could lead to undesirable consequences. Rush gave Indigenous use of a meat's own juices as the only flavoring and the lack of a fixed meal schedule as examples of the dangerous irregularity that could appear if one only followed nature.[61] He noted how Indians fell ill through exposure to the variable elements, limited physical barriers between humans and the environment, and built settlements too close to streams and rivers with their associate miasma.[62]

---

58   Rush, "An Inquiry," 14.

59   Demos, *The Unredeemed Captive: A Family Story from Early America*; Chaplin, *Subject Matter: Technology, the Body, and Science on the Anglo-American Frontier, 1500–1676*.

60   Rush, "An Inquiry," 8. Tribes in what is now the Northeastern part of the United States frequently smoked food to preserve it, Meyer, "Why Did Syracuse Manufacture Solar Salt?," 195–209.

61   Rush, "An Inquiry," 9.

62   Rush, "An Inquiry," 16.

Stanhope Smith wrote with a similar eye to the danger of dampness near Indian dwellings and associated it with difference in skin color.

> The American Indian inhabits an *uncultivated forest*, abounding with *stagnant waters*, and covered with a luxuriant growth of *vegetables which fall down and corrupt on the spot where they have grown*. He generally pitches his wigwam on the side of a river that he may enjoy the convenience of fishing as well as of hunting. The *vapor of rivers*, therefore, which are often greatly obstructed in their course by the trees fallen, and the leaves collected in their channels, the *exhalations of marshes*, and the *noxious gases* evolved from decaying vegetables, impregnate the whole atmosphere, and give a deep *bilious tinge to the complexion of the savage*.[63]

Smith argued that the whole of the American atmosphere produced bilious diseases. The bilious climate led to liver secretions that altered skin-tone, not unlike jaundice. This, he implied accounted for the difference in skin color between American and European-descended people. Indigenous Americans in this view were literally ill all the time with a disease Rush considered characteristically American, as discussed in chapter 6. Anglo-Americans only escaped the change (and only in part) from mediating cultural practices that put distance between themselves and dangerous nature. Rush, on the other hand, took a different route to explaining complexion, but one that also emphasized the lack of protection Native cultures provided. He appealed to outdoor living, sun tanning, and skin-painting to explain the difference. He argued that the skin of American Indians was not originally darker than the skin of Europeans, but rather had tanned from habit and custom just as European laborers tanned in the sun.[64] Both men, however, attributed physical difference in skin color to the Indian's lack of separation from the humid and varied geography.[65]

Skin color aside, Rush used similar arguments to explain disease in Native North Americans and why he thought it different from that experienced by European-descended people. Rush argued that the Indian lifestyle predisposed communities to specific diseases, most notably from irregular and variable environmental circumstances.

---

63 Emphasis added, Stanhope Smith, *An Essay on the Causes of the Variety of Complexion and Figure in the Human Species*, 151.

64 Rush, "An Inquiry."

65 Rush, 13; Smith, *An Essay on the Causes of the Variety of Complexion and Figure in the Human Species*, 7, 49–51.

We need only recollect the custom among the Indians, of sleeping in the open air in a *variable climate*; the *alternate action* of heat and cold upon their bodies, to which the warmth of their cabins exposes them; their long marches; their excessive exercise; their *intemperance* in eating, to which their long fasting and their public feasts naturally prompt them; and, lastly, the vicinity of their habitations to the banks of rivers, in order to discover the empire of diseases among them in every stage of their lives. They have in vain attempted to elide the general laws of mortality, while their mode of life subjects them to these remote, but certain causes of diseases.[66]

Unlike White Americans, Rush thought Native people did less to mitigate the impact of climate on their bodies. This exposed them to a host of disease-triggering irregularities. They were people without "improvement."

Rush perceived native people living in the lands considered by Euro-Americans as too "wild" to be inhabited and too subject to highly variable stimuli in the atmosphere. As such, he argued that Indian customs tried to mitigate the effects of heat and cold upon the body by hardening and strengthening. This may have limited, in his view, susceptibility to small impressions but ultimately did little to protect bodies again strong disease. In a somewhat confusing use of the term "natural" he claimed that death and disease appeared in their natural state among native populations. Rush wrote, concluding the section on Indian diseases that, "[h]aving thus pointed out the natural diseases of the Indians . . . we may venture to conclude that FEVERS, OLD AGE, CASUALTIES, and WAR are the only natural outlets of human life."[67] Not too far removed from this state, the poor laborers and rural White farmers exhibited some of the same traits that Rush and others associated with Indians. They developed darker skin and appeared immune to gout and nervous diseases, diseases of "civilization."[68]

Rush's discussion of the British was much shorter than that of Native Americans, however it follows the same general pattern discussed above. In both cultures, unnatural practices had the greatest effect on the health, appearance, and diseases of individuals. For children, tight clothing, improper education, and damaging food predisposed them to disease both in infancy and later in life. Rush similarly complained about the effects of fashion (again clothing that was too tight) and idleness on elite women.[69]

---

66 Emphasis added, Rush, "An Inquiry," 16.
67 Rush, "An Inquiry," 20.
68 Rush, "An Inquiry."
69 Rush, "An Inquiry," 31.

Meanwhile, civilization and what sounds like class inequality brought new diseases to working men from "idleness and intemperance among the rich, and of hard labour and penury among the poor!"[70]

Despite the differences between British and Native American bodies, Rush maintained in 1774 that colonists could learn from the "successes" and "failures" of each group. His text, and footnotes added in the 1790s, clearly inform the reader that the information provided could be useful for the future, not only a curiosity for the present. Rush's interest in culture, maturity, and climate is related to early work in anthropology conducted by Scottish intellectuals.[71] Like his general interest in stadial theory discussed above Rush largely fell into line with his contemporaries while bringing their ideas into a distinctly American context.

Finally, the essay also shows how gender and culture worked together to construct ideas about race. In nonwhite cultures, menstruation acted as a data point for understanding a different society. Prior to their famous expedition across the North American continent, Benjamin Rush, like Thomas Jefferson, sent Merriweather Lewis and William Clark a list of ethnographic

---

70 Rush, "An Inquiry," 32.

71 Wood, "The Natural History of Man in the Scottish Enlightenment," 89–123; Jonsson, *Enlightenment's Frontier: The Scottish Highlands and the Origins of Environmentalism*; Schiebinger, "Skeletons in the Closet: The First Illustrations of the Female Skeleton in Eighteenth-Century Anatomy," 42–82; Berry, "'Climate' in the Eighteenth Century: James Dunbar and the Scottish Case," 281–92; Wolloch, "The Civilizing Process"; Irving-Stonebraker, "Nature, Knowledge, and Civilization. Connecting the Atlantic and Pacific Worlds in the Enlightenment"; McCosh, *The Scottish Philosophy, Biographical, Expository, Critical, From Hutcheson to Hamilton*, 263. Spanish intellectuals in the sixteenth and seventeenth centuries also took an interest in human physical and cultural difference: Earle, *The Body of the Conquistador: Food, Race and the Colonial Experience in Spanish America, 1492–1700*; Cañizares-Esguerra, "New World, New Stars: Patriotic Astrology and the Invention of Indian and Creole Bodies in Colonial Spanish America, 1600–1650," 33–68. Theories of climate and culture include Montesquieu but also a much older tradition: Montesquieu et al., *The Spirit of Laws, Vol. I*; Gates, "The Spread of Ibn Khaldûn's Ideas on Climate and Culture," 415–22; Gerbi and Moyle, *The Dispute of the New World: The History of a Polemic, 1750–1900*; Glacken, *Traces on the Rhodian Shore: Nature and Culture in Western Thought from Ancient Times to the End of the Eighteenth Century*; Rockman, "New World with a New Sky: Climatic Variability, Environmental Expectations, and the Historical Period Colonization of Eastern North America."

questions to "ask the Indians."[72] He included several specifically related to female bodies, for example, the ages at which women start and cease menstruation, typical age at marriage, and duration of breast-feeding. Presumably by comparing this information with that of white Americans and better-known American Indian cultures, Rush believed himself capable of assessing the cultures and climates of the Northwest.

It is unclear if Rush received answers to his questions or ever took up the specific issue of the Louisiana Purchase again. Nevertheless, he did continue to discuss the general effects of "civilization" on women's bodies in lectures and personal notes. In the case of labor and gender, Rush formed strong opinions on the best balance to maintain female health. He chided both "civilized" and "uncivilized" nations for their gendered division of labor: in the case of the former only men worked and in the latter women bore the brunt of labor. He followed this information with the admonishment that "[b]oth are wrong. Men & Women were made to work together in different ways."[73] Occupation was key for the health of any individual and thus any family, community, or nation in turn. By finding fault with both high European culture and Native work patterns (or rather Anglo-American interpretations of Native work patterns), Rush contributed to a growing idea that the United States would produce a better society than either, civilized but not decadent.

Rush believed cultural differences fundamentally altered bodies and that these alterations were most easily assessed in women's bodies, since they underwent cyclical changes that could be compared and measured, especially in the cases of menstruation and childbirth. He characterized Indigenous masculinity as centered around the vigorous activities of hunting, swimming, and war. The "tone" of the nerves that resulted from this activity led to general good health among Indian men.[74] Among both men and women Rush attributed additional rituals aimed at shaping and strengthening the body, notably "painting, and the use of the cold bath." The use of grease, paint, and cold baths (often in sickness alternated with sweating) were common attributes Europeans and white colonists associated with Indian culture. The historian Joyce Chaplin argues that by the late seventeenth century English colonists used such practices to demonstrate how Indians were unfit for the climate

---

72 Vermeulen, "Origins and Institutionalization of Ethnography and Ethnology in Europe and the USA, 1771–1845," 53. Benjamin Rush Commonplace Book (May 17, 1803, and June 11, 1803), APS, Mss.B.R89c.

73 Benjamin Rush, Commonplace Book 21, July 1792, APS, Mss.B.R89c.

74 Rush, "An Inquiry," 10–12.

of North America compared with themselves.[75] Such a sentiment does not appear in Rush's work. However, Rush recognized that both native and colonizing societies relied on bodily manipulations and practices to survive in any climate. Nature for Rush was a constant (if well-meaning) enemy, something to be improved and overcome rather than used as a guide. If anything, he believed Indians did less to alter themselves and their surroundings than those of European descent, often to the detriment of the former. This was especially the case with Native American women. Rush believed they created a false masculinity within themselves by strengthening their bodies and engaging in hard labor; the result of which was delayed maturity and low birth rates—a biological underpinning to the emerging trope of the "disappearing Indian."

Rush reasoned that there were strong connections between the labor of Native women, their physical appearance, and physiology. The hard work performed by these women supposedly hardened their bodies, making them appear masculine. This masculine tendency seemed to impact their expression of that most feminine trait of childbirth. Rush claimed that Indian women, as a direct result of their labor, did not begin menstruation until the age of eighteen or twenty, and rarely married before twenty. However, Rush's negative comments regarding American Indian women were not uniform. In one situation, childbirth, their masculine bodies appeared ironically helpful. Rush believed this hardening of bodies resulted in lower menstrual flow and a reduction of pain during childbirth. Despite the disparaging of the masculinization of Indigenous women, Rush found much to praise in his assumptions about their childbirth practices, which eliminated midwives and postpartum confinement.

> Nature is their only midwife. Their labours are short, and accompanied with little pain. Each woman is delivered in a private cabin, without so much as one of her own sex to attend her. After washing herself in cold water, she returns in a few days to her usual employments; so that she knows nothing of those accidents which proceed from the carelessness or ill management of midwives; or those weaknesses which arise from a month's confinement in a warm room. It is remarkable that there is hardly a period in the interval between the eruption and ceasing of the menses, in which they are not pregnant, or giving suck. This is the most natural state of the constitution during that interval; and hence we often find it connected with the best state of health, in the women of civilized nations.[76]

---

75 Chaplin, *Subject Matter: Technology, the Body, and Science on the Anglo-American Frontier, 1500–1676*, 9–14.

76 Rush, "An Inquiry," 10–11.

A century before Rush, Hans Sloane had claimed a similar difference in the health and culture surrounding the practices of women, especially enslaved African and Indian women, in Jamaica.[77] Sloane, like Rush, did not attribute this lack of pain to bodily racial differences, but to differences in the practice of childbirth that resulted in a healthier experience. On the other hand, the excessive artifice associated with European women of fashion led directly to pain and disease. European women, especially of the upper classes, allowed fashion to damage their health. Rush complained at various times about tight laces, uncovered breasts, and heavy wigs and hats. In his "Natural History of Medicine Among the Indians," he wrote of the dangers of "civilized" life, stating that it "rises in its demands upon the health of women. Their fashions; their dress and diet; their eager pursuits and ardent enjoyment of pleasure; their indolence and undue evacuaions [sic] . . . their cordials, hot regiment . . . use of art, in child-birth, are all so many inlets to disease."[78]

Consistent with tradition and stereotype, Rush used the bodies of Indian women to generalize about Native American culture and the American wilderness. In this reading, Native people had, for the most part, adjusted themselves to their environment based on their habits; the proof rested in the toughened and gender-distorting bodies of their women. In contrast, Euro-Americans changed their environment to suit human bodies, a more difficult but ultimately (in Rush's mind) more sustainable and healthier course of action. By learning from bodies—both those he personally observed and those he read about—Rush found information that drove him toward a physiology with hard divisions between the sexes and fluid distinctions between race and ethnicity. His daily work as a physician and educator framed the American system. The next four chapters show how Rush took those physiological ideas and applied them to social, political, and scientific projects.

---

77 Churchill, "Bodily Differences?: Gender, Race, and Class in Hans Sloane's Jamaican Medical Practice, 1678–1688," 438.

78 Rush, "An Inquiry," 31.

Part II

Using an American System

Overview

Part I of this book followed Benjamin Rush's career from student to leader of the American medical profession. Along the way he accumulated experiences that convinced him that the United States required a new medical system, one suited to the bodies, societies, and climates of the republican United States. That system—like many theories of eighteenth-century health—focused on the interconnectedness of bodies and the mental and physical spaces that surrounded them. It also took seriously the idea that the same kind of organization (in this case a broad interpretation of "republicanism") was suitable to both bodies and societies. As Rush became a committed republican, he also saw bodies through that lens. Citizens of a republic required a different kind of medicine than subjects of an empire. Moreover, bodies themselves acted as mini republics. As discussed in chapter 2, different organ systems needed to work together in a dance of checks and balances to keep excitement flowing regularly. Chapter 3 discussed how other physicians acted as sources of knowledge and partners in creating the "American system" and chapter 4 demonstrated how medical practice and ideas of sex and racial difference intersected with Rush's work.

Rush's system, however, has been treated as theoretical to this point. This second part of this work asks the question, how did Rush *actually use* his system? The medical worldview of Benjamin Rush operated in the classroom, the sickroom, and in the public square. The following chapters argue that he did so expansively. The "American System" informed the seemingly disparate projects of Rush's life and medicalized numerous social and political issues. Rush's republic was a self-governing machine in which community members obeyed laws, worked diligently, espoused virtue, and worked together for the greater good: the mental and physical health of the nation. This version of governance by active citizens models the actions of other politically and socially minded physicians of the time, especially Rush's Scottish colleagues and teachers. Rush viewed an American republic that took the principles of voluntary organizations, educational opportunity, and intellectual leadership associated with his Edinburgh experience and moved them from the periphery to the center of national life.[1] Rush promoted these views in general and popular publications throughout the 1780s and continued to tie them to his working understanding of human physiology. In this manner, he slowly developed the physiological system he debuted in the 1790s through his work and research in social as well as physical sciences.

This vision—a utopian one to Rush—incorporated political aims and supported the function of the new government; its purpose, however, went beyond statecraft and struck at the heart of society. He believed the new government was part of revolutionary social change in which men and women took responsibility for their own lives and those of their neighbors. Doing so well required proper education, the distribution of responsibilities among the most able, and a suitable physical and mental environment. Over time, he felt these actions would become "natural" to citizens and create a pseudo-evolutionary progression toward a more perfect human condition.[2] Only strong and well-organized institutions framed in accordance with rational principles could achieve these goals. Rush certainly took his involvement in institutions seriously and belonged to numerous groups designed to further republican and scientific goals including the American Philosophical Society, The Philadelphia Dispensary, The Pennsylvania Hospital, The College of Physicians of Philadelphia, The Academy of Medicine (Philadelphia), Pennsylvania Abolition Society, The Library Company of Philadelphia, American Academy of Arts and Sciences, Columbian Chemical Society, Philadelphia Society of Alleviating the Miseries of Public Prisons, and of course the Society for Promoting Political Inquiries discussed in the introduction to name a few.

Outside the United States he continued to link American intellectual culture to a broader Enlightenment republic of letters through corresponding and honorary memberships in the Philosophical Society of Manchester (England), the Literary and Philosophical Society at Preston (England), and the Royal Humane Society of London. He also promoted the establishment of schools and colleges, including Dickinson College, Franklin College (now Franklin and Marshall College), and the Young Ladies Academy of

---

1   Dingwall, *A History of Scottish Medicine: Themes and Influences,* 110–15.

2   D'Elia, "Benjamin Rush, David Hartley, and the Revolutionary Uses of Psychology," 109–18; Priestley, *Hartley's Theory of the Human Mind, on the Principle of the Association of Ideas; with Essays Relating to the Subject of It;* Hartley, *Observations on Man, His Frame, His Duty, and His Expectations: In Two Parts. Part the First.*

Philadelphia. This is not an exhaustive list of projects, nor do these chapters follow a strict chronology. They do, however, demonstrate a variety of ways Rush tried to use and promote the use of his medical worldview. They also show how the seemingly fractured historiography of Benjamin Rush can be knit together when viewed through the dual lenses of medical history and republicanism. The next four chapters mirror those in Part I. Following chapter 4, chapter 5 discusses how Rush used his ideas surrounding physiology to support new ideas about the role of gender in republics and condemn the institution of slavery (while still upholding damaging ideas about race). Chapter 6 details how Rush's system responded to aliments associated with climate, including the successive outbreaks of yellow fever between 1793 and 1820. The final chapters, chapters 7 and 8, examine specific institutions supported by Rush and how they too reflect the goals—the ultimate goals—of the American system. When writing about hospitals, schools, and the proper conduct of citizens the physiological context was never far from Rush's mind. By using American medicine to shape these ideas, Rush hoped to create a successful American republic.

Chapter Five

Explaining Variation in American Bodies

Each year between 1789 and 1813, Benjamin Rush—like most medical school professors before and immediately after him—began the year with a special introductory lecture. Unlike subsequent topics that varied little from year to year, the introductory lecture changed frequently. Young men gathered to begin their journey into the medical profession framed by discussions that ranged from bedside decorum to a biography of Thomas Sydenham to veterinary medicine. One of the most common topics, however, touched on the operations of the mind and the diseases of the mind. Five out of Rush's sixteen published introductory lectures addressed these topics. The connection between mind and body was—and remains—an intriguing philosophical and physiological question. Most physicians and philosophers of the eighteenth century agreed on some link, but the extent to which the mind was rooted and altered by material concerns and how it operated were debated.[1] For Rush, the question of the health of minds and bodies took on added significance in the new republic. The bodies and especially minds of new citizens needed to be healthy for self-governance. Even those bodies and minds

---

1   Wilson, *Seeking Nature's Logic: Natural Philosophy in the Scottish Enlightenment*; Reid-Maroney, *Philadelphia's Enlightenment, 1740–1800*; Reid, *Essays on the Powers of the Human Mind*; Winterer, *American Enlightenments: Pursuing Happiness in the Age of Reason*; Crichton, *An Inquiry into the Nature and Origin of Mental Derangement Comprehending a Concise System of the Physiology and Pathology of the Human Mind and a History of the Passions and Their Effects, Vol. I.*; Hartley, *Observations on Man, His Frame, His Duty, and His Expectations: In Two Parts. Part the First*; Guerrini, *Obesity and Depression in the Enlightenment: The Life and Times of George Cheyne*; D'Elia, "Benjamin Rush, David Hartley, and the Revolutionary Uses of Psychology"; Haakonssen, *Medicine and Morals in the Enlightenment: John Gregory, Thomas Percival, and Benjamin Rush*.

not associated with governance—women, people of color, and the poor—needed to support the social experiment of the new United States in auxiliary roles as caretakers, workers, and members of smaller communities. Teasing out the way different body-mind systems behaved in sickness and in health could, for Rush, help uncover their appropriate role in the environmentally temperate and politically republican nation.

One of the last essays included in the volume of introductory lectures, "Upon the pleasures of the senses and of the mind" included an appeal to family life as a preserver of health. Rush declared that married men and women lived longer than their single counterparts and lived happier lives. Women in particular were presented as in special need of a family. Subsequently, Rush presented marriage as a treatment for nervous disorders in both men and women. Their bodies (and minds) were different but considered complimentary. The joy of children, he implied, was most acute in mothers. He even concluded with a story of a woman cured of a mental disorder (temporarily) by motherhood, writing "a lady in this city was cured of a madness, by the birth and suckling of a child. Her husband took her child from her lest it should contract its mother's disease; in consequence of which her madness returned."[2]

This dark anecdote nevertheless addresses the heart of Rush's concerns about the health of the United States. To Rush, healthy families were the foundation of the country. Any useful medical system needed to address the specific needs of American families in American spaces. The physical construction of bodies necessarily altered that body's physical relationship to the outside world. With respect to sex, Rush reasoned that innate physical differences between men and women's bodies led to different relationships with the world, pathological and otherwise. For Rush, and others of his generation, bodily differences between the sexes could be found throughout the human body. In lectures on the difference between men and women's bodies and on the peculiarity of female diseases, Rush discussed the different bone densities of women, their more extensive lymphatic systems, larger thyroids, and earlier puberty. He associated each natural physiological difference with the ideal feminine lifestyle, one less prone to stimulation than that of men. Women's bodies abstracted excitement through their lymphatic system and large thyroids.

The success of Rush's system of medicine came from its ability to account for variation. His simple concepts could be adapted by physicians

---

2   Rush, *Sixteen Introductory Lectures, to Courses of Lectures upon the Institutes and Practice of Medicine*, 444.

throughout the country to explain the people and diseases they encountered. In doing this, Rush borrowed arguments from other eighteenth-century physicians and ethnographers. For example, from the Baron de Montesquieu he adopted the idea that heat led to reduced mental capacity. Rush claimed that the heat of North Africa and the Middle East overtaxed the mind and body, which led to the cultural habits associated with those regions as well as what Rush considered a despotic form of government in the Ottoman Empire.[3] Even within a temperate climate, however, the minds and bodies of a population might suffer if starved of the mental activity associated with political engagement, an attack he leveled at *ancien régime* France.[4]

In a young, multiethnic republic with a notoriously unstable climate, Rush wanted to find a formula for success. To do so, he needed to understand the forces that drove human difference and how different "races" and societies persisted in the same region. Using personal anecdotes, informal correspondence, and travel literature, Rush presented an explanation for numerous cultural differences in both the old world and new. Such variation did not create a firm categorical difference between people since proper management

3   Benjamin Rush, Lecture Notes, Rush Family Papers, LCP, Volume 166. For other descriptions of the relationship between weather and culture in the eighteenth and early nineteenth centuries, see Adamson, "'The Languor of the Hot Weather': Everyday Perspectives on Weather and Climate in Colonial Bombay, 1819–1828"; Berry, "'Climate' in the Eighteenth Century : James Dunbar and the Scottish Case"; Montesquieu et al., *The Spirit of Laws, Vol. I*; Harrison, "'The Tender Frame of Man': Disease, Climate, and Racial Difference in India and the West Indies, 1760–1860"; Harrison, *Climates & Constitutions: Health, Race, Environment and British Imperialism in India, 1600–1850*; Johnston, "The Constitution of Empire: Place and Bodily Health in the Eighteenth-Century Atlantic," 443–66; Rockman, "New World with a New Sky : Climatic Variability, Environmental Expectations, and the Historical Period Colonization of Eastern North America"; Staunton, *An Authentic Account of An Embassy from the King of Great Britain to the Emperor of China ... Vol. I*; Willoughby, "'His Native, Hot Country': Racial Science and Environment in Antebellum American Medical Thought," 1–24.

4   Benjamin Rush, Lecture Notes, LCP, Volume 166 and Rush, "An Inquiry into the Natural History of Medicine Among the Indians of North-America; and a Comparative View of their Diseases and Remedies with those of Civilized Nations," 1–68.

of self and society could produce healthy and politically engaged populations in many different climates: if culture were managed appropriately.[5]

Of the many variations Rush considered, three stand out as well-documented examples of his interests and concerns: gender, race, and environment. The first section looks at gender, specifically at the way in which European-descended women were viewed as essential to the republic and how their health was shaped by the nation. The second section revisits Rush's ideas about racial difference in the context of the republic's future, especially in the case of Black, Indigenous, and mixed-raced people and their perceived ability to "become" white. The final section differs from the previous parts and addresses the nature of diseases in American spaces. By considering Rush's "American editions" of British and colonial texts, it argues that he was training readers to adapt received knowledge to unpredictable and republican spaces.

Making Republican Women

In 1800, physician John Vaughan—a frequent correspondent and friend of Rush—published a short lecture he delivered on electricity to the Philosophical Society of Delaware. This kind of publication was not unusual at the time, nor was the subject matter. Public discussions and displays of electricity dated back to the 1740s in North America.[6] However, its dedication is worth noting along with its unusual title "To the Female *Enquirers* of Wilmington." With this dedication, Vaughan critiqued the society's presumed exclusion of women writing:

> In obedience to your request, I now present you with our concluding Lecture of last season; and if I am so unfortunate as to incur the criticism of Old Bachelors and Juvenile Sophists, you must defend me with female rhetoric.
>
> The former tribe of unhappy men, deserve commiseration; and tho' the latter may be influenced by prejudice, they are within the bounds of reason and capable of reformation. Despising, as we do, the slavish manners of Asia;

---

5   For more on the Early Republic's as well as Rush's interest in engineering a better society in the United States, see Finger, *Contagious City: The Politics of Public Health in Early Philadelphia*; Powell, *Bring Out Your Dead: The Great Plague of Yellow Fever in Philadelphia in 1793*; Apel, "The Thucydidean Moment: History, Science, and the Yellow-Fever Controversy, 1793–1805"; Bell, *We Shall Be No More: Suicide and Self-Government in the Newly United States*; Brodsky, *Benjamin Rush: Patriot and Physician*.

6   Delbourgo, *A Most Amazing Scene of Wonders: Electricity and Enlightenment in Early America*.

and boasting the honors of civilization, it is high time that the *rights* of women should be justly estimated, and their *wrongs* redressed:

And notwithstanding a learned society has decreed, that "you are inferior to men in mental qualifications," I with pleasure avow my ambition to merit our literary esteem; and request you to accept this tribute of respect.[7]

Vaughn's dedication clearly put him at odds with some of his contemporaries. However, the idea that women had the interest and ability to appreciate science was not unheard of, even if attending certain groups and public events remained unorthodox. In the years following the American Revolution the education and place of women in society were topics that attracted considerable debate among intellectual circles. The education of women and girls as discussed in chapter 8 dives into the institutional implications of this interest. The present chapter, however, examines the way in which Rush's ideas surrounding physiology and sex difference affected social discussions about the role of women (especially wives and mothers) in a republic. Like his friend Vaughn, Rush has been credited by some historians as progressive with respect to gender. The previous chapter demonstrated the limits of that viewpoint and the centrality of sexual dimorphism—physical differences—between men and women (male and female humans) in Rush's view. Nevertheless, this did not mean he held that women were completely inferior to men or that they should be without clear rights in the United States.

In the 1780s and 1790s, women, as much as men, made and remade the world in an age of medical and political revolution. In women's bodies, Rush saw evidence to suggest that women possessed minds and innate abilities fundamentally different (and ideally complementary) to those of men. This conviction, that female bodies and minds were different from their male counterparts, allowed Rush to conclude that there was a biological foundation for a society in which different genders performed distinct roles. Rush's use of women's bodies to discuss the environment is discussed in more detail below, but here we see the rationale behind it: women's bodies were constructed differently from those of men, experienced different physiological processes, possessed different minds, and therefore expressed illness differently. While men too were thought to be affected by their surroundings women were (1) enough of an "other" to attract attention from medical students and (2) had a biology based on observable regular changes that seemed to alter based on climate and society (most notably menstruation but also pregnancy and childbirth).

---

7   Emphasis original, Vaughan, *The Valedictory Lecture Delivered Before the Philosophical Society of Delaware.*

Returning to Rush's intellectual background, his time in Scotland was likely highly influential. Scottish stadial theory of the eighteenth century argued that greater equality between the sexes was an indication of civilization. This was not total equality or even equality before the law, but an acknowledgment of women's spiritual equality and near equality of mental prowess. Philosophers argued that granting of greater equality by enlightened men to previously subdued, subjected, and ignored women resulted in healthier women. Of course, this did not mean complete equality or equality in all things, as noted in the previous chapter, but it did lead to a reevaluation of the fundamental nature of sex and appropriate gender roles. Some believed that "civilization" freed women from physical labor, tyrannical husbands, and dangerous superstitions and in their place educated women formed ideal intellectual partners for enlightened men. The historical literature abounds with descriptions of, complications of, and alterations to the concept of "republican motherhood" or "republican womanhood"—terms used to characterize the idealized role of white women in the American republic.[8]

Women, from this perspective were defined by their relationships with other members of the family. Mothers were encouraged to view themselves as the first educators of future citizens and encourage thoughtful, rational, and civic-minded children. Wives and daughters, meanwhile, could temper the actions of husbands and fathers and encourage moral decision making. Rush medicalized this idea when pronouncing that among the several differences between male and female minds was that degree to which religious and moral principals were developed. Women, he argued, had a greater natural sense of the deity and were more religious than men by nature. However, they could also be more superstitious and less rational if educated poorly. So, while men needed excitement and required the cultivation of their moral faculties, women needed abstraction and were supposed to work on the development of their rational minds. When in balance families could function as mini republics supporting society as a whole with both mothers and fathers contributing to their children's proper development.

---

8   Kerber, "The Republican Mother: Women and the Enlightenment—An American Perspective," 41–62; Nash, "Rethinking Republican Motherhood: Benjamin Rush and the Young Ladies' Academy of Philadelphia"; Zagarri, "Morals, Manners, and the Republican Mother," 192–215; Branson, *These Fiery Frenchified Dames: Women and Political Culture in Early National Philadelphia*; Wulf, *Not All Wives: Women of Colonial Philadelphia*.

Again, Rush centered families in his physiology and psychology. Like the story at the beginning, he argued in his psychiatry textbook *Medical Inquiries and Observations Upon Diseases of the Mind* (1812) that mental health was strongly correlated with marriage and families. In this instance, rather than a single case study he looked to collective data. Every few years, he asked hospital staff to collect numerical data on individuals in the Pennsylvania Hospital suffering from "diseases of the mind." In April 1812, he included marital status in the questionnaire. The results seemed to confirm his feelings about marriage. The two staff members, Dr. Moore and Mr. Jenny, reported that "of seventy-two insane patients . . . forty-two had never been married, and five were widows and widowers, at the time they became deranged." Rush further interpreted these results suggesting that dangerous amounts of time for morbid speculation and "the want of relief in conjugal sympathy from the inevitable distresses and vexations of life, and for which friendship is a cold and feeble substitute, are probably the reasons why madness occurs more frequently in single, than in married people. Celibacy . . . is a pleasant breakfast, a tolerable dinner, but a very bad supper."[9] In medical contexts at least, Rush never hesitated to note the advantages of physical intimacy between partners. And, as the father of nine children who lived to adulthood, he certainly was no stranger to that kind of intimacy.

For the most part, Rush viewed sexual intercourse (within marriage) as a healthy pastime and one that could curb excessive sexual activity in men and correct constitutional aliments (especially of the menses) in women. It had a clear purpose in maintaining health outside of its role in perpetuating the species. Sex and pregnancy were common prescriptions for women with disordered cycles as well as a host of other complaints. Meanwhile, only men, from Rush's perspective, seemed to suffer from an excess of the "venereal appetite." He connected this "disease" to gluttony, excessive consumption of alcohol, and idleness, all things that either spiked or diminished male excitement. Abstracting women seemed not to suffer from such sedentary habits and were less associated with certain vices (at least the "ladies" Rush focused his attention on). Indeed, marriage is the first "cure" listed for such men.[10]

Discussions of health, balance, and sexuality using republican terms had a place in Rush's classroom as well. In a lecture appealing to health, Rush argued for the maintenance of a healthy level of sexual activity and for the biological correctness of traditional western marriage and sexual practices.

---

9   Rush, *Medical Inquiries and Observations Upon the Diseases of the Mind*, 59–60.

10   Rush, *Medical Inquiries*, 349.

Nature, he argued, determined the correctness of marriage, not man. Of course, he very conveniently saw natural arguments for the socially and culturally acceptable views of sex and marriage practiced by Protestant Anglo-American families. Following from the general idea that marriage was a physical as well as a social good he also prescribed age ranges within which men and women should marry, suggesting that women marry between the ages of sixteen and twenty-four and men between twenty-one and thirty.[11] Rush's own behavior only just met these parameters. He was thirty and his wife Julia Stockton sixteen years old when they married in 1776. Neither polyamory nor celibacy, much less any same-sex relationships, had a place in Rush's worldview.

Other aspects of women's experiences were placed under a medical gaze and discussed with an eye to improving the physical health of female patients. This included both pregnancy and menstruation. The former appears in Rush's writings as a form of illness akin to fever writing, "I have been led to consider the female body as in a diseased state from the beginning of conception to the period of delivery. The disease partakes of many of the symptoms of fever, & is relieved by the remedies used for fevers from other causes. Its effects moreover upon the Uterus are the same, as the effect of disease are when it appears in the form of Inflammation upon other parts of the body."[12] Meanwhile, he presented menstruation as a healthy process that was often and easily corrupted by poor physical or mental health management. The experiences of women in both situations spoke—from the perspective of medical men—to the careful need for medical management and the fact that difference social settings led to different outcomes.

Rush attributed illness during pregnancy and pain in childbirth to a build-up of tension in the body. Essentially, the fetus acted as an extra source of excitement located in one part of the body and altering the function of the remainder. This fits Rush's definition of fever almost perfectly. Citing the supposed use of purges in Turkey during pregnancy, which abstracted excitement and led to less pain, Rush made the case for bloodletting as a means of pain relief and easier childbirth. Venesection could occur both prophylactically and during the birthing process. The practice, he further argued,

---

11   J. Overton, "Notes on Lectures Delivered by Dr. Benjamin Rush," UPenn Kislak, ms. Coll. 225 item 1; William Jackson "University of Pennsylvania Lectures of Benjamin Rush M.D.," UPenn Kislak, ms. Coll. 225 item 21 volume 1.

12   Benjamin Rush "Lectures on Physiology" LCP/HSP, Rush Family Papers, Yi2 7397 F.2 Volume 165, 781.

had been tried by several other doctors of his acquaintance to good effect.[13] The sensitive bodies of "civilized" women (which was synonymous with European or European-descended women), Rush and his fellow medical men argued, tended to lead to more difficult and painful delivery. This was not, interestingly, a sign that women in "civilized" society were unhealthy because they were in pain. It supposedly denoted their higher sensitivity and sensibility—traits that outside the "illness" of childbearing were desirable. The extra abstraction provided by prophylactic bleeding and bleeding during labor removed the excess excitement from the fetus that caused such pain in fine-tuned female bodies.

Similarly, Rush felt that information about women's bodies could be "read" through the menses. First onset of puberty, onset of menopause, and length and frequency of cycles, according to Rush, could all say something about a women's surroundings, health, and society. Among (presumably white) girls in the United States Rush claimed first menses arrived earlier in the hotter (more medically exciting) south and much later in New England. This followed some standard assumptions of the period about the health of temperate climates that meshed with Rush's conviction that regular temperate motions, behavior, and society were most healthful. Both the extreme North and extreme South had their dangers. It also conveniently suggested that his own mid-Atlantic region could be the most healthful. He also hypothesized that work and station or class in life affected its onset and patterns, stating "[i]n women in high life it occurs sooner than in women who labour—more especially—if this labor be performed in the open air." This followed up on a physiological notion that menstruation was yet another tactic for women to throw off excess excitement, a problem faced more acutely by the sedentary lady of "high life" than the laboring woman who abstracted her excess excitement through work.[14] Importantly, Rush made an analogous claim with respect to mental disorders, arguing that people of the poorer classes and less "civilized" cultures do not experience insanity due to the effects of labor and exposure to the elements, which take off the excitement that might otherwise ail the brain.[15] Again much of this points to his desire for moderate behavior, activity, and elevation of the lifestyle of the middling classes of Early America.

That Rush gave special attention to specifically female conditions may not appear particularly unusual or surprising. His differential use of the

---

13   Rush, "Defense of blood-letting, as a remedy in certain diseases," 263–64.
14   Rush, "Medical Lectures," LCP, Vol. 180, 725–26.
15   Rush, *Medical Inquiries and Observations Upon the Diseases of the Mind*, 60.

female body, however, extended beyond the specific discussion of female physiology and fertility and contributed to the adoption of a two-sex model of human difference in the early United States. Rush's ideas regarding the physical natures of women are found peppered throughout his discussion of pathology and therapeutics. In his 1805 edition of his *Medical Inquiries and Observations*, for example, he describes women as having different experiences with certain diseases. He believed their sedentary lifestyle rendered them more susceptible to consumption and their innate attachment to their families made them less likely to travel alone for a cure.[16] Women's dress and behavior limited the prevalence of gout but put them in more danger of thyroid conditions.[17] Even epidemic diseases differed in their expression between men and women based on their physicality. In at least one occasion, Rush uses his views on bodily difference to support his controversial stance on depleting remedies in malignant fevers.

> All these depleting remedies, whether used separately or together, induce such an *artificial debility in the system*, as disposes it to *vibrate more readily under the impression of the miasmata*. Thus the willow rises, after bowing before a blast of wind, while the unyielding oak falls to the ground by its side. It is from the similarity of the natural weakness in the systems of *women, in the West-Indies, with that which has been induced by the artificial means that have been mentioned, that they so generally escape the malignant endemic of the islands*.[18]

Rush followed the lead of colleagues in the Caribbean and East Indies who argued that the lax fibers of women allowed them to survive the dangerous seasoning process.[19] By bleeding patients, especially male patients, Rush could loosen bodies and make them more feminine and prepared to abstract the

---

16 Travel abroad was a common means of treatment for consumption, especially among men, see Rothman, *Living in the Shadow of Death: Tuberculosis and the Social Experience of Illness in American History*.

17 Rush, *Medical Inquiries and Observations: Volume 4*, 228; Rush, "An Inquiry into the Functions of the Spleen, Liver, Pancreas, and Thyroid Gland."

18 Emphasis added, Rush, "An account of the bilious yellow fever, as it appeared in Philadelphia in 1799," 95.

19 Harrison, "'The Tender Frame of Man': Disease, Climate, and Racial Difference in India and the West Indies, 1760–1860," 73; Schiebinger, "Medical Experimentation and Race in the Eighteenth-Century Atlantic World," 380; Seth, "Materialism, Slavery, and The History of Jamaica," 767; Kupperman, "Fear of Hot Climates in the Anglo-American Colonial Experience," 222.

excessive excitement of hot climates. Within the United States, the rationale differed somewhat. The strong impressions that faced American bodies were not always temperature related but could also come from the exciting forces of politics and commerce. The ever-changing attributes of American physical and mental spaces created strong illness (through sudden impressions) and required strong medical intervention to bring bodies and communities back into working order by using strong purges and robust bloodletting.

Of course, most of Rush's focus on the bodies of women centered on the experiences and idealization of middling class and European-descended women. It encompassed those for whom the arguments of "republican motherhood" and "republican womanhood" most directly applied, the wives, daughters, and mothers of voting male citizens. The United States, however, was not economically, racially, or ethnically homogeneous. Despite this, Rush looked toward a future in which gender difference was static but racial difference fluid and even eliminated in favor of middle-class, republican, and European-descended norms.

Race: Benjamin Rush's Views and the United States

In 1789–1790, the historian and clergyman Jeremy Belknap wrote to Rush from Boston to discuss the conditions of Indian communities in his home state of Massachusetts. Contrary to Rush's perception, Belknap favorably reported that several Christian Indian congregations existed in Massachusetts and that on the coast Native Americans proved to be excellent whalers and sailors. Nevertheless, negative descriptions of a mysteriously declining Indian population in the wake of war and rampant alcoholism foreshadowed the nineteenth century stereotypes of the "vanishing Indian" and alcoholism. He happily reported that Rush's essay on ardent spirits (a blockbuster early temperance piece) would make its way to Martha's Vineyard for a largely Wampanoag audience.[20] Both men hoped—alongside figures like Thomas Jefferson—that Native Americans could have a place in the American republic.[21] Rush looked at physical as well as social assimilation as a tool in his arsenal.

Rush's perception of bodily difference ultimately reinforced and provided "scientific" support for distinct racial and gender-based roles in the American republic like those evident in the Belknap correspondence. However, Rush

---

20   Jeremy Belknap (1789–1790) LCP, Rush Family Papers, Benjamin Rush Correspondence, Vol. 30, Box 1.

21   Jefferson, *Notes on the State of Virginia*, 62–71.

himself did not clearly espouse the distinct racial divisions and hierarchies of his nineteenth-century successors. His broad Enlightenment view of mutable racial categories and stadial "improvement" called for White Americans to facilitate physical and social assimilation of Black and indigenous people. Nevertheless, the tools he provided were used for a very different purpose decades later. Rush believed citizenship depended upon conformity to the republican world in which race and gender indicated the appropriate roles for individuals. The republic itself, however, was a big tent. Some of his students, most notably Charles Caldwell, went much farther than Rush could have anticipated. Southern students who flocked to attend Rush's lectures in Philadelphia returned home and helped create a distinct regional medicine that helped foster nineteenth-century scientific and medical racism. Caldwell and his followers countered the Enlightenment's claims of racial fluidity with arguments to support polygenism—the idea the different human races came from separate creations and species. As Christopher Willoughby contends, Rush may have had abolition in mind, but his students found the racial language in his work to support a far more radical conclusion.[22]

This is all to say that "race" remained an unstable category in the first decades of American independence. At the same time, race-based slavery looked to some like it might end (if gradually) in the near future. White commentators openly speculated on if and how Black Americans could become part of a national fabric that was (at least implicitly) by and for European-descended people, not African-descended or Indigenous people. By the 1820s, many white Americans who opposed slavery supported a form of colonization in which free African-descended people would "return" to Africa (despite the fact that a majority of enslaved people in the United States were born in North America by the late eighteenth century) or otherwise settle in the far West or South America. Such observers looked at the British colony Sierra Leone as a model that established its first permanent settlement of Black American loyalists from Canada in 1792. While not specifically opposed to such schemes, Rush kept his focus on the possibility of social and biological assimilation of Black people to white culture. To do so, however, he speculated on how biological differences occurred and if they could be "cured."

This is exemplified by his interactions with Henry Moss, an African American man who probably suffered from what we now call vitiligo, a loss of pigmentation in the skin over time. To Rush, Moss appeared to be turning white. On July 27, 1795, Rush wrote in his commonplace book that he had:

---

22 Willoughby, "'His Native, Hot Country.'"

Visited Harry Moss—an African born in Virginia—his grandfather was an African by birth his grandmother an Irish woman But his father black & his mother mostly so. From years ago he began to grow white first at his finger nails, then on the back of his neck—the parts that were covered & sweated, advanced most rapidly . . . his face slowest—His skin was exactly like a white man—no rubbing accelerated it. The black skin did not come off, but changed. He has two Brother[s] in whom no change has taken place . . . no previous change in his manner of living—has a wife but no children.[23]

The case of Henry Moss appears in Rush's published work as an "example" of the potential "cure" for Blackness even if it could not be articulated. For intellectuals like Rush, Volney, and Samuel Stanhope Smith, committed to the idea of racial fluidity, especially as a means to end slavery, Moss became a key example.[24] For popular audiences, Moss's change was more spectacle than philosophical marvel.[25] As Eric Herschthal notes, Rush held two seemingly contradictory positions on race at the same time. The first was, that slavery was immoral and insupportable, but the second, that citizenship in the American republic belonged to white men.[26] Understanding Black men as somehow congenitally ill could have been a way of trying to reconcile those positions for the majority while even supporting the equality of a few exceptional Black individuals. Rush infamously likened Blackness to leprosy based on several racist stereotypes picked up from colonial literature.[27] While darker skin was associated with leprosy so too, Rush pointed out, was a lack of sensitivity to pain and changes in hair texture, additional traits of Blackness as described by white medical men. In terms of the leprosy-like

---

23   Benjamin Rush, Commonplace Book, APS.

24   Volney, *View of the Climate and Soil of the United States of America: To Which Are Annexed Some Accounts of Florida, the French Colony on the Scioto, Certain Canadian Colonies, and the Savages or Natives*, 407; Smith, *An Essay on the Causes of the Variety of Complexion and Figure in the Human Species*, 92–93; Kidd, *The Forging of Races: Race and Scripture in the Protestant Atlantic World, 1600–2000*, 109.

25   Rush pasted a public advertisement for Moss to be on show in his commonplace book next to his entry on meeting Moss. For more on the public response to Henry Moss and his appearances in American cities, see Yokota, "Not Written in Black and White : American National Identity and the Curious Color Transformation of Henry Moss," 1–6.

26   Herschthal, "Antislavery Science in the Early Republic: The Case of Dr. Benjamin Rush," 296.

27   See Block, *Colonial Complexions: Race and Bodies in Eighteenth-Century America*.

disease of Blackness, Rush believed it was contracted in Africa—due to a hot climate and "savage" living conditions—and perpetuated by the degrading mental and physical conditions of slavery. It could only be mitigated by the end of the practice, which would bring about the eventual elimination of the physical distinction—the transformation of Black bodies into white ones.

Rush was a classic eighteenth-century example of an assimilationist based on Ibram X. Kendi's framework of segregationist, assimilationist, and antiracist.[28] Rush believed discrimination caused perceived racial inferiority on the part of Black people without questioning the idea of inferiority or tenants of white supremacy. Rather, he readily attributed racist ideas about African-descended people to a presumed inferiority of African climates and cultures and the physical and mental degradation of slavery. This made Rush a relatively early antislavery advocate but not someone open to a true pluralist society.

Race, for Rush, was fluid and could be altered with the application of scientific reform. For example, he made no mention of Moss's mixed-race background as an explanation of his "whitening," suggesting the irrelevance of hereditary. Rather, he frequently emphasized the fact that Moss was a free man. Rush also remarked on the fact that the white patches of Moss's skin tended to be under the clothes, protected from the elements, and perhaps more "civilized." Rush also looked for African Americans of clear intellectual talent to promote the idea of racial "improvement" and eventual assimilation in color as well as intellect. He maintained correspondence with James Durham, a Black medical practitioner in New Orleans (formerly enslaved by a Philadelphia physician), and introduced his work to the American Philosophical Society. He also supported Richard Allen's and Absalom Jones's work to establish an African Church in Philadelphia, attending the opening dinner on May 22, 1793, and was in contact with the Black Maryland scientist Benjamin Banneker.[29]

---

28 Kendi, *Stamped from the Beginning: The Definitive History of Racist Ideas in America.*

29 Rush, Commonplace Book, APS, Mss.B.R89c; Benjamin Rush, *An Account of the Bilious Remitting Yellow Fever as It Appeared in the City of Philadelphia in the Year 1793* (Philadelphia: Thomas Dobson, 1794), 113, 322–23; Benjamin Rush to the Pennsylvania Abolition Society (Philadelphia, November 14, 1788), Rush, *Letters of Benjamin Rush,* 497–98; Plummer and Durham, "Letters of James Durham to Benjamin Rush," 261–69. Samuel Miller to Benjamin Rush (1807) LCP, Rush Family Papers, Series I Benjamin Rush Papers, Subseries I Correspondence, Vol. 27.

Meanwhile, as noted in the previous chapter, racial difference between European-descended Americans and Indigenous Americans took a very different cast in Rush's work. There is no suggestion that Rush believed Indians had any peculiar aliment like that associated with Blackness. However, he also started to follow the trope of the "disappearing Indian," assuming that Indigenous people wouldn't be part of the American republic. In the case of Native Americans, his concerns were more abstract. Rush's short essay on Native American health marked a few key points that highlighted the complexity of race, climate, and culture in North America and how the matrix could be manipulated. At its core sat the essential question: if climate influenced culture, as theories like Montesquieu's claimed, could two distinctive societies permanently exist in the same location? Was one inevitably doomed to failure?

On the surface, American citizens and Indigenous people were very similar. White Americans and Indians lived in the same climate, and they ate many of the same foods, especially those derived from plants and animals native to the Americas, like maize and venison.[30] In addition to the similarity of their physical environments, Native Americans and European-Americans had at least one important social trait in common. Both groups consisted mainly of free people and were not (or rarely) threatened with enslavement by the turn of the nineteenth century. This difference was extremely important for Rush. He attributed many of the "inferior" or "pathological" traits associated with people of African descent with the mentally and physically damaging state of slavery as discussed above. Such a difference would not apply to Eastern tribal nations. Even though there were and had been free people of color in North America for generations, the default assumption of white Americans was to treat the terms "slave" and "negro" as synonyms.[31] By the early nineteenth century, free African Americans outnumbered enslaved

---

30 Reliance on American crops was more common the further west one traveled. Although corn grew throughout the United States, Volney noted that farmers cultivated wheat as well until he reached the French settlement at St. Vincennes (Vincennes, Indiana) where maize was the only cereal. Volney, *View of the Climate and Soil of the United States of America: To Which Are Annexed Some Accounts of Florida, the French Colony on the Scioto, Certain Canadian Colonies, and the Savages or Natives*, 145. L.J. Jardine noted the prevalence of venison in American diets with much approval, in Jardine, *A Letter from Pennsylvania to a Friend in England: Containing Valuable Information with Respect to America*.

31 Block, *Colonial Complexions: Race and Bodies in Eighteenth-Century America*.

people in Philadelphia, but many of those individuals had been born into slavery and thus, following Rush's logic, were only beginning to recover from its damaging physical and mental effects. In the second edition of his treatise against slavery, published in 1773, Rush wrote:

> I need hardly say any thing in favour of the Intellects of the Negroes, or of their capacity for virtue and happiness, although these have been supposed, by some, to be inferior to those of the inhabitants of Europe. The accounts which travellers give us of their ingenuity, humanity, and strong attachment to their parents, relations, friends, and country, show us that *they are equal to the Europeans*, when we allow for the diversity of temper and genius which is occasioned by climate. . . . *But we are to distinguish between an African in his own country, and an African in a state of slavery in America. Slavery is so foreign to the human mind, that the moral faculties, as well as those of the understanding are debased, and rendered torpid by it.* All the vices which are charged upon the Negroes in the southern colonies and the West-Indies, such as Idleness, Treachery, Theft, and the like, are the genuine offspring of slavery and serve as an argument to prove that they were not intended for it.[32]

Enslaved people could not control their own bodies. As such, according to Rush, they suffered mental anguish and physical harm due to their unfree status. His students noted that the diseases considered particular to enslaved Africans, like yaws and "dirt-eating," were impossible to separate from slavery and did not (they argued) appear in free people of any race. This did not mean that Rush had any scruples about believing stories of general vice and inferiority spread by slave owners or physicians making a living on North American and Caribbean plantations. He readily cited and read both well-known works like those of Hans Sloane from early eighteenth-century Jamaica as well as reports from colleagues and former students. For example, he apparently shared letters of Moses Bartram Jr. (a former student in South Carolina) to the College of Physicians of Philadelphia in 1791, possibly about the different course of fevers in enslaved people compared to white people. That Rush shared the document surprised and slightly embarrassed the writer, but that embarrassment was about making an unfinished work public, not about its contents.[33]

Rush readily collected anecdotes about people of different races from a variety of sources he deemed reputable. He often reprinted those that stood

---

32 Rush, *An Address to the Inhabitants of the British Settlements, on the Slavery of the Negroes in America, the Second Edition*, 1–2, emphasis added.

33 Moses Bartram Jr. to Benjamin Rush (1791) LCP, Rush Family Papers, Series I Benjamin Rush Papers, Subseries I Correspondence, Vol. XXI.

out to him or added them to his classroom lectures to further a point. This also came up in Rush's response to yellow fever in 1793 when he initially believed Black Philadelphians would be immune to the disorder. Many contemporary practitioners in the Caribbean believed that people of African descent were immune to the disease. Following their lead, Rush encouraged the Black population of Philadelphia to act as nurses during the outbreak, to devastating effect. He later retracted his endorsement of immunity in part but continued to claim that the disease was less harmful in African-descended people.[34] Yellow fever was not the only disease to take on a racialized meaning. Other correspondents reported diseases that affected only one race, using it as an assumed and understood mark of "difference." An 1812 letter from a physician who practiced in New Orleans and Natchez, Mississippi, described opthamlia as a racially defined disease affected by climate. The letter stated that the ailment in the Southwest "was uniformly confined to blacks, who had recently arrived in that country from Africa; and never made its appearance . . . until after they had been some days on the Mississippi."[35] Such assessments were not uncommon and although not produced by Rush were kept by him and may have shaped his thinking about the effects of race on illness.

Meanwhile, in his lecture on the intellectual faculties, Rush concluded by considering the effects of race on the mind. He did not question the assumptions of travel writers that non-European individuals were inferior to Europeans and European-descended people. Rush blithely reported—based on the writing of the "pedestrian traveller" Mr. Stewart—that Indigenous men had "dull and disgusting sameness of mind [which] characterizes all savage nations." Nevertheless, he emphasized the cultural differences rather than innate racial differences, noting that "weakness is as much the effect of the want of physical influence upon their minds, as a disagreeable colour and figure are of its action upon their bodies."[36] Again, Rush clearly reinforced ideas of racial difference while trying to distance himself from anything that could hint at polygenesis. His causal and uncritical use of racial categories (and racial stereotyping) reinforced ideas of difference rather than break them down.

---

34 Rush, *An Account of the Bilious Remitting Yellow Fever, as It Appeared in the City of Philadelphia, in the Year 1793*, 97.

35 G. E. Pendergeast to Benjamin Rush (1812) LCP, Rush Family Papers, Series I Benjamin Rush Papers, Subseries I Correspondence, Vol. 13.

36 Rush, *Sixteen Introductory Lectures, to Courses of Lectures upon the Institutes and Practice of Medicine*, 116–17.

Strangely, however, Rush seemed to contradict himself again by noting a sort of mental hybrid vigor among mixed race people. He concluded the essay (one that was mainly on the effects of the body on mind, not a specific treatise on race) with a somewhat out-of-place musing on the intellectual strengths of some people based on ancestry.

> It is possible, the strength of the intellects may be improved in their original con-formation, as much as the strength of the body, by certain mixtures of persons of different nations, habits, and constitutions, in marriage. The mulatto has been remarked, in all countries, to exceed, in sagacity, his white and black parent. The same remark has been made of the offspring of the European, and North American Indian . . . marriages of Danish men, with the East India women, produced children, that had the countenances and vigorous minds of Europeans. . . . It is probable, the qualities of body and mind in parents, which produce genius in children, may be fixed and regular, and it is possible, the time may come, when we shall be able to predict, with certainty the intellectual character of children, by knowing the specific nature of the different intellectual faculties of their parents.[37]

While Rush might have argued that this reflects specific differences between individuals, his choice to focus on mixed-race children is important. It shows his familiarity with using and upholding the developing racial language of the eighteenth and nineteenth centuries. Cases like especially intelligent children of African and European ancestry could even bolster antislavery activities while creating a pathway to racial essentialism in the next generation of physicians.

In addition to accounts of disease Rush also readily collected examples of that "genius" described above. Descriptions of exceptional people of color, are equally characteristic of Rush's work and ideas surrounding the future of American society. He readily corresponded with African-descended people both in the United States and beyond. One man, J. Edward Jesup of St. Christopher (St. Kitts and Nevis), wrote a friendly letter to Rush in 1791 noting his safe arrival home, hurricane damage on the island, and the box of oranges sent with the letter. In all respects, it's a perfectly unremarkable note from a foreign correspondent in Rush's collection. However, it stands out due to a note made by Rush on the back of the page identifying the author as a "free negro."[38] Jesup was an exception but part of a group of men who were important exceptions that "proved" Rush's assimilationist theories.

---

37 Rush, *Sixteen Introductory Lectures,* 117.
38 J. Edward Jesup to Benjamin Rush (1791) LCP, Rush Family Papers, Series I Benjamin Rush Papers, Subseries I Correspondence, Vol. VXXI. Parish records of the year 1743 for St. George on St. Christophers indicate that a Colonel

As noted above, in Philadelphia Rush financially and publicly supported Allen and Jones in the establishment of the African Episcopal Methodist Church in 1793. The two men were also his key contacts and supporters to enlist Black Philadelphians to assist as nurses, blood-letters, and grave-diggers during the yellow fever epidemic that same year. Following the epidemic, Rush not only praised the efforts of the community (especially their civic mindedness) but also relied on the medical expertise of Black healthcare workers. In letters to Julia Rush, Benjamin gleefully noted very large numbers of patients who survived the fever through bloodletting. These numbers (sometimes in the hundreds) were too high to include the work of Rush and his students alone. The corroborating evidence likely came from Black bleeders reporting back to Rush directly or through Allen and Jones who mentioned the success of the practice in their own account of the epidemic in similar terms with similar numbers.[39]

Meanwhile, within the formal medical profession, Rush corresponded with an African-American practitioner in New Orleans, Dr. James Durham. Durham was born into slavery in Philadelphia (although it is unclear when) and at some point, was sold to Dr. John Kersley Jr., who moved to Louisiana (when it was a Spanish territory). Durham attained his freedom and began practicing medicine with a specific focus on diseases of the throat. Because Louisiana was part of the Spanish Empire Durham could not legally practice as a physician without formal credentials unavailable to him in the colony. Nevertheless, from an Anglo-American perspective Durham did have the appropriate qualifications to call himself a colonial physician—experience, apprenticeship, and positive accounts of his skills—and was treated by Rush accordingly. Rush and Durham maintained a professional correspondence between 1789 and 1802 and Rush used Durham as a public example

---

Edward Jessup had "his Negroe woman Elizabeth" baptized on November 20. It seems possible that the J. Edward Jesup who corresponded with Rush was their son. *Caribbeana being Miscellaneous Papers Relating to the History, Genealogy, Topography, and Antiquities of the British West Indies.* Vol. 1, Vere Langford Oliver Ed. London: Mitchell Hughes and Clarke (1910), 359.

39 Benjamin Rush "To Mrs. Rush (Philadelphia, September 6, 1793)," *Letters of Benjamin Rush,* Vol. II, 653; Jones and Allen, *A Narrative of the Proceedings of the Black People, during the Late Awful Calamity in Philadelphia, in the Year 1793: And a Refutation of Some Censures Thrown upon Them in Some Late Publications,* 17.

of African-American ability in talks before abolitionist groups.[40] Although Jesup, Allen, Jones, and Durham were all racialized as Black men, the end of slavery opened opportunities for them. They created communities and a professional standing, which seemed to suggest the possibility of a United States without slavery and without a permanent division between the races, backed by Rush's medical ideas.

Slavery in Rush's view created and perpetuated physical and psychological inferiority, which could only be corrected by the end of the practice. Nevertheless, enslaved African Americans did not, in Rush's view, equal the humanity and sensibility of their free African ancestors or free African American descendants. Generations of slavery, in his mind, would take generations to undo, but potentially lead to the literal whitening of the population.[41] From this perspective, Rush viewed Black Americans as inferior to their white counterparts, but the blame for it fell on the shoulders of white America. Although slavery was being gradually phased out and made illegal in most Northern States, including Pennsylvania in the wake of the Revolution, the institution remained in place in New York (gradual abolition began 1817 and abolished 1827) and New Jersey (gradual abolition began 1804) as well as the nearby "border" states of Maryland and Delaware until the Civil War. Rush thought poor living conditions, dangerous work environments, and a separate culture prevented African Americans from attaining "health" but did so while reiterating racist stereotypes, which floated around the Anglophone Atlantic.[42] Rush's support of emancipation efforts and correspondence with African American intellectual and religious leaders can be explained as support of the institutional changes that might end "Blackness" as a "disease." One of his students, Elijah Griffiths, recorded in his notebook that Rush had stated," I imagine, that their color arose in the first place from the leprosy; & that they exhibit all or most of the signs of that disease, a big lip, flat nose & the offensive smell they emit from their bodies, indicate the

---

40   For more on Durham and his relationship with Rush, see Plummer and Durham, "Letters of James Durham to Benjamin Rush"; Wynes, "Dr. James Durham, Mysterious Eighteenth-Century Black Physician: Man or Myth?," 325–33.

41   For more on science, race, and abolition, see Delbourgo, "The Newtonian Slave Body: Racial Enlightenment in the Atlantic World," 185–207; Schiebinger, "Medical Experimentation and Race in the Eighteenth-Century Atlantic World."

42   Seth, *Difference and Disease: Medicine, Race, and the Eighteenth-Century British Empire.*

presence of leprosy, together with nervous insensibility" and that Rush had witnessed a case of a white girl abandoned and living in squalor who took on characteristics of Blackness.[43]

How, in Rush's view, would African Americans become part of the greater United States? The answer was essentially one of assimilation to whiteness, both social and (possibly) biological. In this Rush differs little from Americans who have called for assimilation of a variety of marginalized groups, including European immigrants. The nineteenth and twentieth centuries saw Irish, Italian, and Jewish Americans among other ethnic and religious groups "become white." In the twentieth centuries the pernicious "model minority" narrative surrounding Asian immigrants and Asian Americans did similar work of praising "assimilation" while perpetuating racial categories and permanent "otherness." Rush used the example of individuals like Henry Moss, James Durham, Absalom Jones, Richard Allen, J. Edward Jesup, and Benjamin Banneker as examples of an analogous process.

Making American Medical Readers

In addition to questions about how gender and race would shape the American Republic, Rush also looked to the medical profession itself as something that needed to be Americanized. Received medical literature was crucial, but not necessarily appropriate for all places in the country. Once again, Rush's ideas sat uneasily between an impulse to see a unique American national identity and connecting to larger, universal themes inspired by the Enlightenment. On the one hand it is tempting to look at Rush's project of American medicine alongside something like his acquaintance Noah Webster's quest for American language. A new national identity needed a medical language and texts suited to the American physical and social situation. On the other hand, however, Rush wanted to use his American setting to uncover something much broader and universal. The United States might be unique, but that uniqueness could be a way of finding new universal truth about disease, bodies, climates, and even religion, as discussed further on. To return to the language analogy, this puts Rush closer to men like William

---

43 Elijah Griffiths, "Notes from Dr. Rushes [sic] Lectures (1797–1798)," CPP, 10a 106, Vol. II. A similar account is found in: John Stevenson, "Notes from Doctor B. Rush's Lectures delievered [sic] in the University of Pennsylvania commenced 27 Nov: 1797," CPP, 10a374, Lecture 39. Rush also believed standard leprosy was a hereditary disease—another perceived connection to Blackness, George F. Lehman, "Student lecture notes," CPP, 10a 239, Vol. I.

Thornton or Volney, who sought universal and rational alphabets.[44] In that cauldron of Enlightenment and nationalism Rush forged a view of medicine that was explicitly tailored to the American condition but not ignorant of broader implications. His American Editions of British medical texts explore this tension well.

Sitting at the center of a growing network of professional contacts and patient correspondence, Rush had access to and mastery over an enormous amount of medical knowledge. Connecting the dots and using that knowledge to create a working medical theory for American practitioners remained his goal. Ultimately, Rush collected information about health, disease, weather, and geography in order to treat American bodies in a variety of spaces and communicate those practices to his students. One of the clearest examples of America in intellectual limbo and the importance of geography to medical knowledge is the existence of specially denoted "American Editions" of British and colonial medical works edited by Rush. Similar projects, like Charles Caldwell's 1805 translation of Jean Senac's *A Treatise on the Hidden Nature, and the Treatment of Intermitting and Remitting Fevers,* were also translations from French or Latin into English. Even texts originally in English, however, underwent a translation process as the crossed the Atlantic. Because America was not Britain Rush needed to translate texts from English into American for his audiences, noting where to follow and where to break from classic medical texts based on social and biological differences. Editing choices, additional prefaces, and discursive footnotes trained the reader to interpret the text from a new perspective, typically that of an American citizen in North America as opposed to a French or English subject in Europe.[45]

Rush first used the phrase "American Edition" in the 1780s to identify American imprints of William Cullen's *First Lines on the Practice of Physic.*[46]

---

44   Lepore, *A Is for American: Letters and Other Characters in the Newly United States,* 52–58.

45   The designation "American Edition" indicated that its original place of publication lay outside the United States but that it was being reprinted locally, often with editing or comments by a well-known American. The genre did not apply only to medical texts. Law books like William Blackstone's *Commentaries* were similarly reprinted for American audiences. Blackstone, William and Robert Bell, *Commentaries on the laws of England By William Blackstone, Esq. Vinerian Professor Law and Solicitor general to Her Majesty: In four Volumes: Reprinted from the London copy, page for page with the last edition,* America [Philadelphia]: Printed for the subscribers (1771).

46   Cullen and Rush, *First Lines of the Practice of Physic, for the Use of Students, in the University of Edinburgh, Vol. I.*

At that point his only addition to the text came in the form of a preface praising his preceptor and the book. The content of the volume did not change
much from the smuggled-in British version to the wartime American edition. This was typical for "American Editions" in general. The designation in
the eighteenth and early nineteenth century simply denoted that a book was
an American imprint of a text. Changing too much would defeat the presumed purpose—making money by selling an already popular or important
text. American readers (usually) didn't want an adulterated product. In post-
war letters to Cullen, Rush discussed the great importance that *First Lines*
had in the American military hospitals during the revolution. He claimed
that "[i]t was read with peculiar attention by the physicians and surgeons
of our army . . . Thus, sir, you see you have had a hand in the Revolution
by contributing indirectly to save the lives of the officers and soldiers of the
American army."[47] Cullen's work shaped the way Rush understood the deep
connections between bodies and spaces and the role of the physician, in this
case military physician, in disciplining those bodies and spaces.

By the early nineteenth century, however, Rush had fully broken with
Cullen's nervous physiology in favor of his more expansive system of
excitement carried out through the nerves, blood vessels, and lymphatics
Considering this, his "American Editions" of the nineteenth century took
on a new character and purpose: to train readers in the new American sys-
tem of medicine by highlighting or altering specific passages. Between
1809 and 1815 he published editions of George Cleghorn's *Observations
on the Epidemical Diseases of Minorca From the Production, Inhabitants, and
Endemical Distempers of Minorca*, William Hillary's *Observations on the
Changes of the air, and the concomitant epidemical diseases in the island of
Barbadoes*, Sir John Pringle's *Observations on the Diseases of the Army*, and
The Works of Thomas Sydenham M.D., on Acute and Chronic Diseases. He
planned to do so with other books as well. In his commonplace book on
April 21, 1810, Rush noted that he "read Pringle's books with a reference
to publishing notes upon them . . . finished [James] Lind on the disease of
warm climates, read for the same purpose"; he finished notes on Pringle on
June 8.[48] Although the Lind book never reached the publisher, the topic fits
well with Rush's other American editions. Each included an extensive commentary and spelled out the connections Rush believed he made between the
original work and his own. Moreover, they demonstrate that although Rush

---

47   Rush, "To William Cullen, Philadelphia, September 16th, 1783," in Letters of
      Benjamin Rush, 311.
48   Rush, *The Autobiography*, 289, 291.

believed local knowledge to be paramount, one could still learn by comparison to Britain and her warm-weather colonies. Rush took information from non-American spaces and clearly noted where, when, and how, such information could be used to understand the diseases and conditions faced by his countrymen.

All of Rush's "American Editions" discuss the intersection of disease with place and situation. By highlighting where these spaces were similar or different to the United States Rush provided a framework for readers to assess spaces and illnesses on their own—specifically, the young medical men he taught and subsequently ushered into medical careers far from Philadelphia. In this way they acted as pedagogical texts, showing American medical men how to make the most out of otherwise flawed texts.[49] Unlike *First Lines,* they do not fit into the category of textbook. Sydenham, for example, largely presented sets of observations on annual epidemics. Pringle, Cleghorn, and Hillary each recounted their experiences in clearly delineated times and spaces. Their specificity appears to undermine any general relevance they might have for the equally distinct American states. Nevertheless, Rush presented his American Editions as important contributions to American medical literature. He dedicated each edition to the medical students at the University of Pennsylvania and the United States of America, highlighting their intended use as a pedagogical tool. By the end of his career most of Rush's students came from and returned to places their preceptor had never visited, much less practiced medicine in. These circumstances encouraged Rush to teach students how to adapt medical ideas to new environments rather than simply how to treat patients in an existing one. The American Editions demonstrated the kind of work Rush had in mind.

Rush's first attempt at this new form was an 1809 American edition of *The Works of Thomas Sydenham.* Sydenham's observations of epidemics and empiricism fit well within Rush's ideal of physician behavior even when he tended to reject specific therapies. In the preface Rush introduced the great man by saying that there are both many things worthy of praise and many instances of error. Among the latter were Sydenham's rejection of theory, belief in contagion with respect to plague, and reliance on botanical medicines. Nonetheless, students were also primed to read the work of a genius of the seventeenth century.

---

49 Naramore, "Recommended for 'Frequent Perusal' and 'Improving the Science of Medicine': Benjamin Rush's American Editions and the Circulation of Medical Knowledge in the Early Republic."

His histories of acute disease; his details of the laws of epidemics; his intuitive discernment of old diseases, entangled in new ones; his defence [sic] of cool air, and of depleting remedies, to which millions owe their lives; his sagacity in discovering the precise time, and manner of administering his remedies, and the difference of his practice in the same disease in different seasons, constitute a galaxy of medical knowledge, and . . . rare assemblage of discrimination and combining talents, which have elevated him above the claims of the century and nation in which he lived, and rendered him the physician of all ages and countires [sic].[50]

This is the Sydenham that Rush emulated when he recorded and analyzed his observations of annual epidemic diseases. The above observations are also those that Rush found most useful in understanding and combatting illness and tried to emulate in his own habits of recording epidemic diseases rather than Sydenham's own intentions.[51] Rush's system would add reason to the empirical work of his predecessor. Where Sydenham described the merging of one disease into another or the changes over time, Rush applied theory. Like the letters he received from across the country and journal articles he read, Rush used Sydenham as a means of accessing general laws of disease that could be applied to specific, regional, situations.

Rush felt that the laws uncovered in Sydenham's discussion of the plague provided the most information for the rejection of nosology, the classification of diseases, which he felt hampered medical progress. Previous translators of Sydenham (from Latin to English), John Swan (1742) and George Wallis (1788) also included discursive footnotes and preface. Contrary to Rush, however, they praised the seventeenth-century physician's observations that they marked the beginning of medical nosology.[52] Rush bucked this

---

50 Sydenham and Rush, *The Works of Thomas Sydenham, M.D., on Acute and Chronic Diseases: With Their Histories and Modes of Cure*, vi.

51 The connection between Rush and Sydenham's bleeding practices is also commented on in Waring, "The Influence of Benjamin Rush on the Practice of Bleeding in South Carolina," 230.

52 Thomas Sydenham, *The Entire Works of Dr. Thomas Sydenham: Newly Made English from the Originals: Wherein the History of Acute and Chronic Diseases, and the Safest and Most Effectual Methods of Treating Them, Are Faithfully, Clearly, and Accurately Delivered.*, ed. John Swan, 1742; Thomas Sydenham and George Wallis, *The Works of Thomas Sydenham, M.D. on Acute and Chronic Diseases; Wherein Their Histories and Modes of Cure, as Recited by Him, Are Delivered with Accuracy and Perspicuity. To Which Are Subjoined Notes, Corrective and Explanatory* (London: G.G.J. and J. Robinson, W. Otridge, S. Hayes, and E. Newbery, 1788).

convention and argued the exact opposite. For Rush, Sydenham was important because his work could be used to end nosology. The blending of symptoms Sydenham witnessed made far more sense to Rush if "disease" were a general state of being rather than one of several hundred discrete "diseases." Amended to Sydenham's description of the similarities between plague and erysipelas, Rush writes that Colin Chisholm's erysipelas appeared in the West Indies just before an outbreak of yellow fever, indicating that they had the same root cause. He then attributed the change of symptoms to the change of season rather than disease. Rush thereby used Sydenham (with assistance from Chisholm) to argue that plague, erysipelas, and yellow fever are all different manifestations of the same "disease" and merely driven to different presentations.[53] Most evident in Rush's adoption of Sydenham's epidemiology is the primacy of the atmosphere as setting the stage for epidemic diseases. Despite individual variations, epidemics suggested the existence of a general change in the air that affected whole populations in both Sydenham and Rush's accounts.

Diseases in similar locations, presenting similar symptoms, or similar times of the year might be helpful as one-to-one comparisons. However, Rush demonstrated that different illnesses could be useful as comparisons only if the natural history of both relevant instances were well understood. In still other instances Rush noted the sections his readers could safely ignore. For example, he argued that Sydenham's scorbutic rheumatism did not occur in the United States, thus giving the reader reason to discount it as an important piece of medical knowledge.[54] Despite the variable forms that comments could take, Rush kept his audience in mind: American medical students and young doctors. The editions helped knit together medicine in the United States in direct comparison with practice in other parts of the world.

Rush was not only interested in the work of physicians living in temperate regions analogous to his own Pennsylvania. As noted above, tropical locations were especially important because they helped address the variation within American climates and yellow fever. The fever in the United States will be discussed in greater detail in the next chapter. However, it is worth examining the way in which Rush centered the fever in a broader literature before focusing on the specifics of Philadelphia in 1793. The disorientation of a tropical fever in temperate Philadelphia was likely all the greater considering the fact that yellow fever was not a novel ailment, just a misplaced one. In

---

53 Sydenham and Rush, *The Works*, 56.

54 Sydenham and Rush, *The Works*, 191.

1809 Rush published an American Edition of George Cleghorn's *Observations on the epidemical diseases of Minorca. From the year 1744 to 1749*. With respect to the book's value, he wrote in the dedicatory preface that:

> The following work contains a greater mass of practical knowledge in a small compass, than any book perhaps of the same kind in medicine. . . . Its merit consists chiefly in the number and importance of its facts, which afford the surest passport of a medical book to present and future generation[s]. The notes which I have added to this first American edition of this valuable work, are intended to point out a few of its errors, but chiefly to impress those remarks, upon your minds, which accord with the diseases a mode of practice that are common in the United States.[55]

This preface reinforces the value Rush placed on American editions for himself, and his readers. The volume's value lay in its "mass of practical knowledge" and the "number and importance of its facts." Rush's notes, meanwhile, directed the reader to the most important sections, facts, and observations. The value of medical texts, therefore, came from the quality of observable facts rather than the analysis of a great physician.

Rush's most congratulatory observations began in chapter 2 where Cleghorn wrote in a manner that emulated Sydenham's descriptions of epidemics. As with Sydenham, Rush both noted Cleghorn's observational skills and translated facts into his own medical mindset. In the case of bilious fevers, for example, Rush agreed with Cleghorn that in both the United States and Minorca children often became ill with *cholera infantum* prior to the outbreak of the clearly bilious epidemic. On the other hand, despite Cleghorn's argument to the contrary, Rush used the description of bilious fever in Minorca to argue for a proximate atmospheric rather than an exciting contagious cause. In a note, Rush wrote that "[t]hey [bilious fevers] spread only from the action of an impure atmosphere, and never extend beyond its influence." This description accounted for the fever's narrow geographic distribution and the cessation of illness with the onset of cold weather. Contagious diseases, like smallpox, spread in all seasons and only required human bodies to support and carry the morbid matter.[56] Ultimately, only Cleghorn's empirical observations mattered to Rush. Cleghorn's analysis, that

---

55   Cleghorn and Rush, *Observations on the Epidemical Diseases of Minorca from the Year 1744 to 1749 to Which Is Prefixed A Short Account of the Climate Productions, Inhabitants, and Endemical Distempers of Minorca*, iii.

56   Cleghorn and Rush, *Observations*, 80.

the bilious fever's contagion spread from person to person, was quickly and quietly dismissed by the American authority.

Just as he had with Sydenham and Cleghorn, Rush simultaneously praised and criticized William Hillary's work on the climate and diseases of Barbados and set the boundaries of applicability in a dedicatory preface.

> The physician, to whose patience and labour we are indebted for performing that useful task by means of the following work, was a pupil of the celebrated Dr. Boerhaave. . . . It is true, some of the theories he adopted, from his illustrious master, have been discovered to be erroneous, but the facts he has recorded in his history of weather, and of its effects upon the symptoms, and cure of diseases, will be true, in like circumstances, in all ages and countries, nor will they be affected in their importance or utility by any of the successive revolutions which may take place in the principles of our science.[57]

This preface specifically critiqued Hillary's theoretical background as a student of Herman Boerhaave. With that warning stated, however, Rush directed his readers to attend to the facts presented "in [Hillary's] history of the weather and of its effects upon the symptoms and cures of diseases." Hillary's study, like the other American editions, came from a previous medical generation. Rush was updating as well as altering the text in search of American utility. He included descriptions of diseases and therapeutics in terms of air and weather changes. Like the collection of facts, Rush had a use for the empirically derived treatments for disease as another blank canvas from which he could develop medical theory. Hillary prefaced the second part of the book noting "[a]s I have in the preceding observations taken notice of all the most material changes of the air and weather, and of such alterations as happened in their concomitant epidemical diseases: I shall in the following essays, indevour [sic] carefully to observe, and strictly to trace out, and follow nature, both in the descriptions of the diseases, and their symptoms."[58] The "following essays" describe a number of specific diseases Hillary encountered during his time in Barbados. Many of his essays, including "Of the Putrid Bilious Fever, Commonly Called the Yellow Fever," were similar to illnesses encountered by Rush in the United States.

---

57   Hillary and Rush, *Observations on the Changes of the Air, and the Concomitant Epidemical Diseases in the Island of Barbadoes. To Which Is Added A Treatise on the Putrid Billious Fever, Commonly Called the Yellow Fever; and Such Other Diseases as Are Indigenous or Endemical.*

58   Hillary and Rush, *Observations*, 101.

Hillary, like Rush, proposed venesection as a common treatment for warm weather diseases and in instances when bodies appeared to be at a low rather than high state of fever. A short, footnoted statement from Rush summed up his feelings on the subject: "See here! a striking proof of the safety and advantages of bleeding in a depressed state of the system, and of being guided by 'acuteness of pain' instead of a full or tense pulse."[59] Rush used Hillary to support his own opinions on the use of venesection, or bloodletting in most fevers in the United States. In Hillary's work Rush believed he saw a unity of disease akin to the theory that he wanted to advocate in the United States.

In the American Editions Rush presented Sydenham, Cleghorn, and Hillary as models for how a well-trained physician could adapt his knowledge and skills to fundamentally different disease environments. Their careful observations of their surroundings, both cultural and natural historical, could be emulated by American doctors, both in the east and, presumably, the new western territories. Between these examples and Rush's additions to the main text, American medicine could grow out of careful and widespread observation of unique spaces. This placed American medicine in a similar position to British colonial medicine, which was busy innovating and producing knowledge of spaces distinct from Britain. Mark Harrison cogently argues that these practitioners actually drove the progressive narrative of medicine that emerged during the eighteenth century.[60] Rush and his colleagues were engaged in a similar progressive project with the added impetus of creating a national identity.

That drive to craft an identity encouraged Rush to ask how spaces could be constructed to improve American health. Although present on the individual level in these editions, this movement toward management of places reached its zenith in the final America edition: John Pringle's *Observations on the Diseases of the Army* (1810). As with the previous editions, Rush's Edition of Pringle begins with a bold address to its potential readership.

> Behold! gentlemen, another attempt by your preceptor to transplant a vigorous and fruitful European plant into the soil of our country; or, in other words, behold, in the following American edition of sir John Pringle's Observations upon the Diseases of the British Army, an attempt to increase and diffuse medical knowledge in the United States from a source to which physicians and learned societies have done homage in every part of the world.[61]

---

59   Hillary and Rush, *Observations*, 49.

60   Harrison, *Medicine in an Age of Commerce and Empire: Britian and Its Tropical Colonies.*

61   Pringle and Rush, *Observations on the Diseases of the Army*, iii.

The image of transplantation is especially poignant in the American editions. Rush was familiar with the science of botany and the difficulty of successful transplantation over a long distance. The metaphor calls attention to the idea that students needed to take care when reading and using foreign information in the United States.[62]

As with the other American Editions, Pringle fit into the same broad circles as Hillary, Cleghorn, and Sydenham.[63] Specifically, Rush highlighted the connections between Boerhaave's Leiden, physicians from dissenting religious backgrounds, the Scottish Universities, and Rush's American Edition authors. Pringle was no exception. His formal education took place in Scotland and the Netherlands in connection with Gerhard van Sweiten (Boehaave's student and commentator). He then taught philosophy at the University of Edinburgh before taking a post with the British Army, which inspired *Observations on the Diseases of the Army*. While he was away, Cleghorn took over his university courses, again demonstrating the intellectual fluidity of the Scottish university and association between medicine and philosophy.[64] Much later, a young Benjamin Rush was personally introduced to the renowned Pringle in London in 1769. The meeting left a favorable impression on the young Rush, who recounted it in his autobiography.[65]

A shared intellectual background was not the only connection Rush had with Pringle. Pringle's military background also struck a chord with Rush who served in the Continental Army during the American War for Independence. Both during and after the conflict, Rush relied on his experiences in military hospitals and regional travel to support his theory and practice. From firsthand experience, association with British military physicians like Pringle, and his friendship with John Morgan, Rush developed strong opinions on the management of military hospitals. As surgeon-general for the middle department of the Continental Army, Rush spent much of 1777

---

62 Schiebinger et al., *Colonial Botany: Science, Commerce, and Politics in the Early Modern World*; Zilberstein, "Inured to Empire: Wild Rice and Climate Change."

63 With respect to Sydenham, Pringle was compared to the English physician in his used of fact and adherence to the experimental principles of Francis Bacon. Pringle and Rush, *Observations*, xii, xxv.

64 Pringle and Rush, *Observations on the Diseases of the Army*.

65 Rush and Biddle, *A Memorial Containing Travels Through Life Or Sundry Incidents in the Life of Dr. Benjamin Rush, Born Dec. 24, 1745 (Old Style) Died April 19, 1813*, 32.

on the road inspecting hospitals and wrangling supplies. Rush left the Army after a short tenure, discouraged by his experience, but he remained deeply interested in the role a medical department could play in military life.

Rush's military background had several effects on his view of Pringle. First, he used Pringle as another node in an important international network of highly respected British physicians who came of age when both the first British Empire and Edinburgh's medical school were at the height of their powers. As an Edinburgh graduate, chair-holder at a Scottish-inspired medical school, and citizen of a new republic with imperial ambitions,[66] Rush still wanted to associate himself with that legacy. Second, a part of the legacy that Rush wanted to associate himself with was that of careful observation and a medicine that connected bodies and their surroundings. Third, despite respect and near reverence for the elder physician, Rush did not hesitate to modify and reinterpret Pringle to better support his own efforts. Lastly, and distinctly related to Pingle's work, Rush drew on his own military experience during the American War for Independence.

In the author's preface to *Observations on the Diseases of the Army*, Pringle made it clear he wanted to address two audiences with the work: medical and military.[67] Based on his experiences in the Low Countries (Belgium and the Netherlands) during the War of Austrian Succession (1740–1748) and Scotland during the Jacobite Rising of 1745, he set out a number of principles for maintaining the health of armies. Despite some poor conditions being unavoidable, Pringle argued that it was "incumbent on those who have the command, to make such provision as shall enable the soldier to withstand most of the hardships incident to a military life."[68] Such modifications included shading camps in hot weather, ensuring that men slept in their tents at night, distribution of "under waistcoats" for cold months, and strong shoes to prevent damp feet.[69] In a period in which more men died of disease than combat, Pringle strongly believed that keeping communicable illness at bay was a concern of any officer or quartermaster, not only physicians.

The original book is part medical treatise and part instruction manual. Pringle taught officers and quartermasters how and where to set up a healthy camp, what supplies the soldiers required, and how to instruct enlisted men

---

66 Thomas Jefferson, see Cogliano, *Emperor of Liberty: Thomas Jefferson's Foreign Policy*.

67 Pringle and Rush, *Observations on the Diseases of the Army*, xxxiii–xxxviii.

68 Pringle and Rush, *Observations*, 83.

69 Pringle and Rush, *Observations*, 84.

to behave and maintain personal hygiene. The physician, on the other hand, might learn about certain fevers, conditions under which patients might best recover, and how best to advise military and civilian governing bodies on the maintenance of healthy populations. War offered an unusual opportunity for eighteenth-century physicians. In military camps and hospitals patients fit into a fairly narrow category of person: they lived under similar conditions and were compelled to follow physician orders. Such experiences forced doctors to think about health as a communal rather than an individual virtue and held the possibility of applicability to civilian practice. Pringle himself applied the lessons of *Diseases of the Army* to health in British cities and even experimented in London. Diseases could become communicable in conditions that favored putrefaction, like poorly ventilated hospitals and prisons.[70] For Rush, the lessons taught in all four American editions were to carefully observe surroundings, compare and contrast with known locations, and apply facts to theory for the best practice possible.

Three years after Rush's death one of his students, Ohio physician and medical geographer Daniel Drake, seemingly followed his preceptor's footsteps in cautioning colleagues about the danger of variation. In an article outlining the disease and climate of Cincinnati he wrote, "The variations of atmospheric temperature are more potent cause of disease, than either extreme" and "[v]ariations of temperature, particularly changes from *heat* to *cold,* are sometimes the *exciting* causes of intermitting and other fevers, produced by marsh exhalation." As with Rush variation held danger to the system, yet also like Rush, Drake suggested that such danger could be mitigated by altering a person's immediate environment through "clothing, lodging and fires."[71] The need to change spaces on the frontier to preserve the mental, physical, and social health of White settlers is peppered throughout medical writing of the period. In another piece that was Rush-inspired, Gideon C. Forsyth described the deplorable conditions of early settlers in the Ohio valley the same year Rush published his first American editions: 1809. He counted fevers, exposure, and homesickness, which could be permanently remedied only by better housing and cultivation. In this assessment Forsyth shifted from the description of a region to the reciprocal pathology of place and people identified by Volney in similar settings.[72]

---

70   Hamlin, *More Than Hot: A Short History of Fever,* 114–18.

71   Drake, "Medical Topography."

72   Forsyth, "Geological, Topographical and Medical Information Concerning the Eastern Part of the State of Ohio; by Dr. Gideon C. Forsyth, of Wheeling; in

Throughout the books, Rush compared foreign diseases with those of the United States. Although the diseases went by different names, Rush showed his readers how and where to garner useful information from otherwise climatically distinct diseases. Through careful observation of one's own location and wide reading from abroad (viewed through the lens of Rush's system) young American doctors could better treat the patients and diseases they encountered no matter where they ended up practicing in the new nation. Variations in space and bodies were a challenge in the United States. But the biggest challenges occurred when the delicate system of bodies, environments, and societies broke down, resulting in epidemic disease.

Two Letters of Dr. A.C. Willey, of Block-Island; and by Him Communicated to the Editors," 350–58.

Chapter Six

Confronting Climatic Ills

Benjamin Rush grew up as a city boy. He spent most of his childhood in the expanding large town that was mid-eighteenth-century Philadelphia and remained in the city as an adult. Living and working in a city, however, did not mean Rush was completely comfortable with the effects of urban spaces on American health. Indeed, like others of his era he worried that cities damaged human bodies over time. Health in turn, of course, could have a direct impact on the function of a family, community, and ultimately republic. As cities grew so too did the ubiquitous health and environmental concerns. Rush argued that "civilization" produced artificial and complicated diseases among the British and city-dwellers as early as 1774.[1] Rush's colleague and sometimes rival, William Currie, concurred in his description of the United States, writing that the close proximity between people and buildings made locations more complex and as a consequence, diseases more dangerous. In response to the claim from a correspondent that Boston's diseases were different from those of the surrounding countryside, Currie reasoned that disease existed "in all large cities where the houses are built close together, and the occupations of the inhabitants are unfavorable to exercise; and the more so, as they recede from habits of temperance; especially where luxury and fashion take the lead of reason and common sense." He contrasted this lifestyle with that of the farmer who through labor "acquires vigour of body and resolution of mind . . . [and who] respires a salubrious air."[2]

Currie did not exaggerate when he described the close quarters of working-class inhabitants of American cities. In Philadelphia most families lived in small row-houses of three rooms: a front work room, a back room,

---

1   Rush, "An Inquiry into the Natural History of Medicine among the Indians of North-America; and a Comparative View of Their Diseases and Remedies with Those of Civilized Nations," 38-39.

2   Currie, *An Historical Account of the Climates and Diseases of the United States of America and of the Remedies and Methods of Treatment . . .* , 5.

and an upstairs room. At the same time, many others lived in alleys that cut through the original grid pattern. This created a much denser city center than the one William Penn envisioned in the late seventeenth century for his "country town".[3] When describing the city at the turn of the nineteenth century Rush claimed that it extended three miles up and down the riverfront, but penetrated only a half-mile westward toward the Schuylkill at its widest. Meanwhile the most populous street, by Rush's reckoning, sat only a few feet above the waterline.[4] These parameters made for a very high population density. The crowded nature of the city certainly did not aid in its health. Meanwhile citizens who had the leisure to care for their health often did not and fell into indolent and "fashionable" behaviors, including unhealthy forms of dress, dueling, and a lack of exercise. For different reasons, Rush argued, both the rich and the poor lived sedentary lives damaging to their future health.[5] British physician William Cadogan similarly called out his countrymen for cultivating disease with their lifestyle. He wrote that most physical and moral evils "we most undoubtedly bring upon ourselves by our own indulgencies, excesses or mistaken habits of life."[6]

Rush addressed his concerns early in his essay "An Inquiry into the Natural History of Medicine among the Indians of North-America," discussed in chapter 4. For the purpose of the present chapter, the oration's most powerful points came in the form of instructions for managing a temperate republic, which required thoughtful and delicate balance. Two contrasting paragraphs highlight the distinctions.

> The diseases introduced by civilization extend themselves through every class and profession among men. How fatal are the effects of idleness and intemperance among the rich, and of hard labour and penury among the poor! What pallid looks are contracted by the votaries of science from hanging over the "sickly taper!" How many diseases are entailed upon manufactures, by the materials in which they work, and the posture of their bodies! What monkish diseases do we observe from monkish continence and monkish vices! We pass over the increase of accidents from

---

3　Warner, *The Private City: Philadelphia in Three Periods of Its Growth*.

4　Rush, "An Account of the Climate of Pennsylvania, and Its Influence upon the Human Body," 74–75.

5　Beatty, *Nervous Disease in Late Eighteenth-Century Britain: The Reality of a Fashionable Disorder*, 169.

6　Cadogan, *Dissertation on The Gout, and All Chronic Diseases, Jointly Considered, As Proceeding from the Same Causes; What Those Causes Are; and A Rational and Natural Method of Cure Proposed*, 1.

building, sailing, riding, and the like. War, as if too slow in destroying the human species, calls in a train of diseases peculiar to civilized nations.[7]

Despite this dark outlook on the health of those in the learned professions Rush did not think ill health was inevitable. While the poor had little choice, the middling ranks of society and the elite could adjust their lifestyles without forgoing the benefits of "civilization." A healthy American republic depended on this self-reflection and self-disciple for the success of the nation.

> The blessings of literature, commerce, and religion were not *originally* purchased at the expense of health. The complete enjoyment of health is as compatible with civilization, as the enjoyment of civil liberty. We read of countries, rich in every thing that can form national happiness and national grandeur, the diseases of which are nearly as few and simple as those of the Indians. We hear of no diseases among the Jews, while they were under their democratical form of government, except such as were inflected by a supernatural power.[8]

This point was vital to Rush's larger project, which argued that republican governments were naturally and even divinely ordained for health and productivity. He went on to list modern countries that managed to balance health and civilization, including China, Scandinavia, and the New England states.[9] Nonetheless, diseases of civilization—those that emerged from poor management rather than a "natural" disturbance of excitement—started to bear down on the Americans. Rush lamented that "[o]ur bills of morality . . . show the encroachments of British disease upon us. The NERVOUS FEVER has become so familiar to us, that we look upon it as a natural disease," consumption spread rapidly, and "[t]he HYSTERIC and HYPOCHONDRIAC DISEASES, once peculiar to the chambers of the great, are now to be found in our kitchens and workshops. All these diseases have been produced by our having deserted the simple diet and manners of our ancestors."[10] The situation would only deteriorate. After 1793, yellow fever garnered the most attention from American physicians who debated the aliment's origins, spread, cure, and additional causes. Most considered the fever natural in very hot

---

7   Rush, "An Inquiry into the Natural History of Medicine among the Indians of North-America; and a Comparative View of Their Diseases and Remedies with Those of Civilized Nations," 32–33.

8   Rush, "An Inquiry," 58.

9   Rush, "An Inquiry," 59.

10 Rush, "An Inquiry," 57.

climates, but it was a new feature of the mid-Atlantic starting in the 1790s. Its appearance suggested that there was either an invasion of a foreign disease or that American cities had changed so rapidly that the deadly ailment could be generated locally. Rush ascribed to the latter view, in which a disease of climate became a disease of poor management and botched "civilization."

This chapter examines two very different diseases that garnered the attention of Rush and his close colleagues in the early nineteenth century. Yellow fever became a disease of the urban North and East for a generation, challenging the idea that American cities could be healthy. On the other hand, endemic goiter, a disease of the West, tapped into worries about the health and success of new American settlements. Was the republic suited to either extreme or would both require careful health mitigation by Rush or Rush-trained experts? Rush's answer would likely have been a resounding yes. These opposites on the disease spectrum demonstrate exactly what the American system was supposed to prevent and mitigate. Moreover, they represented ailments not exclusive to the United States, but ones that presented themselves differently in North America than in other regions. This alteration spoke not only to the perceived uniqueness of the United States, but also demonstrated the broader utility of American knowledge. If Americans had something new and fundamental to say about yellow fever or goiter, their knowledge would be on equal footing with that produced in Europe or more "exotic" colonial locations.

Revolutions in the Atmosphere

In 1803, Rush received a letter from Moses Guest, a tanner living in New Brunswick, New Jersey. Like many of Rush's correspondents the author was not a physician but an ordinary citizen with medical news to share. Guest, who had never met Rush, noted that he would not have had the courage to write, "had I not been informed of the very great exertions you have frequently made in alleviating the sufferings of the Citizens of Philadelphia when sickness and death were staring you in the face, and it might truly be called the time to try mens [sic] souls."[11] Guest was making a reference to the yellow fever outbreaks that plagued the city of Philadelphia, and other towns on the east coast of the United States, beginning in 1793 and recurring until around 1820 north of the Chesapeake before fading away and becoming a regional southern disease. In Philadelphia alone, 1793 was

---

11   Moses Guest (1803), Library Company of Philadelphia (hereafter LCP), Rush Family Papers, Benjamin Rush Correspondence, Volume VI.

followed by epidemic years in 1797, 1798, 1802, and 1805. Other years did not see epidemic disease but isolated cases often appeared in Rush's notes and case books. Guest's reference to Thomas Paine's *The Crisis No. 1* was aptly chosen. Like the winter of 1776 the annual exposure to deadly epidemic disease was not for the "summer soldier" or "sunshine patriot." Doctors and patients alike faced down a deadly disease that threatened lives, livelihoods, and the future of the republic's largest cities.

When Rush is remembered as a physician it is often for his dual "heroic" actions during the fever; advocacy for "heroic" therapeutics (copious bloodletting and use of calomel) or his heroism for remaining at his post throughout the crisis of 1793, even falling ill himself. Despite variation in historians' portrayals of Rush and his therapeutics, the vast majority of literature on yellow fever looks at the disease as a disease. Scholars assume that a single distinct entity invaded American space in the 1790s and brought conflict and chaos in its wake. While important and valuable perspectives, they skirt around the core issue of the fever for Rush and many other Americans who looked at the epidemics as a problem of geography and unstable landscapes. As discussed in previous chapters, Americans worried about their unstable climate and its consequences. Yellow fever was an extreme consequence. It is less important to document American yellow fever as modern yellow fever than to understand it as a challenge to the future success of the United States.

Nevertheless, before continuing it is useful to take a moment and consider the nature of yellow fever infections and transmission. Yellow fever is a viral hemorrhagic infection endemic to tropical regions, including parts of West Africa and South America that were in regular commercial contact with the United States during Rush's lifetime. The virus enters the human (or nonhuman primate) body via a bite from a female *Aedes aegypti* mosquito. Although year-round populations of *Aedes aegypti* were not possible in the eighteenth-century United States the insects were regularly imported through coastal and transatlantic trade. Once inside a human body the virus can replicate, be picked up from the bloodstream from another bite, and the cycle begins again. This mosquito-to-human chain of transmission was not directly understood until the twentieth century, leaving room for etiological speculation in Rush's time. The disease did not clearly move from person to person or spread into the countryside, but it also did not clearly arise from the same local causes all the time. Not only was the cause difficult to ascertain, but diagnosis is also tricky.

Once infected with the yellow fever virus, the patient develops a slate of generic "flu-like" symptoms, including fever. After about a week, symptoms subside. For many people that is the extent of the illness. However, between

15 and 20 percent of infected people develop a second intoxication stage with the characteristic, and deadly symptoms of yellow fever. Later symptoms include yellowing of the skin and eyes (jaundice), high fever, internal bleeding, vomiting blood (which appears very dark), renal failure, and problems with the central nervous system.[12] Many of these symptoms were specifically noted by eighteenth- and nineteenth-century physicians. The black vomit associated with hemorrhage was especially noteworthy and a key diagnostic criterion for yellow fever alongside jaundice. Mortality rates from this second stage may be as high as 60 percent in modern outbreaks, such as that in Sudan in 2012. While there is a vaccine for yellow fever now, treatment of unvaccinated patients focuses on symptoms; there is no specific cure.[13]

Clear statistics on the fever in North America are impossible to recover for the late eighteenth and early nineteenth centuries. Most towns and cities did not keep regular bills of mortality, especially smaller communities in the Mid-Atlantic and South. Although remembered as an urban disease in this era, contemporary accounts from small towns throughout the region regularly appeared in medical journals at the turn of the nineteenth century. Nor can historians always say with certainty that a specific case or outbreak was yellow fever as we understand it today. Some outbreaks may have been different fevers or a mix of yellow fever and other ailments. Nevertheless, it is clear that something changed after 1793 and the frequency of violent fevers identified as yellow fever increased dramatically north of the Chesapeake.

It is difficult to exaggerate the fallout from the yellow fever crisis and how deeply it shaped Americans' sense of self. In addition to the sheer loss of life, the epidemic struck the political, social, and intellectual capital of the new nation. To a population that equated health with social, political, and geographic "improvement," an epidemic was a sign that the republic was mismanaged on every level.[14] The outbreak in 1793 in Philadelphia proved to be only the beginning of a disease pattern for the United States. That year hot and dry weather dominated in Philadelphia, which encouraged city residents to stockpile water in open backyard barrels. At the same time the city's population swelled to include a few thousand white refugees and the people they enslaved fleeing Cap-Français, Saint-Domingue (Cap-Haitien,

---

12 Paules and Fauci, "Yellow Fever—Once Again on the Radar Screen in the Americas," 1397–99.

13 Markoff, "Yellow Fever Outbreak in Sudan," 689–91.

14 Harrison, *Medicine in an Age of Commerce and Empire: Britian and Its Tropical Colonies*, 254; Coleman, *Yellow Fever in the North: The Methods of Early Epidemiology*; Humphreys, *Yellow Fever and the South*.

Haiti). On the voyage from the Caribbean Island, they may have brought a stowaway pathogen.

The yellow, also called the bilious remitting, fever commenced in August and according to contemporary accounts (including Rush's personal estimates) killed between 4,000 and 5,000 Philadelphians. By the time the frosts arrived in late October, killing the mosquitos, close to 10 percent of the city's population was dead and thousands of others had fled into the Pennsylvania and New Jersey countryside.[15] Early in the epidemic a confused and frightened Rush wrote to his wife Julia, stating that the ailment caused "a scene . . . , which reminded me of the histories I had read of the plague."[16] Like the plague in medieval and early modern Europe, yellow fever dominated the disease landscape of the young American republic in a violent, visible, and swift manner.

Even after the fever itself passed, the memory of it lingered in Philadelphia. In late 1793 Rush reported that bilious symptoms continued to affect survivors in their normal winter ailments. This followed what he expected as a reader of Sydenham. Epidemic diseases like plague or yellow fever came from strong atmospheric conditions, which tainted the expression of other diseases like smallpox, measles, and influenza. Recovery from the fever could take months and the physical signs of illness haunted the streets well into the winter. On the domestic side, homes needed to be purified of any lingering miasmata (or contagion, depending on an individual's philosophy), an act that visibly changed homes. Some residents fumigated with niter to purify the air, others buried or baked furniture to remove any lingering effluvia. In a particularly dramatic act, some survivors threw bedding and clothing into the Delaware River.[17] In letters home from the relative safety of New Jersey, Julia Rush expressed anxiety throughout the epidemic over the winter clothes she had left behind and the miasmata Rush and his pupils brought into the house.[18] In a postscript to her letter from September 24, she noted

---

15   Rush counted 4,044 deaths using personal and churchyard records. Rush, "An Account of the Bilious Remitting Yellow Fever, as It Appeared in Philadelphia in the Year 1793," 181; Moseley, *Medical Tracts*, 209.

16   Benjamin Rush, "To Mrs. Rush (Philadelphia, August 25th, 1793)," *Letters of Benjamin Rush*, ed. L.H. Butterfield (Princeton, NJ: Published for the American Philosophical Society by Princeton University Press, 1951), 640–41.

17   Rush, "An Account of the Bilious Remitting Yellow Fever, as It Appeared in Philadelphia in the Year 1793," 193–94.

18   Julia Rush to Benjamin Rush (October 24, 1793), APS, Julia Stockton Rush Collection of 20 Letters, Mss.B.R894.

that "I am so agitated that I can scarcely write intelligibly"; the body of the letter was without paragraph markings and rushed from one concern to the next. Even unstated, her fear would have been evident to her husband.[19] Death stalked the place. Three out of Rush's five students died that summer, Rush nearly died, his mother was ill, and his widowed sister Rebecca Rush Wallace succumbed to the fever while keeping house and nursing the sick. In 1794 the Rushes moved to a new house, perhaps in an attempt to leave the memory, if not the miasma, of fever behind, as much as it was meant to accommodate a growing family.

In a decade rife with anxiety from the rise of partisan politics, revolutions in France and Haiti, and fear of anarchy, yellow fever in the 1790s both added to the constellation of worries and appeared as a physical manifestation of the country's situation. Americans noticed that something had changed in the regional disease landscape. Their healthy country felt threatened and unhealthy regions became death traps, especially those that held effluvia (dangerous gasses from human bodies) in the built environment. In a letter to Rush in 1796, New Yorker E.H. Smith wrote, "I doubt whether it would be possible to generate or import, either the one or the other [yellow fever or low fever], into well built & well-ventilated Towns, whose inhabitants were temperate & cleanly."[20] Locations could prevent or exacerbate the fever. Smith provided an example in the case of Newburyport, Massachusetts, where he claimed the fever "which has been so fatal this very summer . . . originated from the putrefaction of a large quantity of Mackerel."[21] Low and marshy ground (characteristic of a damp continent) harbored yellow fever, like it did any other autumnal intermittent or remittent fever; the addition of something that could rot was catastrophic. In other regions heat and humidity may have been enough. For example, in 1810, Rush's former student Robert P. Archer wrote from Chesterfield, Virginia, that he considered himself "bound" as Rush's pupil to report local cases of fever in low-lying areas of the county.[22] This also suggests that he felt bound to encounter fever.

Jan Golinski addresses the general anxiety of Americans and argues that yellow fever fundamentally changed the way they thought about their

---

19   Julia Rush to Benjamin Rush (September 24, 1793), APS, Julia Stockton Rush Collection, Mss.B.R894.

20   E.H. Smith (1796), LCP, Rush Family Papers, Benjamin Rush Correspondence, Vol. XV.

21   Ibid.

22   Robert P. Archer (1810), LCP, Rush Family Papers, Benjamin Rush Correspondence, Vol. I, Box 2, Folder 19.

climate. In his assessment, yellow fever was important as an atmospheric disease. General confidence about the United States and its healthy air plummeted after 1793; as Golinski puts it, "[s]ome writers suggested that the atmospheric constitution had suffered some kind of corruption. . . . Others insisted that the air had been contaminated by noxious influences brought to American shores," and nearly everyone agreed the air was the problem.[23] Rush was no exception and championed the corruption argument. He claimed that a "revolution in the atmosphere" was the root cause of the disease, likening it to patterns of disease described by Sydenham. These "revolutions" were hypothetical but powerful ideas about the composition of the atmosphere. Human or geological actions could, Rush felt, alter the balance of gasses in the air and trigger disease through the imbalanced excitement. When diseases threatened the population, they indicated to those who believed the disease was imported and those who thought it was produced locally, that something had gone awry with their immediate environment. His choice of words reminds us that revolutions of all kinds were considered unstable and even dangerous if managed improperly.

Within a few years, Rush cast yellow fever as the new normal, the new version of the old autumnal fever(s) driven to higher malignancy by improper waste-management and chemical "revolutions in the atmosphere." The fever in this sense was not specific to the tropics or completely new, but the standard unified fever he spoke of in his lecture, supercharged by a poor environment. Like Sydenham's "epidemic constitutions," which Rush considered an essential source, these "revolutions" resisted medical management and were likely produced by geological activity, like earthquakes and volcanoes releasing as yet unknown chemicals into the global atmosphere.[24] Decades later, Rush's former pupil and successor to the chair of theory and practice at the University of Pennsylvania, Nathaniel Chapman (1780–1853) described the disease in strikingly similar terms. He wrote, "from 1793 to 1805, there was an universal distemperature of the atmosphere pervading, in various degrees, this immense continent, and annually, the fever broke out in several of our cities, attended by all the phenomena of a wide spread morbid influence."[25] During the time of "universal distemperature," articles in early American

---

23   Golinski, "Debating the Atmospheric Constitution: Yellow Fever and the American Climate," 150.

24   Sydenham and Rush, *The Works of Thomas Sydenham, M.D., on Acute and Chronic Diseases: With Their Histories and Modes of Cure.*

25   "Nathaniel Chapman to Nicholas Chervin, 17 May 1821," CPP, MSS 2/0141-01.

medical journals showed an interest in events like earthquakes and their potential relation to disease.[26] As was the case with weather reports, doctors actively sought evidence that would connect geological activity with human health and continued to do so into the nineteenth century. This included the adoption of new instrumentation like the eudiometer, which measured the proportion of different gasses in the air. Rush's contemporaries worried about carbon dioxide (sometimes referred to as "fixed air") specifically due to its association with decomposition and therefore disease and decay.[27]

Importation of the disease on cargo ships from the sickly Caribbean was one explanation, poor management of cities in the wake of social and atmospheric revolutions was another. Neither hypothesis initially garnered enough support to be the clear winner. Rush was a founding figure of a medical narrative in which the seemingly epidemic yellow fever was merely an expression of the ordinary endemic American autumnal fever. He argued that the disease was not imported and (sometime after 1794) that it could not pass from one person to another.[28] The locally produced illness, he claimed, was a more severe variant of the annual autumnal fevers, which allowed him to argue (1) that "yellow fever" was not a new or specific disease, and (2) that this variant of bilious fever appeared in epidemic and nonepidemic forms based on personal constitutions, proximity to effluvia, and regional or global atmospheric constitutions. Others like Currie and publisher Matthew Carey protested that the fever—especially the first outbreak in Philadelphia—was imported and passed from person to person.

---

26 Hugues, "Rapport fait aux Citoyens Victor Hugues et Lebas Agens particulierd du Directoire Executif aux Isles du Vent, par la Commission etablie en vertu de leur Arret du 12eme Vendemiaire, l'an 66eme de la Republic"; Ramsay, "Extracts from an Address delivered before the Medical Society of South-Carolina"; Webster, "On the Connection of Earthquakes with Epidemic Diseases and on the Succession of Epidemics"; Macrery, "A Description of the Hot Springs and Volcanic Appearances near the Washita, or Black River, in Louisiana"; Mease, "Review: Geological Account of the United States."

27 Boott, *Memoir of the Life and Medical Opinions of John Armstrong ...: To Which Is Added an Inquiry into the Facts Connected with Those Forms of Fever Attributed to Malaria or Marsh Effluvium, Volume 1*, 234–35; Vaughan, *The Valedictory Lecture Delivered Before the Philosophical Society of Delaware*, 26–28.

28 Rush's earliest accounts of the fever are ambiguous and lean toward supporting its ability to pass from human to human. Rush, *An Account of the Bilious Remitting Yellow Fever as It Appeared in the City of Philadelphia in the Year 1793*; Rush, "Dr. Rush's Directions, for Curing and Preventing the Yellow Fever."

Rush's main rival in the debates, Currie, claimed that yellow fever had been a sporadic, imported visitor to North America for nearly a century by 1793. He reported that Philadelphia and Charleston experienced their first outbreaks in 1699, Boston in 1693, and New York in 1702. Currie used these dates to argue against Rush's local production argument—seventeenth-century American cities were small and could not produce the required urban filth—and support for a French theory. This alternate theory stated that yellow fever originated in what is now Thailand in the 1680s. From Asia, the argument went, a British Man-of-War brought the fever to Martinique, where it found a new endemic home.[29] On the other side of the argument, Caldwell ignored early examples of yellow fever and addressed only the current epidemics. He claimed that urbanization had changed the atmosphere by increasing the heat of city centers to produce a local tropical climate. This local torrid zone promoted the violent and more frequent outbreaks.[30] The deadly combination of a charged atmosphere, hot weather, and plentiful organic matter ready to putrefy made American cities prime targets for fever. Philadelphia—and most of the mid-Atlantic—did not fit comfortably within a healthy "temperate" zone. The region's weather swung between extremes and supported the diseases of many climates. Cold winters and hot humid summers shifted the definition of "temperate" in the North American context to one that was more variable and less stable than in Europe, analogous to the threats and promise of republican government. Proximity to the Caribbean and a robust coastal trade meant that the climatic spectrum of the United States could easily overlap with their southern neighbors. If the atmosphere changed, the geographies of both places suffered.[31]

As early as 1793, supporters sent Rush evidence to try and confirm this local view of yellow fever, which by its very geography challenged preconceived notions of the epidemic. Physician Francis Bowes Sayre of Crosswicks,

---

29   Currie, "Facts and Arguments in Favour of the Foreign Origin and Contagious Nature of the Pestilential or Malignant Yellow Fever, Which Has Prevailed in Different Commercial Cities and Seaport Towns of the United States, More Particularly since the Summer of 1793," 181–96; Boott, *Memoir of the Life and Medical Opinions of John Armstrong …: To Which Is Added an Inquiry into the Facts Connected with Those Forms of Fever Attributed to Malaria or Marsh Effluvium, Volume 1,* 245–46.

30   Caldwell, *Medical & Physical Memoirs, Containing Among Other Subjects a Partiuclar Enquiry into the Origin and Nature of the Late Pestilential Epidemics of the United States,* 8–15.

31   Smith, *Ship of Death: A Voyage That Changed the Atlantic World.*

New Jersey, provides a particularly good example of such evidence. In the late autumn of 1793, Sayre sent the following case to Rush.

> My patient Mr. Abbott, whose case I stated to you a few days after I had written that of his wife, [died] two hours after I left him, on the day on which I wrote. Since the death of those two persons, I made every inquiry, and engaged their friends to do the same, in order to discover whether they had been exposed to the infection, by any communication with persons or goods from Philada; and the result of these inquiries is, that they *neither of them had been from home previous to the wife's attack—that they had reed; no goods of any kind either from the city or from any persons coming from thence* and that they had not seen any one from that place for many weeks. *The situation of Mr. A's house is peculiar and unlike that of any other in the neighbourhood,* being placed on the dulivily [sic] of a hill facing the north—some thick woods on the west and a considerable rising ground round with an orchard to the south. At the foot of the hill, on the side of which the house is situated, is the beginning of a large tract of meadow much of which is in a rude and very unimproved state. *How far the exhalations from this marshy ground together with the almost total exclusion of the South and west winds,* which are almost the only winds we had thro' the later part of summer, may have anasiwned [sic] the disease in these instances I leave you to judge—*The remainder of the family were immediately removed—no persons took the infection from them that I ever heard of.*[32]

The Abbots serve as an example of how the disease was not necessarily epidemic and that it was neither infectious nor imported. These were key arguments for Rush, both in the fact that they connected the disease with the local environment and that they suggested concrete geographic causes that might be remedied.

The Abbot case was unusual but emphasized the power of local knowledge and an increasing interest in controlled or nearly controlled environments to test out medical theory. They lived in a unique geographic location with a house positioned near a marsh or meadow (an excellent source of dangerously exciting miasma). High ground and trees around their dwelling blocked prevailing winds that might have swept the disease agent away and trapped it around the home instead. Malignant marsh miasma, in this reading, permeated the bodies of Mr. and Mrs. Abbot, blocked the circulation of "excitement," and created the diseased state. The fact that other family members escaped the ailment by moving further cemented the notion that the fever (in individual instances) remained confined to strict geographies and

---

32   Emphasis added, Francis Bowes Sayre (1793), LCP, Rush Family Papers, Benjamin Rush Correspondence, Vol. XV.

was not passed from person to person. Crosswicks, just east of Bordentown, New Jersey, is less than 50 miles from the former location of the Arch Street Warf, the 1793 fever's metropolitan epicenter. This was too far to contract the disease from Philadelphia but close enough to know about and worry about its impact. Other cases suggested that Americans believed the disease ravaged cities, towns, and rural retreats much further afield. The terror of yellow fever grew over time and became rooted in its routineness rather than its strangeness. American medical periodicals described a sharp increase in the number of yellow fever outbreaks in the 1790s and 1800s, before it retreated from northern cities in the 1810s.[33]

New or only newly dangerous, even Rush knew something was going on with American health in coastal cities that required attention. Epidemics classified as yellow fever affected Americans from Maine to Georgia during this period.[34] If anything, southern towns reported fewer outbreaks in the medical literature before 1800 than mid-Atlantic towns. This reinforced the assumption that yellow fever was an urban disease rather than a sectional one. The mid-Atlantic boasted sizable cities in New York, Philadelphia, and Baltimore, while the South had only Charleston as a port city of any consequence. The domestic news section of the New York-based *Medical Repository* stated in 1798 that,

> The northern, southern and western parts of the Union have chiefly escaped this calamity [yellow fever]. The commercial towns, situated to the eastward of the bay of Chesapeake, and the river Susquehanna, have principally suffered. Portsmouth

---

33   After this point, yellow fever rarely appeared in Philadelphia or New York and took on a new role as a sectional disease, specifically of cities in the South like Charleston and New Orleans. Humphreys, *Yellow Fever and the South.*

34   Benjamin Vaughan noted the fever in Hallowell, Maine, while cities like Waynesborough and St. Mary's in Georgia experienced a similar epidemic. Benjamin Vaughan (1799), LCP, Rush Family Papers, Benjamin Rush Correspondence, Vol. XVIII; Joshua E. White, "Topographical Description of the Country around Waynesborough, in Georgia, with the State of the Thermometer and Weather, for Part of the year 1802. To which is added, some Account of the prevailing Diseases, and a few Observations on Yellow Fever, and on the principal Remedies of Fever," *The Medical Repository*, 3.1 (1806); James Seagrove, "Origin of yellow fever in the contaminated air of a coasting vessel, and of the town of St. Mary's in Georgia; with an enumeration of its symptoms and mortality, and the beneficial effects of volatile alkali as a remedy," *The Medical Repository*, 1.2 (1810).

in New-Hampshire, Boston, New-London in Connecticut, New-York, Philadelphia, and Wilmington in the State of Delaware, besides some other places in inferior degree, have largely shared in this epidemic.[35]

The geography described by the *Medical Repository* authors is predominately that of the mid-Atlantic and southern New England. This assessment matches that of other American publications and printed reports of yellow fever in travelogues and medical journals between 1790 and 1811.

As an educator and growing expert in yellow fever Rush accumulated numerous reports of the ailment and requests for assistance from practitioners across the country. Rush's former pupil Nathaniel Potter (1770–1843), regularly reported on the nature of the autumnal fever in Baltimore and expected information about Philadelphia in return. Some of his reports arrived in Philadelphia with a hint of secrecy. Potter asked that Rush refrain from sharing or publishing the information he sent. He claimed in 1800 that the fever clearly raged around Fell's Point, but that the Baltimore board of health refused to recognize the epidemic.[36] The denial could not last long; ultimately the outbreak claimed the lives of 1,200 people in Baltimore.[37] Writing openly about an officially denied epidemic might have hurt Potter's standing in the community. The city might have been trying to avoid panic, a shutdown of trade, or bad press that might hurt their reputation. Potter did blame cities. He fiercely supported his preceptor's theory of local production. Upon hearing about the Philadelphia season of 1799 Potter wrote that his sympathy for the city would have been greater, "but could I ascribe their affliction to any other causes than their own ignorance & prejudices."[38]

In an 1808 epidemic, again at Fell's Point, Potter noted the disease's variance with the weather, writing that it died down during the September frosts but came back later in the month and still raged at the end of October.[39] In a letter to Rush in 1800, physician James Tongue explained why Fell's Point suffered so severely. He described the neighborhood as:

---

35 "Domestic-Pestilence," *The Medical Repository*, Vol. II, No. 2, 211.

36 Nathaniel Potter (1800), LCP, Rush Family Papers, Benjamin Rush Correspondence, Vol. XIII.

37 Crenson, *Baltimore: A Political History*, 63.

38 Nathaniel Potter to Benjamin Rush (1799), LCP, Rush Family Papers, Benjamin Rush Correspondence, Vol. XIII.

39 Ibid.

[S]everal acres of land which lay between the point and the Town which is over-flowed by the tide when full; and is left naked (as I am informed) when the tide ebbs and leaves to the action of the sun a large quantity of grass which putrefies together with the roots. This in the spring of the year whilst vegetation is active produces health by giving out pure air; but now is an ample source of disease.[40]

The above description supported Rush's 1793 argument that an alteration in the chemical composition of the atmosphere—its constitution—increased the putrefaction rate of a pile of coffee left out on the dockside.[41] Similar effluvia-producing events in subsequent years could be blamed for the illness. Nor was the idea of a disease-ridden city particularly difficult for Americans to imagine. Even small towns possessed enough danger for residents to take notice. In 1803, physician Benjamin W. Dwight described the Hudson River town of Catskill, New York, as a cesspool. The drinking water appeared downright dangerous. Dwight described it as "hard and abounds in hot weather with animalcules . . . and not unfrequently with small worms."[42] Meanwhile the organization, or lack thereof, of the town itself provided an explanation for the disease. He wrote "in addition to the stagnant water in the gutters, &c. . . . not more than two years ago a slaughter-house was opened near the middle of the main street, a little east from the road . . . All the offals [sic] . . . lay there from season to season. . . . In the neighbor-hood of this stink of filth and poison it has, in several instances, been very sickly."[43] The vomit-inducing smell of a slaughterhouse certainly appeared sufficient to harbor more dangerous ailments.

---

40 James Tongue to Benjamin Rush (1800), LCP, Rush Family Papers, Benjamin Rush Correspondence, Vo. XVII.

41 Rush, *An Account of the Bilious Remitting Yellow Fever as It Appeared in the City of Philadelphia in the Year 1793.*

42 Dwight, "Some Remarks on the Origin and Progress of the Malignant Yellow Fever, as It Appeared in the Village of Catskill, State of New-York, during the Summer and Autumn of 1803, in a Letter from Dr. Benjamin W. Dwight to Eneas Monson, M.D. of New-Haven, Connecticut," 109.

43 Dwight, 110. The association between slaughtered animals and illness, especially related to yellow fever, in nineteenth-century America has been discussed in Barnes, "Cargo, 'Infection,' and the Logic of Quarantine in the Nineteenth Century"; Morman, "Guarding Against Alien Impurities: The Philadelphia Lazaretto 1854–1893." General associations between stink, filth, and disease were common in the period and drove reform in the United States and Europe. Harrison, *Climates & Constitutions: Health, Race, Environment*

Although not as stomach-churning as the Catskill scenario, Rush pointed to the dangers of fever-producing city rubbish as a target for governments to improve public health. At other times Philadelphians noted the contamination of wells with wastewater, especially in dry weather.[44] They assumed the chemical impurity of the water (rather than a specific pathogen) incurred disease. The products of putrefaction—that is rot—could damage sound bodies. If a small river town like Catskill could provide such sources of putrefaction, certainly a busy and rapidly growing port city complete with marshy lowlands held the danger in epidemic proportions. The process of putrefaction (abundantly evident in most large towns of the time) clearly altered the state of waste. Why not in living human bodies as well? In this manner, yellow fever was to the United States what nervous diseases had become for Britain, a disease of "civilization," although the former presented a more immediate and deadly problem than the latter. By the end of the eighteenth century the extent of "nervous" disease was considered a potential threat to national security in Britain, yellow fever was an analogous threat to the United States.[45] As the country's largest city and temporary capital, Philadelphia's susceptibility to the American plague reinforced the association between urban squalor, immorality, and disease. This combination of flaws dangerously resonated with the future of the country as a whole.[46]

Rush's opinions remained strong in the United States through the early decades of the nineteenth century. In 1833, Francis Boott (1792–1863) concisely described the conditions he deemed necessary for epidemic yellow fever:

---

and British Imperialism in India, 1600–1850, 176; Barnes, The Great Stink of Paris and the Nineteenth-Century Struggle against Filth and Germs; Hamlin, "William Pulteney Alison, the Scottish Philosophy, and the Making of a Political Medicine"; Hamlin, "Predisposing Causes and Public Health in Early Nineteenth Century Medical Thought," 43–70; Mitman, "In Search of Health: Landscape and Disease in American Environmental History," 184–210.

44   Philadelphia's high water table, crowded living conditions, and shallow wells made contamination inevitable and encouraged the storage of rain water as a source for drinking, bathing, and cooking. Finger, Contagious City: The Politics of Public Health in Early Philadelphia.

45   Beatty, Nervous Disease.

46   Currie, "Facts and Arguments." For a discussion of the debate, see Apel, Feverish Bodies, Enlightened Minds: Science and the Yellow Fever Controversy in the Early American Republic.

This form of fever requires the cooperation of four concurring causes: viz., malaria; a state of atmosphere like that so often insisted upon by Sydenham, favouring [sic] the development of epidemic diseases; a high temperature; and that predisposition of body which is connected either with a sudden change from a high to a low latitude, or with a great range of temperature from winter to summer.[47]

These are not Rush's words, but they certainly fit his assumptions about how a combination of geography, weather, and personal constitution allowed the disease to appear.

While initially controversial, the environmental approach became the standard line by the 1820s. This transition is illustrated by the work of French physician Nicholas Chervin (1783–1843). Chervin arrived in Philadelphia in 1822 to learn about yellow fever, nine years after Rush's death. He sent a short survey to local physicians and asked if, in their opinion, the fever was or was not a disease passed from one person to another (i.e., contagious) and if it was produced locally or imported from tropical climes. Around twenty Philadelphia physicians responded and nearly all of them agreed on the cause of the fever. Only Samuel Powel Griffiths—a student of Rush's in 1790 and 1791—broke with the majority and argued that the disease was introduced annually from the tropics and spread from person to person.[48] Doctors in the city ascribed to the view that the fever was locally produced, and non-contagious, which Rush supported in the 1790s. They argued that victims fell ill when noxious organic effluvial from marshes or rotting matter (which abounded in early nineteenth-century cities) entered their systems and threw them out of equilibrium to devastating effect.

Philadelphians had reason to believe this theory. The elimination of sources of effluvia and inspection of "dangerous" cargo after 1800 correlated with a reduction in yellow fever's frequency and severity in the city.[49] Such a stance had become characteristically American by the 1820s, and the opposite of the prevailing wisdom in Chervin's native France, which experienced only sporadic outbreaks. The answers collected, however, are less important than the purpose of the study. Chervin wanted to learn about yellow fever

---

47   Boott, *Memoir of the Life*, 232.

48   "Samuel Powel Griffiths to Nicholas Chervin, 8 May 1821," CPP, MSS 2/0141-01. Rush Student Lists, LCP, Rush Family Papers, Series I Benjamin Rush Papers, Subseries VII Professorship at University of Pennsylvania, Vol. 106.

49   For a discussion of Philadelphia's management and definition of "dangerous" cargo, see Barnes, "Cargo, 'Infection,' and the Logic of Quarantine in the Nineteenth Century."

from the source and that meant learning from Americans and extensive travel in the Western hemisphere. Despite strong opinions on the fever on both sides of the Atlantic, Chervin associated the epidemic with the Caribbean and United States of America.[50]

Despite the urban terror of yellow fever in New York, Philadelphia, and Baltimore, Rush's correspondence and contemporary journal literature tell a different story. Small towns like Catskill and rural retreats like the home of the Abbots near Crosswicks could also harbor the dreaded American fever. Rural as well as urban Americans worried about new and more violent summer fevers. Charles Caldwell cited the North Carolinian Dr. Harris, who argued that fevers had become more dangerous in the 1790s.[51] These accounts help explain why yellow fever could be viewed as a disease of the American environment, not just an imported ailment brought to port cities. Its links to multiple geographies meant that the common denominator between individual ill bodies was not trade links to the Caribbean or even crowed conditions. It was American dampness, an unfortunate accident of charged atmospheres, and a lax approach to personal and municipal hygiene, which allowed fever to rage in the minds of many Americans.

Yellow fever and Philadelphia act as an ideal case study to explore Rush's vision of epidemic disease. He relied on specific examples in Philadelphia, often related to yellow fever, to support his general theoretical concepts about the unity of fever and ubiquity of effluvia in the United States. Yellow fever shook Americans' pride in the health of their country and reminded them how easily they could emulate the unhealthy characteristics of European urban squalor or suffer from the dangers of hot climates. Cities like Philadelphia exhibited both. They were urban spaces embedded in toxic atmospheres and damp, dangerous places. Even those physicians who believed international trade and refugees from the Caribbean brought the plague saw the danger as a warning about the future of American society.

---

50 For a discussion of Chervin's biography and results by city, see Waserman and Mayfield, "Nicolas Chervin's Yellow Fever Survey, 1820–1822," 40–51. Chervin also published his findings after returning to France, Chervin, *De L'Opinion Des Médecins Américains Sur La Contagion Ou La Non-Contagion de La Fievre Jaune, Our Réponse Aux Allégations de MM. Les Docteurs Hosack et Townsend de New-York, Publiées, l'an Dernier, Dans La Revue Médicale La Gazette De France et Le New-York.* For more on yellow fever in Europe, see Coleman, *Yellow Fever in the North: The Methods of Early Epidemiology.*

51 Caldwell, *Medical & Physical Memoirs, Containing Among Other Subjects a Partiuclar Enquiry into the Origin and Nature of the Late Pestilential Epidemics of the United States,* 138.

Growing Pains

Sudden death was not the only way disease served as a proxy for understanding the toxicity of the American environment. Rural and western Americans were far more likely to encounter agues, remitting and intermitting fevers (of the "usual" kind), dysenteries, and endemic goiter than yellow fever. Nevertheless, such "ordinary" ailments could do damage. In *The Health of the Country*, Conevery Bolton Valenčius notes how antebellum settlers of the Old Southwest and Lower Mississippi Valley a generation after Rush discussed the relative health of their geography based on physical cues (like dampness) and disease cues, typically "ague."[52] A generation before Valenčius's settlers crossed the Mississippi, endemic goiter worried physicians, boosters, and migrants to the trans-Appalachian west. Unlike yellow fever, a disease of "civilization," these Americans encountered the dangers of isolation and strong geographic influences.[53] By the 1820s, some believed that "civilization" itself was enough to cure one of these pernicious ailments: goiter.[54]

Goiter was not a disease unique to the United States, but unique in how and where it appeared within them, which made it like yellow fever. Both diseases existed elsewhere but they also came to characterize American people and places. Rush, and others drew on a robust trans-national goiter, or bronocele, literature to compare their findings. That broader literature also explains why chronic endemic goiter frightened Americans: its association with inherited mental debility and physical disability. Rush did not write extensively about goiter, but letters about the disease and the thyroid more generally indicate his role as an educator and acknowledged expert on medical geography. His influence, if not his imprint, can be felt.

In 1801, W. Brackenridge, a doctor in Pittsburgh, Pennsylvania wrote to naturalist, physician, and Rush's colleague Benjamin Smith Barton in Philadelphia on that very subject. The letter responded to a short book Barton had written on the prevalence of goiter in North America, *A Memoir concerning the Disease of Goitre as it prevails in Different Parts of North-America*

---

52   Valenčius, *The Health of the Country: How American Settlers Understood Themselves and Their Land.*

53   Onuf, "Liberty, Development, and Union : Visions of the West in the 1780s." Fear of "savagery" and white Americans turning away from "civilization" has a long history going back to early colonization and remained strong into the eighteenth century. Demos, *The Unredeemed Captive: A Family Story from Early America*; Chaplin, "Natural Philosophy and an Early Racial Idiom in North America: Comparing English and Indian Bodies," 229–52.

54   Naramore, "Making Endemic Goiter an American Disease, 1800–1820," 24.

(1800). Like many letters between colleagues at the time, Brackenridge wrote to both praise Barton's work and offered his comments and advice. He appreciated Barton's attention to the topic, although he did not agree with Barton's hypothesis as to goiter's cause, "miasmata," the same general source Rush blamed for yellow fever. Nevertheless, Brackenridge emphasized the importance of facts Barton had gathered and the urgent need to find a cure for goiter in the west.[55] Near the end of the letter he wrote "[a]s the population of this country increases the malady [goiter] becomes extensive—and is felt. It is a serious drawback. Humanity is greatly interested in the investigation of the cause and ascertaining a preventative or cure."[56]

Barton's work spoke to a larger literature on endemic goiter and provoked not only epistolary reaction, but formal consideration in book reviews and American medical publications.[57] Rush, meanwhile, received pleas for assistance regarding the ailment and its danger, including a letter from E. Daugherty of Morgantown, Virginia (West Virginia) who asked the Philadelphian "wether [sic] you. . . . Discovered any cure for the Goitre a complaint the women are very much troubled with in this country and are Very anxious to be relieved from it."[58] Goiter led Rush to think about the gendered nature of disease and placed him in an active dialogue with his peers, including Barton.

The disorder piqued Barton's curiosity, particularly its peculiar geography in the United States. Goiter was endemic in the United States and appeared in geographies that bore little resemblance to its common haunts in other parts of the world, especially in Europe. In the United States goiter presented itself as a condition of the west. On the continent swelled thyroid glands appeared in mountainous regions like the Alps. Even in England, hilly

---

55　Barton cited the low terrain and prevalence of remitting fevers in central New York as well as goiter and thought they might share an exciting cause. Benjamin Smith Barton, *A Memoir Concerning the Disease of Goitre as It Prevails in Different Parts of North-America* (Philadelphia: Printed for the author by Way & Groff, 1800), vii.

56　W. Brackenridge to Benjamin Smith Barton (1801), Benjamin Smith Barton Correspondence, American Philosophical Society.

57　Schultz, "Review: A Memoir Concerning the Disease of Goitre, as It Prevails in the Different Parts of North-America," 47–53; Caldwell, *Medical & Physical Memoirs, Containing Among Other Subjects a Partiuclar Enquiry into the Origin and Nature of the Late Pestilential Epidemics of the United States.*

58　E. Daugherty to Benjamin Rush (August 13, 1803), LCP, Rush Family Papers, Benjamin Rush Correspondence, Vol. IV.

Derbyshire was most associated with the aliment, called "Derby-neck" by the locals. Elevation clearly played a very minor role (if any) in American goiter. In the United States the iodine deficiency that created the ailment was correlated with distance from the coast. Access to ocean fish and sea salt—two important natural sources of iodine—dwindled over distance. From New York's Mohawk Valley westward, incidence of the condition rose. Barton observed it in the 1790s during a summer trip to learn about the state's plant and animal life. In 1797 he wrote about the disease in a letter home to Rush stating, "I saw several cases of the disease called Goitre [sic]. It is a common complaint, both among the whites and Indians.—I cannot make up my mind respecting its cause: but I do not entertain a doubt, that the disease is somehow connected with the water of the country."[59] Barton reached a receptive audience. Rush was already interested in the role of glands and their connection to mental and physical health, including the thyroid, as discussed in chapter four. In 1795, for instance, a former Edinburgh classmate Rigby Brodbelt shared his son's dissertation on bronchocele published the previous year, assuming interest on Rush's part.[60]

At the turn of the nineteenth century British and continental literature benefited from several decades of interest in the geography of goiter and associated cretinism—severe developmental disability. In such cases, goiter served as one symptom of a general disorder defined by physical deformities of the skull and low cognitive ability. Most believed that goiter in the extreme or congenital forms of the ailment led to this unusual form of "imbecility" observed in Alpine Europe. By the time Barton visited Central New York, Britons on the "Grand Tour" had identified alpine valleys in northern Italy, Switzerland, and the Pyrenees as regions of endemic bronchocele and cretins. By the nineteenth century the association became so strong that tourists to the picturesque valleys could purchase postcards or illustrated books depicting the disease. British physician Benjamin Moseley (1742–1819)—a physician Rush cited and admired in connection to yellow fever—noted that on a trip to Italy "[i]n the hopital della Carita [in Turin], there was scarcely one female, from the age of four or five years, to the oldest woman, exempt from more or less of it [goiter]."[61]

---

59   Benjamin Smith Barton to Benjamin Rush (1797) LCP, Rush Family Papers, Benjamin Rush Correspondence, Vol. XXVII.

60   Rush, "An Inquiry into the Functions of the Spleen, Liver, Pancreas, and Thyroid Gland." Rigby Brodbelt to Benjamin Rush (1773 and 1775) LCP, Vol. IIa, Box 5, Folder 60, and Vol. XXV.

61   Moseley, *Medical Tracts*, 255.

Modern epidemiology explains the divergent patterns of goiter based on iodine deficiency. Iodine is a key component in the thyroid hormones triiodothyronine (T3) and thyroxine (T4). Together these hormones play a vital role in human growth and metabolism. Low T4 levels or hypothyroidism can lead to fatigue, slow metabolism, and depression, while higher than normal levels—hyperthyroidism—can lead to a faster metabolism, faster heart rates, and in severe cases becomes toxic. Levels are maintained in healthy bodies through a feedback loop with the pituitary gland at the base of the brain. If T4 levels are low the pituitary gland produces thyroid-stimulating hormone (TSH), which triggers hormone production in the thyroid. TSH production decreases if levels are normal or high.[62] However, this system is tricked in cases of low environmental iodine. If you don't consume enough iodine in your diet your thyroid cannot produce enough T4, which in turn triggers TSH production. The thyroid keeps getting the message to make more hormone by growing and is not told to stop. The result is an enlarged thyroid or goiter. Neither the American West nor Europe's mountains possess a naturally occurring supply of the vital element required for healthy thyroid function. In nature, environmental iodine is most common in the oceans. As a result, sea salt, ocean fish, and seaweeds all have high levels and make excellent sources of natural dietary iodine. Meat, eggs, and some vegetables also contain iodine but at lower levels.

Rush, Barton, and their contemporaries, however, were unaware of iodine's existence, let alone its role in goiter production or human metabolism. French chemist Bernard Coutou first described iodine in 1811 with additional work performed by English chemist Humphrey Davy (1778–1829) in 1813. English physician William Prout (1785–1850) first associated the element with goiter in 1816, three years after Rush's death, and claimed to cure some patients. Although physicians borrowed folk remedies, which included iodine-rich items, as specific cures like burnt sea sponges for centuries, prior to the element's "discovery" the specific connection to the ocean remained obscured.[63] As with yellow fever the uncertainty surround-

---

62　Chung, Hye Rim, "Iodine and Thyroid Function," Annals of Pediatric Endocrinology & Metabolism, 19.1 (March 2014): 8–12; "Iodine," Linus Pauling Institute Micronutrient Information Center, www.lpi.oregonstate.edu (accessed August 10, 2022).

63　Gibson, "Remarks on Bronchocele or Goitre," 66; Greenwald, "Observations on the History of Goiter in Ohio and in West Virginia," 280; Leoutsakos, "A Short History of the Thyroid Gland," 268; Schultz, "Review: Memoir Concerning the Disease of Goitre," *Medical Repository of Original Essays and*

ing goiter's cause, cure, and prevention opened space for Rush to apply the logic of his system.

In the United States, the fear of goiter did not come from the present events, but the future. It was a worrisome and unstable entity for the first generation of Americans. Goiters did not kill, but they did produce visible signs of unhealthiness of a region and possibly future degeneration.[64] For an intellectual elite already hyper-aware of any charges of deficiency from Buffon's *Histoire Naturelle* and other European natural philosophers, any hint of "degeneration" came across as threatening. This anxiety was all the stronger in light of the association between goiters and "cretinism," a form of developmental disability. Horace Bénédict Saussure (1740–1799) noted in his travels through the Alps that the most evident symptom of cretinism was goiter writing, "Le signe extérieur le plus ordinaire de cette malade est un engorgement das les glandes du col, qui proudit les tumerus connues sous le nom de *goîtres/* The most common external sign of this disease is a swelling of the glands of the neck, which produces the tumor known by the name of *goiter.*"[65] In an account of his travels in Switzerland, British traveler William Coxe hinted at the danger the disorder brought to regional character.

> With respect to manufactures; there are *none of any consequence*: and indeed the *general ignorance of the people is no less remarkable than their indolence*; so that they may be considered, in regard to knowledge and improvements, as *some centuries behind the Swiss*, who are certainly a very enlightened nation. The peasants seldom endeavor to meliorate those lands where the soil is originally bad; nor to draw the most advantage from those, which are uncommonly fertile: having few wants, and being satisfied with the spontaneous gifts of nature, they enjoy her blessings without much considering in what manner to improve them.[66]

Coxe's comments highlight two concerns: the "ignorance" and the "indolence" of the people. The lack of "improvement" to the land and satisfaction with a state of nature echo similar stereotypes Euro-Americans ascribed to Native Americans and deemed "savage." Could goiter and eventual

---

Intelligence Relative to Physic, Surgery, Chemistry, and Natural History, 157; Niazi et al., "Thyroidology over the Ages," 95–100.

64 Valencius, *The Health of the Country: How American Settlers Understood Themselves and Their Land.*

65 Translation by author. Saussure, *Voyages Das Les Alpes: Précédés d'un Essai Sur l'histoire Naturelle Des Environs de Geneve,* 292.

66 Emphasis added, Coxe, *Travels in Switzerland. In a Series of Letters to William Melmoth, Esq. from William Coxe, M.A. F.R.S.F.A.S. ...* 396–97.

"cretinism" hasten a descent into "savagery?" Not only did goiter appear in some locations at a higher rate than others, but some scholars thought that the disease could become progressively worse and lead to increased rates of cretinism over generations. In North America, goitrous regions and "Indian Country" were often one and the same. In his 1810 journey to the Great Lakes, English botanist Thomas Nuttall recorded and expected to see cases of goiter as soon as he reached western Pennsylvania.[67] Given Rush's promotion of improvement and skepticism of both nature and savagery it would have been easy for him to make a link between goiter, mental degradation, and loss of "civilization." Accounts like Barton's demonstrated the prevalence of the illness among all ethnic groups, including the "savage" Native Americans, the group exposed to such conditions longest. On an individual level Rush often connected swollen thyroids with mental health concerns.

A dysfunctional thyroid, for example one enlarged by goiter, opened one up to the possibility of hysteria, mania, or death from an unprotected brain. When citing Francis Rigby Brodbelt's 1794 Edinburgh dissertation on bronchocele Rush noted that the inhabitants of Derbyshire, England experienced enlargements or pain in the thyroid as a result of increased excitement from running or strong emotions.[68] Rush learned of this dissertation from the author's father, Rigby Brodbelt, who wrote to Rush as noted above, stating "my Son (who is not in his 25th year) graduated in September last at Edinburgh after studying in that University upwards of seven years. His Thesis is on the Bronchocele, and if I do not say with too partial an Eye I think it a very good one."[69] The younger Brodbelt presumed that this increased pain came from an already overtaxed system by the disease and malfunctioning gland. An already enlarged thyroid was already overworked and therefore could not contend with additional blood flow. The excitement of the rush of blood could, in this situation, bypass the thyroid and reach the vulnerable brain unimpeded. A whole community afflicted with thyroid swellings was at risk of any sudden collective change. Rush noted that his own thyroid patients suffered greater disturbances of the mind than those with normal glands. It remains unclear how often "cretinism" appeared outside specific geographic regions or if Rush treated cretins in either private practice or the hospital. Nevertheless, he was well aware of the condition and its severity in some bodies. In his 1807 essay on the spleen, liver, and thyroid

---

67 Thomas Nuttall diary (1810), American Philosophical Society, Mss B N96.
68 Rush, "An Inquiry," 28.
69 Rigby Brodbelt (1794), LCP, Rush Family Papers, Benjamin Rush Correspondence, Vol. IIa, Box 5, Folder 60.

gland, Rush wrote, "[t]he bronchocele of the Cretins is generally accompanied with imbecility of mind."[70]

By the 1810s, the American medical community treated Rush as an expert on the intersection of thyroids and mental health. The organs were at the crux of multiple things that interested Rush: gender, the mind, and the environment. In 1809, W. Winter Dunnington, a physician in Port Tobacco, Maryland, recounted his attempts to cure a "Miss Grey" of fever and mania with special attention paid to her thyroid noting that it was "considerably enlarged." A year later she appeared cured, but Rush's recommendations are not recorded.[71] In another instance Rush received a letter from South Carolina recounting three cases of *globus hystericus*, or an acute swelling of the thyroid gland in cases of mental distress. Physician J. Mactide wrote in 1811 presuming that Rush was (1) an expert in mental disorder and (2) specifically interested in the thyroid and its connection to mental health. The first case study provides the most specific information and is recorded here in full:

> "Elizabeth Hardcastle, a mulatto woman, received a refined education in England & lived in affluent circumstances for many years in St Stephen's parish So. Carolina. About the 45th year of her age an event occurred which was calculated to rouse her feelings in an extraordinary degree. A man who had lived with her for several years as a husband, determined much against her will to separate from her, & for this purpose had packed up his effects in a chest & placed it in an open carriage before her door. Experiencing the strongest mental agitation she fixed her eyes on the chest & to her imagination it represented the coffin of her friend. Under this impression she swooned away but was immediately roused by a sense of suffocation or rather of being choked. She felt her throat & found an unusual, large tumour, filling the space between the promun adami & the sternum & extending considerably on both sides of the trachea. She was accidentally found in this state by a physician a few hours after the event, and through much at a loss he endeavoured to relieve her. The tumour gradually subsided to a certain degree but ever after exhibited, plainly circumscribed, the thyroid gland, enlarged, & retaining its characteristic shape. She lived about 10 years after this occurrence, & she always experienced the sudden enlargement of the tumour, & sensation of choking when invaded by mental depression."[72]

---

70   Rush, "An Inquiry," 28.

71   W. Winter Dunnington to Benjamin Rush (1809 and 1810) LCP, Rush Family Papers, Series I Benjamin Rush Papers, Subseries I Correspondence, Vol. IV.

72   J. Mactide (1811), LCP, Rush Family Papers, Series I Benjamin Rush Papers, Subseries I Correspondence, Vol. XI.

The disorder attributed to Hardcastle, *globus hystericus*, specifically associated the thyroid gland with mental disorder. In a time of severe stress, doctors assumed the thyroid swelled and altered the function of the brain by restricting blood flow. The events leading up to Hardcastle's distress are vague but tragic. Her mind and body suddenly malfunctioned. It seemed as if her thyroid attempted to slow the damage to no avail. Importantly, Mactide included racial language in his description of Hardcastle's ailment and that of one of his other case studies; in a third, Mactide did not identify the race of his patient but based on her designation as "a respectable lady" without any qualifier we can presume she was white.

Racial language typically appears in American case studies from this era (at least in the case of nonwhite patients). What is remarkable in this letter and other cases of thyroid disorder is that racial difference does not seem to bear on diagnosis or presumed susceptibility to thyroid disorder. It does little other than to denote the social circumstances of the three women: white and privileged; biracial, free, and wealthy; and Black and enslaved. In his 1800 book on the subject of endemic goiter Philadelphia physician Benjamin Smith Barton argued that goiter appeared more frequently in women than in men from four different ethnic groups: Dutch-American women long settled in Central New York, Oneida women from the region, recently arrived Anglo-American women, and recently arrived women at the Brothertown settlement of New England Indians.[73] Gender seemed to be a factor in thyroid ailments, but race did not seem to have an overarching role. Women, it appeared, needed special consideration in cases of endemic goiter and acute psychiatric distress. Locating specific threats and altering the environment, therefore, became important avenues of research.

Throughout the transatlantic goiter literature multiple theories existed to explain the condition's geographic specificity, if not its physiological effects. Water was considered the most frequent culprit. Specifically, William Coxe wrote in his *Travels* that he believed calcareous minerals (from limestone) in local water sources led to obstructions in the body, which caused the swelling. Surgical studies by Haller and Morgagni found stones or calcium deposits in thyroids, which seemed to support the argument as well.[74] Moseley argued that temperature was the real culprit and lamented that the ailment

---

73   Barton, *A Memoir Concerning the Disease of Goitre as It Prevails in Different Parts of North-America*, 8–10.

74   Barton, *A Memoir*, 27, 32; Coxe, *Travels in Switzerland. In a Series of Letters to William Melmoth, Esq. from William Coxe, M.A. F.R.S.F.A.S.* ... , 401–3.

could not be cured, only prevented by keeping the chests and necks of women warm by proper clothing.[75] Similar worries appear in American goiter literature in reference to women and women's fashion. Jonathan Dorr postulated that goiter arose from cold temperature and the association of the lips, genitals, breasts, and thyroid. Therefore, when women did not sufficiently cover their chests in cold regions (he was describing northern New York and Vermont), the thyroid swelled.[76]

With this context in mind consider Barton's surprise to find the condition in relatively flat Central New York. His work on goiter charted the ailment's prevalence across space, gender, and species in the region. It also critiqued previous theories regarding the cause of goiter and presents an alternative explanation with implications for both America and Europe.

The transatlantic aspect of the project is evident from the dedicatory preface to German naturalist Johan Frederick Blumenbach (1752–1840).[77] Unlike most of his American colleagues Barton maintained an active correspondence with physicians and naturalists in German as well as in French and English following his education in German universities.[78] Barton noted that goiter was not an exclusively American disease, but that its appearance differed based on place. This difference, he believed, could have serious consequences for American treatment of the disease and knowledge about its probable cause.

> As the disease of Goitre [sic] is extremely common in some parts of Germany, and in other parts of Europe, the philosophical physicians of those countries will not deem it an incurious point to examine . . . what affinity there is between the soil, the climates, and exposure of the European districts in which this disease prevails, and the soil, the climates, and exposure of those countries of America in which it also prevails. If the facts contained in my memoir should serve to throw any light upon the nature of this complaint, I shall think the time which I have employed in the investigation has not been altogether misapplied.[79]

---

75   Moseley, *Medical Tracts*, 263.

76   Dorr, "Facts Concerning Goitre, as It Occurs in the Towns of Camden, Sandgate, and Chester, within the States of New-York and Vermont; and Conjectures Concerning Its Cause," 143.

77   For a full account of Barton's training and character as a student, see Whitfield J. Bell, "Benjamin Smith Barton, M.D. (Kiel)," *Journal of the History of Medicine*, 1971, 200.

78   Barton Correspondence, American Philosophical Society.

79   Barton, *A Memoir*, v.

Beneath the polite dedication Barton set up the context in which he wanted to discuss American goiters; related to, but possibly different from, European accounts of the disease. Finding the commonality in conditions that would trigger the physiological response of goiter meant taking a critical and comparative look at geography. Barton's observations began with a collection of local information about the goiter. Following a narrative approach, he described his initial interest in the disorder's prevalence in the region. He claimed to have noticed goiters on two Oneida women in the Western Mohawk Valley. This sparked his interest and with minimal inquiry he learned that endemic goiter could be found not only in the American Indian populations, but also in Dutch New Yorkers, and recent migrants from Connecticut heading west.[80]

Unlike Alpine descriptions of the disorder, which included instances where it was congenital, Barton's goiters affected adults almost exclusively. Beyond age exclusivity, however, the ailment readily crossed cultural and even species lines. Like "ague," Barton's goiter existed within the local geography and left its physical mark on livestock as well as humans.[81] Unlike yellow fever, which some physicians argued affected white people more severely than those of African descent, endemic goiter was not a racially dependent disease, or even one mitigated by a process of "seasoning." Although typically associated with hot climates the process of "seasoning" by which newcomers to a region suffered from local diseases while their bodies adjusted only to be resistant afterwards, influenced thinking in most of the United States into the nineteenth century.[82] All people, regardless of ethnic or racial background seemed equally subject to the disorder. Variation only existed in terms of gender, and Barton's observations confirmed similar European accounts. Wherever it prevailed, endemic goiter was a disease of women, as noted above in Moseley's hospital observations. Whatever the source of goiter, it clearly appeared tied to specific geographic locations and strongly influenced female constitutions. Strangely, the exact type of geography proved elusive.

Barton's study challenged the prevailing assumption in medical and lay literature from Europe that endemic goiter was a disease of mountain valleys, or

---

80 Barton, *A Memoir*, 6–8.

81 Barton, *A Memoir*, 12.

82 Nash, *Inescapable Ecologies: A History of Environment, Disease, and Knowledge*; Valencius, *The Health of the Country: How American Settlers Understood Themselves and Their Land*, 2002; Wilson, "Fevers and Science in Early Nineteenth Century Medicine," 386–407.

at least high elevations. American goiters certainly appeared in river valleys, but not in exclusively mountainous regions, which eliminated the snow-melt hypothesis.[83] Furthermore, while Pittsburg and Vermont met the qualification of a mountain valley of the kind theorists like Saussure associated with trapped and vitiated air, the flat military tract of New York State or low regions along the Wabash River in the Indiana Territory did not.[84] In none of these places did water come from snowmelt or ice, which some associated with the disease, and air moved freely, precluding any alteration of the atmosphere in enclosed and isolated areas. Lacking any better explanation Barton turned to the ever-present miasma, a characteristic of damp American regions.

In 1801, the *Medical Repository of Original Essays and Intelligence Relative to Physic, Surgery, Chemistry, and Natural History* reviewed Barton's work on goiter. It began with a common theme to Barton, Rush, and many others: the sheer vastness and variability of the United States.

> In a widely extended country, reaching from the confines of Acadia to the limits of Florida, there exists a great variety of climate. And in the range from the ocean to the stream of the Mississippi, the diversity, occasioned by alteration of latitude, is exceedingly increased by intervening and local circumstances, which checquer [sic] the scenes and the seasons in a remarkable manner.[85]

Volney presented a similar view of the country, if in less enthusiastic terms: "the United States include the extremes of all the countries I have mentioned [Egypt, Morocco, China, France, Tartary, etc.]."[86] He preceded it with the ominous note that "it will be obvious, that this extensiveness of territory is in

---

83   Wilmer, *Cases and Remarks in Surgery: To Which Is Subjoined, An Appendix, Containing the Method of Curing the Bronchocele in Coventry*, 237.

84   Saussure, *Voyages Das Les Alpes: Précédés d'un Essai Sur l'histoire Naturelle Des Environs de Geneve*, 299. The same topography which made the region a good choice for building the Erie Canal two decades later. Barton, *A Memoir Concerning the Disease of Goitre as It Prevails in Different Parts of North-America*, 54–55.

85   Schultz, "Review: A Memoir Concerning the Disease of Goitre, as It Prevails in the Different Parts of North-America," 47.

86   Volney, *View of the Climate and Soil of the United States of America: To Which Are Annexed Some Accounts of Florida, the French Colony on the Scioto, Certain Canadian Colonies, and the Savages or Natives*, 5.

reality a cause of weakness at present, and does not promise to be a source of union in future."[87] How was such diversity to be managed? Could it?

No one specifically brought up the image of a "city upon a hill" in the wake of the yellow fever outbreaks or news of goiter in the west, but the sentiment applied. If the United States fell victim to disease its future promise would be compromised. Americans in the 1790s feared their country would not thrive as a well-regulated republic populated with self-sufficient, moral, and healthy citizens. Disorders like endemic goiter and yellow fever represented the potential dangers of an understudied environment and the limitations of imported knowledge. In light of all this a pessimistic attitude could be forgiven. However, despite the challenges, significant optimism remained. Although eighteenth- and early-nineteenth-century Americans believed their environment shaped them, they also believed they could shape their environment.

Within his purview as a man of science and medicine Rush became convinced that one way forward was to revamp the American medical system. Caldwell echoed this sentiment and argued "[s]ince the year ninety three [sic], a memorable revolution has occurred, in the type and state of fevers, in many parts of the United States. The event has, necessarily, given rise to a corresponding revolution in their medical treatment."[88] By doing away with what they considered incorrect theories and an overcomplicated educational system American doctors would be better prepared to manage their country. The continued collection of information on disease, climate, and geography by trained eyes would better explain the unique challenges Americans faced and hint at ways to ameliorate the destructive forces of nature. In the east, careful management of bodies and institutions would shape men (and women) into "republican machines" fit for their new world and new society. Medicine and her allied sciences might show the way forward. By the 1820s, some thought that had succeeded. Yellow fever retreated from the North and goiter appeared on the way out as well. Effective iodine treatments helped, but some in Pittsburgh suggested a different answer. They believed that the incidence rate was lower simply due to urbanization and "civilization" in the West. Had he lived to see such changes Rush may have felt himself and the system of medicine he promoted vindicated.

---

87 Volney, *View of the Climate*, 4.
88 Caldwell, *Medical & Physical Memoirs, Containing Among Other Subjects a Partiuclar Enquiry into the Origin and Nature of the Late Pestilential Epidemics of the United States*, 138.

Chapter Seven

Care, Curing, and Prevention in American Institutions

Despite Benjamin and Julia Rush's best efforts to raise healthy and useful children, tragedy struck the family in 1807. Their eldest son John shot and killed a fellow naval officer named Benjamin Turner—a friend "as dear to him as a brother"—in a duel. Shocked by what he had done, John fell into a deep depression recorded as an "insanity." His grief (and probable feelings of guilt) led him to neglect his health and hygiene and even attempt suicide, according to reports sent to the Rush family. This pattern persisted through 1808 and part of 1809. Suddenly, John appeared to recover and had returned to duty by the time Benjamin sent a letter to John Adams on the subject on August 14, 1809.[1] By this point, the letters between the two men were deeply personal and often touched sensitive subjects. It is unlikely that Benjamin would have lied to one of his closest confidants on the matter.

John's recovery, however, proved temporary. Shortly thereafter, in February 1810 at the age of 33, John Rush became his father's patient at the Pennsylvania Hospital in Philadelphia, still suffering from depression and delirium. The young man was incarcerated in a specialized wing for those suffering from "diseases of the mind," which Benjamin had lobbied for almost two decades earlier.[2] John never recovered, developing psychosis within a few years of his depression, and died in the hospital on August 9, 1837. At that point, he believed himself to be a successful Louisiana planter and the hospital a plantation. Visitors claimed that he walked up and down

---

1   "To John Adams from Benjamin Rush, 14 August 1809," *Founders Online*, National Archives, accessed April 11, 2019, https://founders.archives.gov/documents/Adams/99-02-02-5414.

2   Carlson and Wollock, "Benjamin Rush and His Insane Son."

the yard each day surveying his "property."[3] While his attempts at self-harm subsided within a few years John never regained his sense of self and hospital staff never deemed him recovered enough for release. Like many others who suffered from acute and chronic ailments of the mind in the nineteenth century, an institution became his whole world.

To his father, John's illness and decline demonstrated the risks of reckless living, dueling, and a lack of self-control that could damage individuals and societies. The high hopes he and Julia harbored for John in his childhood—a brilliant medical career to carry on his father's work—fizzled before collapsing with his illness. In hindsight, they may have pointed to John's stubborn behavior as a child, card-playing at Princeton, inability to settle into a career, and drinking to explain his eventual end. From Rush's perspective his son, like other patients, fell ill through a dangerous lifestyle, tragic event, or hereditary predisposition, which demonstrated the limits of good education and good parenting. Bodies did not always work well either physically or mentally. For the case of diseases of the mind, the hospital became the space associated with the correction of illness and preparation for patients to reenter active republican society whether they were ultimately released to the care of family or not.

This chapter looks at Rush's connection with the medical institutions of Philadelphia and the way they fit into his larger concerns about American society. His interest in and care of hospitalized patients is not often emphasized, but it played a key role in his ideas surrounding a medical republic. As indicated in chapter 1, Rush was always interested in what can broadly be considered the public's health. The most vulnerable members of the public, in body and mind, found their way to medical institutions like hospitals and dispensaries. The broader community, meanwhile, could be protected from illnesses like those discussed in the previous chapter, through preventative medical action directed by collections of physicians. This chapter addresses both kinds of institution—physical spaces of care and collections of like-minded physicians—and Rush's role in the post-Revolutionary War development.

Hospital and Dispensary Practice

The Pennsylvania Hospital significantly predated Rush's leadership in the Philadelphia medical community. Benjamin Franklin and physician Thomas

---

3   For a detailed account of John Rush's illness see Evans, "Notes Taken From Dr. Rush's Lectures upon the Institutes and Practice of Medicine and on Clinical Cases, Vol. I."

Bond worked together to establish a voluntary hospital for the "worthy poor," in 1751. They located the building on what was then an empty block on the edge of the city. By the time Rush was studying medicine under Redman, Bond served as a hospital physician and gave clinical lectures on the premises, a practice Rush took over in the 1790s.[4] Before the American Revolution, the hospital was the only institution of its kind in British North America. It served as a provincial version of London hospitals like St. Thomas's or Guy's, which catered to the poor and trained medical students like Rush. Voluntary Hospitals served as a place of last resort and no one who could afford to be cared for at home entered the wards. Donations financially supported the institution and younger staff doctors, and patients often required a letter of recommendation to receive treatment. In a response to the Reverend Ashbel Green in 1803, Rush outlined the process, instructing him to "send your poor neighbor to the Hospital about 11 o'clock or a little before that hour. I will attend there and plead his cause (with your note in my hand) with the managers."[5] By the end of the century, however, a major exception arose to counter this narrative: treatment of patients suffering from "diseases of the mind."

Rush began working with hospital patients as an associated physician in 1789 (the same year he began lectures in the theory and practice of medicine) and quickly became a leading figure in early American psychiatry. He leveraged his access and decades of experience to inform his research on "diseases of the mind" and test new methods of care and treatment. As noted above, Rush believed human bodies and minds were inextricably linked, so it stood to reason that political events, like the American Revolution, altered mental and physical health. Diseases of the mind were associated both with psychological and physiological irregularity and as such appear to have been used as a window into the general mental health of the nation. Increased mental distress connected to political instability, for example, could point to dangers inherent in the political system.

The hospital experience differed considerably between somatic and psychiatric patients in Philadelphia. Those suffering from "diseases of the mind" came from all classes of people and occasionally traveled to receive treatment from the increasingly famous Rush. Dr. Allison, a minister from Maryland, fell into this category. Allison's wife and brother-in-law, J.A. Buchanan of Baltimore, sent him to Rush in 1801. The exact nature of his mental distress

---

4   Rosenberg, *In the Care of Strangers: The Rise of America's Hospital System*, 18–19, 22–23.

5   Benjamin Rush to Ashbel Green (April 26, 1803), *Letters of Benjamin Rush, Vol. II*, 863.

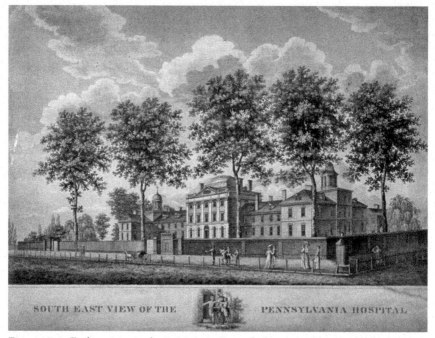

Figure 7.1 Early nineteenth-century image of the Pennsylvania Hospital with the additional wing for psychiatric patients. Public Domain, National Library of Medicine.

was not recorded by Rush or his family members. However, a series of letters from Buchanan to Rush from 1801 into 1802 describe Allison's decline and treatment inside and outside the hospital.

Treatment included familiar therapeutics for all disease, including bloodletting and calomel to produce a "salivation." Rush would have prescribed such remedies to deplete the amount of excitement in the body in preparation for building up healthy excitement during convalescence. Allison apparently complained about this treatment afterwards and lingering damage to his mouth, but did not "question the goodness of your [Rush's] intentions." The next letter from Buchanan, however, contained bad news. Physical illness again reduced Allison's mental health to the point at which Buchanan doubted recovery, writing, "I wish to God that something could be done to compose his mind, for the only alleviation now sought for by his afflected [sic] friends, is to render his Exit peaceful & composed—if you Sir can contribute to the attainment of this desirable End it will afford much consolation to the Friends & Connections of your unhappy Patient." A peaceful end required a receptive mind, but it seemed Allison's mind was not prepared and could not be suitably prepared for death. Perhaps he was unable to grasp the immediate danger to his life. Mental and physical illness mixed to the distress of all involved. Rush made a note on the back of the last letter recommending Allison's decayed teeth be extracted and prescribing "Syrup of Galls terdic—with Vs: [venesection]: also Laud: [laudanum]: glysters."[6] Again, these remedies do not differ from the kinds of treatment recommended for most strong fevers at the time.

Despite this therapeutic similarity, Rush firmly believed that unlike diseases of the body, diseases of the mind required isolation and hospital care. Family and friends—however well-meaning—were more likely to cause distress, he argued, than promote relief. Reminders of homes or businesses could prevent recovery as could feelings of shame or a desire to conceal the illness. Poorly designed hospital visitation was no better. While many hospitals and asylums of the eighteenth century allowed the public to visit, Rush feared that such practices damaged mental health both inside and outside institutions. The mere reputation of hospitals as places of lurid visitation could lead to tragedy. Rush shared one case in which "the dread of being exposed and gazed at in the cell of a hospital by an unthinking visitor . . . is one of the greatest calamities a man can anticipate in his tendency to madness. The apprehension of it was so distressing to a young gentleman in this city in a fit of low spirits, that he prevented it, by discharging the contents of a loaded musket through his brain."[7] The fear of becoming an object and othered in his community (at least according to Rush) was so intense that suicide was the result.

Buchanan's letters about Allison make another important point about the assumptions of hospital practice. In an early letter, he noted the sense of social shame and surprise from members of the community that surrounded Allison's hospitalization. He wrote, "when I placed him under your care . . . I have had to combat, the clamours & prejudices of many whose sensibility was shocked at the term 'Hospital,' viewed as a residence for a person so highly esteemed as Doctor Allison—I have thus far Braved their opposition, but the tash [sic] is too painful." As indicated by Buchanan, most people

---

6   J.A. Buchanan to Benjamin Rush (1801–1802) LCP, Rush Family Papers, Series I Benjamin Rush Papers, Subseries I Correspondence– Vol. II, Box 6, Folders 7–14.

7   Rush, *Medical Inquiries and Observations Upon the Diseases of the Mind*, 236.

thought of hospitals as a place inappropriate for someone of the middling or upper classes. Those with means and families to care for them simply did not go to hospitals when physically ill, they stayed in their own sick rooms. This probably came from associations with the kind of somatic patients' hospitals treated during this time. Patients with physical ailments were almost entirely members of the urban poor. Anyone who could afford treatment at home or get by with trips to the outpatient dispensary did so. Those in the hospital also required letters of reference to prove they were part of the so-called "worthy poor" and known to the community. Sailors were a rare exception but even then, separate federally funded Marine Hospitals were constructed in the 1790s specifically to provide care for men far from their homes and patrons.[8] Patients could not come to the hospital if they were incurable or suffering from a known contagious infection either. In large hospitals like those in London and even the Pennsylvania Hospital, patients were also used to train medical students with or without consent. Patients received "free" care but gave up many of their rights in doing so. These rules were standard for most municipal or voluntary hospitals in the United States and Great Britain in the eighteenth and early nineteenth centuries.[9]

In addition to treating patients at the Pennsylvania Hospital, Rush brought students into the institution. As was often the case with Rush, he used the lecture hall as a space to articulate his medical opinions most clearly. In 1802, he used the opening lecture of the year to describe in detail the kind of building best suited for a hospital in the Middle States (Pennsylvania, Delaware, Maryland, and New Jersey). Amos Evan's notes stated that hospitals needed to be on high ground with a southern exposure and good access to fresh water. Evan's wrote that "the Dr lays great stress upon air and water," something very believable coming from Rush.[10] Other aspects of the lecture focus on the kinds of illness that were common in hospitals. Prevention of typhus was especially important. The "low" fever of typhus (or typhoid) was occasionally referred to as "ship," "hospital," or "gaol/jail" fever, due to its prevalence in enclosed spaces. In his American edition of William Hillary's *Observations on the Changes of the Air, and the Concomitant Epidemical Diseases in the Island of Barbadoes,* Rush addressed typhus in a footnote stating "[t]he typhus fever when of long duration often generates a matter that produces

---

8   Duffy, *The Sanitarians: A History of American Public Health,* 159.

9   Rosenberg, *In the Care of Strangers: The Rise of America's Hospital System.*

10   Evans, "Notes Taken From Dr. Rush's Lectures upon the Institutes and Practice of Medicine and on Clinical Cases, Vol. I."

a fever. It has been called the 'contagion of excretion.'" Hospitals, jails, and ships were all confined spaces where—if poorly designed—inhabitants were bound to come into regular contact with the excretion of their fellows.[11]

To prevent the spread of disease Rush took care to note the desired material construction of institutions. Rush recommended clean air and water, and especially clean and airy attic spaces to prevent the ailment from sweeping through the vulnerable bodies and minds of the hospital.[12] Even's also noted that Rush recommended lime-coated attics and large but relatively few windows on the ward (to better regulate temperature), and that "the fever wards should have earthen or ground floors; and all the wards arranged so as that the tenents (sic) of them may not incommode each other."[13] Much of this expertise likely came from Rush's time managing military hospitals during the Revolutionary War and his later association with the Pennsylvania Hospital starting in the 1780s. Students like Evans had the opportunity to walk the wards with their preceptors and experience a variety of ailments treated in the institution.

Besides the hospital, Philadelphia did have an additional source of medical care available outside the private marketplace. The Philadelphia Dispensary treated far more people, mostly in an outpatient capacity (and for free), than the hospital. Established in 1787, it was a model republican institution in which Rush's hand was evident. Like the hospital it worked within the concept of care for the "worthy poor" only. Those with a reference from a dispensary subscriber (financial supporter) could receive free health care. Like many charities of the era donors provided funds via a subscription campaign that ran as a who's who of Philadelphia society. Those who signed on—which included married women under their own names for the first time in the history of Philadelphia philanthropy—donated money, acted as references, and were publicly recognized for their service. The whole point was to reduce the stigma of free medical care for the poor while providing a worthy cause for the city's enthusiastic republican supporters.[14]

---

11   Hillary and Rush, *Observations on the Changes of the Air, and the Concomitant Epidemical Diseases in the Island of Barbadoes. To Which Is Added A Treatise on the Putrid Billious Fever, Commonly Called the Yellow Fever; and Such Other Diseases as Are Indigenous or Endemical*, 44.

12   Evans, "Notes Taken From Dr. Rush's Lectures upon the Institutes and Practice of Medicine and on Clinical Cases, Vol. I."

13   Evans, 5.

14   Pencak, "Free Health Care for the Poor: The Philadelphia Dispensary," 25–52.

In a later edition of his essay on the medicine and health of "Indians" (after the creation of the dispensary), Rush included a footnote indicating the good work of dispensaries and his preference for them over hospitals for many diseases, noting, "Philosophy and Christianity alike concur in deriving praise and benefit from these excellent institutions . . . for in what other charitable institutions do we perceive so great a quantity of distress relieved by so small an expense."[15] The expense may have been small to subscribers, but the power dynamics of the hospital remained. Those "worthy poor" who frequented the dispensary required patronage from subscribers and therefore expected to perform some deference to social superiors. Meanwhile, in terms of health care, the dispensary, like the hospital, allowed doctors to try out new therapeutics on the poor, dependent, and often Black patients.[16] While the dispensary provided an important service, the benefits were not necessarily distributed equally.

Nevertheless, the dispensary turned out to be so important to the public's health that it appears in a lecture Rush gave on causes of death in curable diseases, in other words preventable deaths. He praised the dispensary movement as a means of ending this sad trend. If the poor could see a doctor sooner rather than later and see one on a regular basis, he reasoned, surely the health of the community would improve. Rush wrote, "it would be an improvement in charity, if a certain number of physicians could be supported at the public expense . . . to attend those persons whose narrow and appropriated incomes prevent their applying for early and constant medical aid."[17] His call for public support of healthcare came from the same political and intellectual spaces as the dispensary itself. As Rush continued, "dispensaries . . . have been the means of saving many lives. They would be more useful, if physicians were rendered so independent by governments as to devote their time exclusively to them." In this instance "independent" is used to suggest financial security. A government paycheck so doctors could care for their own families while dedicating their professional lives to the care of the poor. The thought did not become a full-fledged plan, but again points to the centrality of community health for Rush and the possible role of public support

---

15 Rush, "An Inquiry into the Natural History of Medicine among the Indians of North-America; and a Comparative View of Their Diseases and Remedies with Those of Civilized Nations," 84.

16 Pencak, "Free Health Care for the Poor: The Philadelphia Dispensary"; Benjamin Rush "On Sore Legs," M I&O Vol. 1, 230; Benjamin Rush "On Dropsies," M I & O Vol. II, 110.

17 Rush, *Sixteen Introductory Lectures, to Courses of Lectures upon the Institutes and Practice of Medicine*, 78.

for healthcare. In fact, he was so enthusiastic about the promise of the institution that he directly connected it to the kind of institutions humans could look forward to at the Millennium, or period surrounding Christ's second coming. Mixing religion, prophesy, promise of the future, and polities he enthusiastically wrote:

> A late French writer, in his prediction of events that are to happen in the year 4000, says, 'That mankind in that aera shall be so far improved by religion and government, that the sick and the dying shall no longer be thrown, together with the dead, into splendid houses [hospitals], but shall be relieved and protected in a connection with their families and society.' For the honour of humanity, an institution destined for that distant period, has lately been founded in this city, that shall perpetuate the year 1786 in the history of Pennsylvania. . . . There is a necessary connection between animal sympathy and good morals.[18]

Not only could health care help states and individuals, but it might also bring society closer to God.

Despite his overarching praise for the dispensary as a moral institution, Rush reinforced the idea of hospital practice for one set of ailments: diseases of the mind. According to Rush's system, it was the role of the physician to correct damage to the system wrought by outside forces. In a fever—yellow fever—physical corrections like bleeding, low diet, and cheerful company might be called for as well as the careful supervision of a physician during the patient's convalescence. In the case of mental derangement, however, home might not be an ideal location for such careful observations, especially if the home, business, or family contributed to the derangement. The hospital allowed that work to happen in a far more controlled environment than the home. Meanwhile isolation also "protected" the healthy from the example of the insane and vice versa. It was at its core a disciplined space designed to prevent a tragedy. Rush's ideas for the Philadelphia Hospital, especially his assumption that modern life caused madness, laid the foundation for nineteenth-century asylum care.

Healing Diseases of the Mind

In the United States, political revolution and perceived social instability made the threat of madness feel immediate and continued to vex specialists

---

18   Rush, "An Inquiry into the Influence of Physical Causes upon the Moral Faculty," 119.

into the nineteenth century.[19] Rush worried that instability in society would lead directly to the instability of minds. Increased reports of suicide, political demonstrations, and rebellions against the government in the 1780s and 1790s fueled such fears.[20] In his 1786 oration on the moral faculty, Rush went so far as to suggest that dangerous behaviors be kept secret so as to prevent mimicry. Suicide was one of his chief concerns. He wrote "I believe [suicide] is often propagated by means of newspapers. For this reason, I should be glad to see the proceedings of our courts kept from the public eye, when they expose or punish monstrous vices."[21] Rush also supported a movement to provide life-saving devices near bridges and rivers where people were known to take their own lives.[22] Richard Bell's work on suicide in the Early Republic shows that the papers did not take Rush's advice and sensationalized accounts of such deaths were printed and reprinted in multiple cities.[23]

---

19   Bell, *We Shall Be No More: Suicide and Self-Government in the Newly United States*; Bell, "The Moral Thermometer: Rush, Republicanism, and Suicide"; Vallee, "'A Fatal Sympathy': Suicide and the Republic of Abjection in the Writings of Benjamin Rush and Charles Brockden Brown," 332–51.

20   For more on the perception of suicide in the early republic, see Finger, "An Indissoluble Union: How the American War for Independence Transformed Philadelphia's Medical Community and Created a Public Health Establishment," 17; Webster, "American Science and the Pursuit of 'Useful Knowledge' in the Polite Eighteenth Century, 1750–1806," 148; Herschthal, "Antislavery Science in the Early Republic: The Case of Dr. Benjamin Rush," 281; Altschuler, "From Blood Vessels to Global Networks of Exchange: The Physiology of Benjamin Rush's Early Republic From Blood Vessels to Global Networks of Exchange," 222. Rush famously feared what he termed "anarchia," a social disease of too much liberty and certainly associated with social unrest in the years following independence. Benjamin Rush, *An Inquiry into the Influence of Physical Causes upon the Moral Faculty: Delivered before a Meeting of the American Philosophical Society, Held at Philadelphia, on the Twenty-Seventh of February, 1786*, ed. George Combe (Philadelphia: Haswell, Barrington, and Haswell, 1839), 22.

21   Bell, *We Shall Be No More: Suicide and Self-Government in the Newly United States*.

22   Bell, "The Moral Thermometer: Rush, Republicanism, and Suicide," 316.

23   Benjamin Rush, "An Account of the Influence of the Military and Political Events of the American Revolution upon the Human Body," in *Medical Inquiries and Observations*, 2nd ed. (Philadelphia: J. Conrad & Co., 1805), 277.

Rush's republicanism valued liberty and self-government but feared the health effects of long-term strife and instability. For all his support of British radicals and well-written essays by men of letters, overly emotional actions were out of the question. In an essay on the influence of the war and political change on American bodies and minds Rush wrote, "[t]he scenes of war and government that it introduced, were new to the greatest part of the inhabitants of the United States, and operated with all force of *novelty* upon the human mind."[24] That "novelty" could be equated to a burst of stimulating excitement. Among soldiers and officers, he reported that passions of excitement, fear, and love of country lead to "patience, firmness, and magnanimity with which the officers and soldiers of the American army endured the complicated evils of hunger, cold, and nakedness."[25] In *Diseases of the Mind* Rush described what sounds like self-medication with a variety of substances, including excessive alcohol consumption among those suffering from some variety of pathological distress (either described as hysteria or hypochondriasis). In modern terminology we might point to PTSD or some other lingering effect of a traumatic experience. In Rush's words this happened when, "after [a person] has completely put off all its hysterical symptoms, the patients fly for relief to such stimuli as act upon the body, in order to counteract the insupportable pressure of distress."[26] Distress or trauma from warfare is not explicitly mentioned in this scenario, but it is difficult to imagine that it could not have been one cause for such behavior, especially considering the connection Rush drew between war and substance abuse in other settings.[27]

Independence caused permanent alteration to the minds and health of people living in the United States. At the end of the American war, Rush claimed those who favored revolution experienced joy and cure from hysterical distempers (and one case of death from happiness), whereas loyalists suffered hypochondriasis or other depressive disorders.[28] War, for soldiers and civilians, was a source of excitement, which had both healthy and pathological consequences. The trauma of war's violence, illness, and depravation left scars on the American people. Some of those ailments persisted long after the war ended. In 1812, Stephen W. Williams, a physician in Deerfield,

---

24 Rush, 286.

25 Rush, 287.

26 Rush, *Medical Inquiries and Observations Upon the Diseases of the Mind*, 90.

27 Carlson, "Benjamin Rush on Revolutionary War Hygiene" 627.

28 Thacher, "Bond, Thomas, M.D.," 177.

Massachusetts, wrote to Rush about the case of Joshua and Caleb Clapp, twin brothers who served as captains in the Continental Army. Both brothers suffered from melancholia after the war ended and eventually committed suicide within ten days of each other. Williams wondered if it was their constitutions or experiences that led to their tragic end. He also noted that the men's mother and sisters suffered from derangement as well. This suggested some hereditary disposition, but the lingering effects of the war were not discounted as an important cause.[29]

Rush may have pointed to both constitutional and circumstantial causes in the case of the unfortunate Clapp brothers. Some bodies were ill-suited to certain kinds of stimulus. Families shared similar physical and possibly mental constitutions through some hereditary principle Rush could not quite articulate. Nevertheless, it was clear that some disorders ran in families. Their internal vibrations, especially the delicate and (in healthy people) harmonious vibrations of the brain, could be knocked into fatal irregularity with the application of the wrong psychological or physiological stimulus. Fear, war, physical depravation, or the act of killing another human being could have permanently damaged the Clapps in the same way that a duel damaged the mind of John Rush. Constitutions also altered, based on life-experience. The horrors of war shape young men incorrectly, leaving them fragile and vulnerable to disease.

Rush was not alone in making connections between body and mind. Associations between mental and physical health featured prominently in early modern medicine. Enlarged spleens, for example were commonly associated with hypochondriasis and depressive symptoms.[30] Rush's mentor

---

29   Stephen W. Williams to Benjamin Rush (1812), LCP, Rush Family Papers, Benjamin Rush Correspondence, Vol. XX.

30   Rush cited Prost in his essay on the spleen, liver, and thyroid and owned two volumes by the French physician Noyes, "The Transformation of Hypochondriasis in British Medicine, 1680 – 1830," 281–98; Berrios, "'Febrile Anxiety' by Robert James (1745)"; *A Catalogue of the Medical Library, Belonging to the Pennsylvania Hospital: Exhibiting the Names of Authors and Editors, in Alphabetical Order, and an Arrangement of Them Under Distinct Heads. Also, a List of Articles Contained in the Anatomical Museum; A* (Philadelphia, 1806); Rush, *Medical Inquiries and Observations Upon the Diseases of the Mind,* 157; Rush, "Pathological and Practical Remarks upon Certain Morbid Affections of the Liver," 92. Rush also had access to the work of Willis and James at the Pennsylvania Hospital Library and cited Willis in his own psychiatric work. Noyes, Berrios, Catalogue, Rush Diseases 157, Rush

Cullen, meanwhile, centered all of physiology on the nerves, which directly connected to the brain. From a more spiritual perspective, Rush could also draw on the wisdom of his preceptor John Redman, who imparted a sense of skepticism about the ability of human reason.[31] The idea that mental faculties could deceive or be corrupted in healthy and ill individuals is an additional necessary component to developing Rush's theories of diseases of the mind. This background shows in Rush's ideas about the deep connections between the mind, brain, and physical body. Similarly, his French contemporary Philippe Pinel (1745–1826) worried about what digestion and eating habits might contribute to mental health.[32] Building on these earlier theories, Rush approached "diseases of the mind" as any other illness caused by irregular functions or structures in key bodily systems, with a focus on the nerves, blood vessels, glands, and lymphatics.

Meanwhile, political, social, and economic distress similarly peppered the literature as causes of mental derangement. This provided important precedent for arguments about the American Revolution and mental health. In eighteenth-century Britain observers pointed to the perceived connection between economic distress and mental health, citing the bursting of the South Sea Bubble in 1720 and high admissions rates to the Bethlehem Hospital as an example. Similarly, worries appear in Rush's commonplace book during a financial panic in 1792 in which many Philadelphians lost money in poorly valued stocks. Political instability was not the only threat in a revolutionary country.[33]

After the revolution Americans worried about both the long- and short-term effects of public political engagement on mental health, as well as political order. Rush's system, which emphasized regulated excitement and predictable physiological motion, recommended a careful balance between healthful political participation and dangerously unstable spectacle or revolt. This careful and at times contradictory desire is evident in his politics, in which Rush hovered in a middle ground between the hierarchical federalism

---

Liver 92, Williams, "Stomach and Psyche: Eating, Digestion, and Mental Illness in the Medicine of Philippe Pinel," 358–86.

31   Reid-Maroney, Philadelphia's Enlightenment, 101.

32   Rush and Biddle, *A Memorial Containing Travels Through Life Or Sundry Incidents in the Life of Dr. Benjamin Rush, Born Dec. 24, 1745 (Old Style) Died April 19, 1813*, 134–35.

33   May, *The Enlightenment in America*, 208–11.

and more egalitarian republicanism in the 1780s and 1790s.[34] While not all inhabitants of the new republic suffered from "diseases of the mind," Rush considered their care central to the success of the American experiment. In a letter addressed to the Managers of the Pennsylvania Hospital in 1810, he laid out plans to better address the growing number of patients treated for mental illness. He noted that:

> As great improvements have taken place in the treatment of persons in that melancholy situation within the last thirty years, I beg leave to lay an account of them before you as far as I have been able to obtain them from the histories of asylums for mad people in foreign countries, as well as from my own experience during five and twenty years' attendance upon that class of patients at the Pennsylvania Hospital.[35]

By this point, the Pennsylvania Hospital earned a reputation for the care of the "insane" or "deranged." This reputation meant that unlike patients on the general wards those suffering from "diseases of the mind" came from across the country and from every walk of life.

As evidenced by his American and international correspondence Rush garnered a reputation as an expert in the care of the insane as a result of his hospital connections. Patients, worried family members, and physicians wrote frequently, seeking in-home care and in one instance a prospective asylum keeper wrote requesting advice for his institution. Frederick A. Vandyke of New Brunswick, New Jersey, appealed to Rush and his colleague, Philip Syng Physick, for advice on constructing and running a private madhouse. Such institutions started to supplement the work done in public facilities and hospital as the nineteenth century progressed.[36] Between 1797 and 1812 Rush received requests from at least 35 families and four physicians in ten states and the District of Columbia specifically to admit patients to the Pennsylvania Hospital for psychiatric disorders. The case of a Mr. Dunbar of New Haven, Connecticut, reported by physician Eli Ives demonstrates the manner in which heredity and circumstance were thought to lead to madness.

---

34 Benjamin Rush, "To the Managers of the Pennsylvania Hospital (September 24, 1810)," in *Letters of Benjamin Rush, Vol. II*, ed. L.H. Butterfield (Princeton, NJ: Princeton University Press, 1951), 1063–64.

35 Weimerskirch, "Benjamin Rush and John Minson Galt, II. Pioneers of Bibliotherapy in America.," 510–26.

36 "Frederick A. Vandyke to Benjamin Rush (1811)," LCP, Rush Family Papers, Benjamin Rush Correspondence, Vol. XXXI.

[Dunbar] Became deranged last Febr the disease came upon him gradually he had been six or eight years since affected in the same way. . . . The family is predisposed to mania, his father has been deranged before him. Mr. Dunbar was educated at [Yale] studied law which he has practiced for 7 years past. Within two years past he has distracted his attention between the practice of the law, farming, speculating & a few months before he became quite deranged his mind was occupied on religion.[37]

Dunbar suffered both from a trait passed down in his family and triggered by the stress of his profession, poor investments, and excessive religious activity. All of these causes appear in Rush's textbook and were not considered uncommon, just distressing. Isolation, in Rush's view, would help restore Dunbar's mental health away from the stimuli that caused his illness. Close observation by the hospital staff, in an ideal setting, was supposed to help put the mind right. Dunbar's fate is unknown, however many patients did recover, or recover enough, to return to their families. Most people admitted in the 1790s and 1800s did not end their days in the hospital.

While there, however, patients experienced a very different kind of care compared with the family-based social medicine of most somatic disease. Isolation was the defining feature of the construction and maintenance of the hospital building itself. The Pennsylvania Hospital in the early nineteenth century remained a single building situated in a wooded block formed by 8th, 9th, Spruce, and Pine Streets. At the time of its construction in 1752 the block was far from the core of Philadelphia. Time progressed and the city moved west, eventually surrounding the previously pastoral hospital, which made the walls and landscaped spaces within them all the more important for maintaining ventilation and isolation. The original building still exists and remains set back from the road and behind a wall with gardens in between; a small respite from the bustle of twenty-first century Philadelphia. In the 1790s patients suffering from "diseases of the mind" were separated from others in the hospital. Like most eighteenth-century voluntary hospitals, patients were rarely separated based on diagnosis. Categorization and separation, alien from the general wards, became characteristic of Rush's little kingdom of mental health. In the 1810 letter to the hospital managers, he included additional recommendations for the treatment of the "insane." Rush's letter called for even greater separation in designated buildings based on gender and the severity of "derangement." For recovering or convalescing

---

37   Eli Ives to Benjamin Rush (1811), LCP, Rush Family Papers, Benjamin Rush Correspondence, Vol. VIII.

patients, he suggested that amusements be provided for psychiatric patients (adjusted to their social status and gender) as well as mental stimulation from book-reading and conversation with "an intelligent man [or] woman."[38] These activities modeled the regular stimulation required for health and promoted amusements that would build good citizens. In essence he wanted to create ideal and individualized sick room experiences as best he could under the circumstances. He also replicated and reinforced gender, class, and race-based behavioral expectations.

The organization Rush proposed both borrowed from innovations of European asylums and described features soon to become characteristic of nineteenth-century institutions. As an example of the former, he suggested providing cells with close-stools half-filled with water to prevent additional infection from the feces. Rush attributed this innovation to Dr. Clark of Newcastle, England. The modified close-stools prevented effluvia from feces to spread through the air and cause illness. Before the adjustment, Rush claimed that human waste was responsible for the death of hospital attendant George Campbell as well as the perpetuation of mental illness for untold numbers of patients from the damaging stimulus of effluvia.[39] This again connected mental and physical illness with environmental management. More generally, he suggested separating patients based on their degree of madness and gender as well as isolating patients from visitors. All of these ideas had counterparts in the large hospitals of France and private British madhouses.[40]

In addition to reading, Rush sought firsthand accounts of treatment in British asylums and hospitals including the large London hospitals—St.

---

38   Rush, "To the Managers of the Pennsylvania Hospital (September 24, 1810)," 1064.; Rush, 1065.

39   Digby, *Madness, Morality, and Medicine: A Study of the York Retreat, 1796– 1914*; Tomes, "The Domesticated Madman: Changing Concepts of Insantiy at the Pennsylvania Hospital, 1780–1830," 271–86; Tomes, *The Art of Asylum-Keeping: Thomas Story Kirkbride and the Origins of American Psychiatry.*

40   This included asylums practicing "moral" treatment like the York Retreat, Castel and Halls, *The Regulation of Madness: The Origins of Incarceration in France*; Scull, *Social Order/Mental Disorder: Anglo-American Psychiatry in Historical Perspective*; Scull, *Madness in Civilization: A Cultural History of Insanity from the Bible to Freud, from the Madhouse to Modern Medicine.* As well as larger institutions Benjamin Rush, "To James Rush (Philadelphia, March 19, 1810)," in *Letters of Benjamin Rush, Vol. II*, ed. L.H. Butterfield (Philadelphia: Princeton University Press, 1951), 1039.

Luke's and Bethlehem (Bedlam)—and the innovative York Retreat famous for its use of the "moral treatment."[41] Writing to his son James—who was finishing his studies in Edinburgh in 1810—Rush included a long list of places the young man should visit before returning to the United States. At the time Rush was preparing his manuscript for what would become *Medical Inquiries and Observations Upon Diseases of the Mind.* With that context it is not surprising that most of the sites on Benjamin's list to James related to mental health. Specifically, the elder Rush wanted to know more about the treatment of both body and mind, writing, "pry into everything that relates to the management both of bodies and minds of the patients that are confined in them."[42] Through James and other transatlantic correspondents Rush maintained a working knowledge of European trends and practices that could be adapted for his own work in the United States, and vice versa.

This informal network allowed men like Rush and Pinel to hear of, and even borrow from each other outside and before formal publication. From at least 1800 onward Rush was part of a transatlantic community of physicians interested in describing and treating mental disorders, which was largely conducted through informal communications and what essentially amounted to medical gossip. Moreover, in the personality-charged debates of Philadelphia medicine Rush could use accounts of such treatments as external endorsement of his practice. "Evidence" of certain work was not always clear and may have been second- or thirdhand. This combined with Rush's bad habit of poor citations makes it difficult to determine just how much he knew about Pinel's work in France or the York Retreat in England outside formal publications. However, it is certainly reasonable to suggest that he was in the loop without neglecting Rush's independent work. Not only did Rush contribute to the new medicine of psychiatry, but he also fit it in to his broader medical system.

Isolation from the world and a blend of physical and mental therapeutic activity characterized early nineteenth-century care for the "insane" and in Rush's view were designed to encourage regular physical function and

---

41 Nancy Tomes suggests that Rush and the managers of the Pennsylvania Hospital arrived at the tenets of "moral management" independently from similar projects in England. Digby, *Madness, Morality, and Medicine: A Study of the York Retreat, 1796–1914*; Reiss, *Theaters of Madness: Insane Asylums and Nineteenth-Century American Culture*; Tomes, "The Domesticated Madman: Changing Concepts of Insantiy at the Pennsylvania Hospital, 1780–1830."

42 Rush, "To James Rush (Philadelphia, March 19, 1810)," 1040.

strengthen the system to better handle the dangerous stimuli of the outside world. After all, patients were not expected to remain hospitalized forever. In terms of physical treatment standard therapies mirrored those for somatic patients and were designed to return regular motion to the circulatory and nervous systems. By the late 1790s Rush thought of mental illness as a form of fever, writing to a former student John Seward that he "late found *copious* bleeding, purging, a salivation, and afterwards the cold bath . . . to be very effectual in the [cure] for recent and acute mania . . . I consider it as a *state of fever.* No wonder that it yields to the common remedies for fever."[43] Bleeding occurred regularly, using the "tranquilizing chair," cooling clays were applied to the head to patients, and swings were designed to encourage circulation. The chair and swings were peculiar to Rush's practice. The former immobilized patients at the wrist, ankle, and chest, preventing excessive and exciting movement. Meanwhile the head was often encased in a box to block out light and sound. This was designed to lower excitement in the body without the constriction of straightjackets and provide access to the body for physicians. In theory these were tools designed to reorient the body toward healthy function in a manner like that proposed for patients suffering from physical illness.

Meanwhile, techniques suggested by Rush and proponents of "moral treatment" in Britain and the United States addressed the mind as a site of medical practice.[44] Rush recommended sensible conversation, reading, and writing as therapies that were directed at the mind. In his letter to the hospital managers, he wrote, "[w]hile we admit madness to be seated in the mind, by a strange obliquity of conduct we attempt to cure it only by corporeal remedies. The disease affects both the body and mind and can be cured only by remedies applied to each of them."[45] Rush also allowed for some psychological trickery to help "cure" patients.

The blending of physical and psychological treatment appears in one particularly disturbing case of a suicidal patient in the early 1790s. Rush attempted to "cure" the man with the terror of death accompanied by physical actions on the part of the hospital attendant. By seeming to give in to

---

43 Emphasis in the original. Tomes, "The Domesticated Madman: Changing Concepts of Insantiy at the Pennsylvania Hospital, 1780–1830," 275.

44 Rush, "To the Managers of the Pennsylvania Hospital (September 24, 1810)," 1064.

45 Rush, *Medical Inquiries and Observations Upon the Diseases of the Mind,* 128.

a "maniac's" desires, Rush claimed the ill person could be brought back to health.

> A maniac in the Pennsylvania Hospital some years ago, expressed a strong desire to drown himself. Mr. Higgins, the present steward of the hospital, seemed to favour this wish, and prepared water for the purpose. The distressed man stripped himself and eagerly jumped into it. Mr. Higgins endeavoured to plunge his head under the water, in order, he said, to hasten his death. The maniac resisted, and declared he would prefer being burnt to death. "You shall be gratified," said Mr. Higgins, and instantly applied a lighted candle to his flesh. "Stop, stop," said he, "I will not die now;" and never afterwards attempted to destroy himself, or even expressed a wish for death.[46]

To a modern reader this account reads as torture. The man was in a position of no power and clearly hurt and terrified. From Rush's perspective, however, this temporary harm was easily justified, disturbing as it might be. Inside the hospital, Rush gathered anecdotes and observations like that of the suicidal man and Mr. Higgins to support his ideas about isolation and a combination of psychological and physical treatment. In a similar case, Rush recorded bleeding a suicidal patient to the point of passing out after telling the man that his request to die was being fulfilled. After bleeding to the point of passing out the patient seemingly recovered his senses the next day.[47] Hospital care required men like Higgins to carry out much of the medical work, especially the physically demanding work of the swings, chairs, and mock-deaths.

In terms of numbers, the "insane" population of the Pennsylvania Hospital was not insignificant in the late eighteenth century and appeared to be on the rise during Rush's tenure. According to information collected by Nicholas Waters at Rush's request, between 1780 and 1787, 106 men and women entered the hospital with diagnosed mental disorders.[48] According to the document, just under 40 women and nearly 80 men had been admitted to the Pennsylvania hospital. The vast majority, 90 percent were diagnosed with mania. Mania, like fever, could be traced to numerous exciting

---

46   Rush, 127.

47   Rush, 25, 47; James Thacher, "Waters, Nicholas Baker, M.D.," in *American Medical Biography: Or, Memoirs of Eminent Physicians Who Have Flourished in America. Vol. II.* (Richardson & Lord and Cottons & Barnard, 1828).

48   "List of Lunatics in the Pennsylvania Hospital (1787)," LCP, Rush Family Papers, Benjamin Rush Correspondence, Vol. XXXI.

causes, from suppressed menses to "disappointment in love."[49] Rush must have found the document useful because he requested additional information in subsequent years. For example, in 1810 and 1812 Rush requested another hospital physician and former student, Frederick Vandyke, to collect information on patients' illness as well as their hair and eye color. The results linked dark hair and light eyes to mental derangement but suggested no mechanism to explain the supposed connection.[50] Rush was grasping for something, perhaps still struggling with the relative influences of nature versus nurture in mental disorder.

Numerous changes in the city and country accounted for the increase in hospital population, from demographic change to the growing reputation of the hospital for treating "mental derangement," to poor or incomplete recordkeeping in the 1760s and 1770s. Nevertheless, using these numbers Rush saw a correlation between mental illness and social upheaval that fit neatly into his view of physiology. Political revolution, economic instability, and general uncertainly contributed to the assumption by many Americans that mental derangement, especially suicide and mania, were on the rise.[51] As noted by Richard Bell, no accurate counts of death by suicide existed in the early nineteenth century, at least not on a consistent basis. Bills of mortality, for example, only existed in cities and in most were erratically kept. However, newspapers frequently printed and reprinted individual instances of suicides and suicide attempts. This publicity produced a public fear of an epidemic.[52] Outside the hospital walls Rush was also engaged in plans to reshape Philadelphia as a whole and in the wake of other epidemics.

Rush's time at the Pennsylvania Hospital resulted in his most lasting literary work, *Diseases of the Mind*, published the year before his death. The book provided the framework for thinking about the mind and how it could become ill. In its pages Rush broke down the faculties of the mind, states of illness, and cases of cure (Figure 7.2). As with his work on physical illness, Rush's organization of mental disorders was designed to be simple and ultimately be

---

49   "List of Lunatics in the Pennsylvania Hospital (1787)," LCP, Rush Family
     Papers, Benjamin Rush Correspondence, Vol. XXXI.

50   Rush, *Medical Inquiries and Observations Upon the Diseases of the Mind*, 64;
     Bell, "The Moral Thermometer: Rush, Republicanism, and Suicide"; Bell, *We
     Shall Be No More: Suicide and Self-Government in the Newly United States*.

51   Bell, *We Shall Be No More: Suicide and Self-Government in the Newly United
     States*, 2–6.

52   Caldwell, *Medical & Physical Memoirs, Containing Among Other Subjects a
     Partiuclar Enquiry into the Origin and Nature of the Late Pestilential Epidemics
     of the United States*, 41.

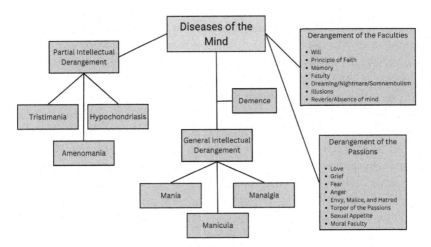

Figure 7.2 Chart showing how Rush understood diseases of the mind. Image by author.

rooted in a single cause: irregular motion in the body. In their turn various causes in persons with variable constitutions led to a wide array of symptoms. Throughout the text he remarked on the concept of regular motion and moderate excitement distributed through several physiological systems (the republican view of the body). Moreover, *Diseases of the Mind*—the first American textbook on psychiatry—remained in print for decades and was translated into several European languages. The republican medicine of Rush became canon in the new field of psychiatry. Rush also shaped the hospital as an institution and created an experimental space to learn about human minds and train the next generation of physicians dedicated to mental health.

The Dream of a Medical Republic

The hospital was a controlled setting. But health in the outside world also required regular management and support. However, cities and towns also suffered from poor health management. In October 1800, after a relatively healthy summer, Rush opened a letter to Thomas Jefferson emphasizing his agreement with the Virginian on the danger of cities. He noted that he viewed them "in the same light that I do abscesses on the Human body, viz., as reservoirs of all the impurities of a community" and noted "[William] Cowper the poet very happily expresses our ideas of them compared with the country. 'God made the country—man the cities.'"[53] If cities were the product of humans and contained errors it was the duty of knowledgeable citizens to correct the mistakes. In the real world neither Rush nor Jefferson could seriously contemplate a country with *no* urban areas or isolated from the world of international trade. The only solution was to fix the cities, drain the "abscesses," and shut down the "laboratories of poison." In such instances medicine became the natural partner of republican government. Medical institutions like Rush's Academy of Medicine of the late 1790s made collective recommendations, pooled research, and formalized the thoughts of an increasingly professional medical community. While the institution's goals were never fully realized—disinterested government and medical infighting prevented unity—it was a serious attempt to apply medical knowledge for the (re)public's health.

After 1793, yellow fever and other seasonal distempers damaged the healthy reputation of American cities compared to European capitals. It appeared that republican or monarchial, cities collected filth, bred miasma, and were plagued with epidemics. The only reasonable response for many was medically informed reform. Rush's student, Caldwell, never one to pull his punches, described all cities and towns as "laboratories of poison" responsible for the poor health of their citizens.[54] Writing in 1801, he described the utter filth present in early nineteenth-century cities and connected such conditions to frequent epidemics. Growing urban areas lacked clean sources of drinking water, sewage, or regular waste removal. A lack of green space artificially increased temperatures in city centers creating "artificial torrid zones." Natural or artificial, the torrid zone, characterized by hot and human conditions, had a bad health reputation. According to Caldwell, the heat and humidity trapped by buildings and pavement led to violent tropical fevers in temperate Pennsylvania and New York that should never have been there.[55]

53　Benjamin Rush, "To Thomas Jefferson (Philadelphia, October 6th, 1800)," in *Letters of Benjamin Rush, Vol. II*, ed. L.H. Butterfield (Princeton, NJ: Princeton University Press, 1951), 824.

54　Caldwell, *Medical & Physical Memoirs, Containing Among Other Subjects a Partiuclar Enquiry into the Origin and Nature of the Late Pestilential Epidemics of the United States*, 9, 40.

55　Barnes, *The Great Stink of Paris and the Nineteenth-Century Struggle against Filth and Germs*; Martin, "Sewage and the City: Filth, Smell, and Representations of Urban Life in Moscow, 1770–1880," 243–74; Hamlin, "William Pulteney Alison, the Scottish Philosophy, and the Making of a Political Medicine"; Hamlin, "Commentary: Ackerknecht and

Although yellow fever was his main target, the Philadelphia of Caldwell's and Rush's time generated diseases of various types, including measles, small-pox, influenza, dysentery, and typhus/typhoid fevers, which left their mark on the city and its inhabitants. Urban living could also have long-term consequences on inhabitants, especially the youngest and most vulnerable to environmental impact. Caldwell claimed that children who grew up in cities were sicker and smaller than their country counterparts.

In a less direct manner, Rush's concern about both physician status and urban epidemics appears in a letter of introduction from 1802. Dr. John C. Otto—a former Rush pupil—carried the letter addressed to John Warren with him on a trip to Boston. At this point Warren, like Rush, was a Revolutionary War veteran and leading figure and medical educator in his city, as a founder of Harvard's medical school.[56] In addressing his colleague, Rush wrote, "Mankind are often said to be members of one family. This should be true in a more especial manner of the members of our profession. The bond of our union should be common studies, common labors, common acts of self-denial, and, when they dare to charge their natives cities with generating pestilential disease, common persecutions."[57] His final note of persecutions and dangers that argumentative physicians could cause for cities exposes Rush's own frustration and anxiety about urban environments and health. Presumably, a brotherhood of American physicians who shared an education, work ethic, and commitment to their vocation could avoid such persecutions. The note says little about Otto's qualifications specifically and Rush appears to have taken the opportunity to share his ideas with a (hopefully) receptive audience.

The United States was not alone in its worry about health and urban land-scapes. Physicians in France, Britain, Russia, and Italy all contended with filth and urban spaces and what that meant for their own countries between the late Middle Ages and early twentieth century. Sanitary policy, medical police, and restricted movement of goods and people through quarantines

'Anticontagionism': A Tale of Two Dichotomies," 22–27; Hamlin, *More Than Hot: A Short History of Fever*, 62, 89–90; Fors, "Medicine and the Making of a City: Spaces of Pharmacy and Scholarly Medicine in Seventeenth-Century Stockholm," 473–94; Porter, *The History of Public Health and the Modern State*.

56 Howard A. Kelly et al., "Warren, John," *American Medical Biographies*, Baltimore: Norman, Remington Co. (1920) 1193–94.

57 Benjamin Rush to John Warren (August 6, 1802), *Letters of Benjamin Rush*, Vol. II. 851.

and lazarettos had a long history in most European states by the time the United States faced similar challenges.[58] While some of these methods were adopted in Philadelphia, this section focuses on the role of professionals and professional organizations as advisory bodies in the young republic, which took on a particularly American character. The voluntary organization was key to the way Philadelphians understood their responsibility as citizens. Banding together, citizen organizations sought to bring reform and improvement to their city as an expression of their republican values.[59] With respect to health, some physicians led by Rush felt an analogous impulse to provide information and recommendations for the city to enforce.

This was especially the case with large disease outbreaks. As discussed in the previous chapter, general filth combined with an epidemic atmospheric constitution (likely chemical in origin) formed the disease effluvia, which in turn invaded and disrupted the healthy action of human bodies. Those who believed in the local production of fever often emphasized the noxious nature of the cities and towns where it took hold. Even physicians who believed that epidemics were imported from tropical climates blamed the same root cause: the poor policing of urban areas. The two groups, "localists" and "importationists," agreed that American cities were poorly protected from disease and that something needed to change. Filth, all agreed, harmed community health and needed to be mitigated by increased medical involvement in public life. This meant, as James C. Mohr has pointed out, a new and robust relationship between the medical profession and legal institutions in the early American republic.[60] Doctors could make recommendations, but legislators and lawyers were required to enforce change.

Four years after the devastating 1793 experience, yellow fever dominated medical discourse and had become characteristic of American diseases.[61] It

---

58   For a discussion of European urban landscapes, disease, and social unrest, see Pencak, "Free Health Care for the Poor: The Philadelphia Dispensary," 33; Cipolla, *Fighting the Plague in Seventeenth-Century Italy*; Calvi, *Histories of a Plague Year: The Social and the Imaginary in Baroque Florence*; Colin Jones, "Plague and Its Metaphors in Early Modern France," 97–127.

59   Ackerknecht, "Anticontagionism Between 1821 and 1867," 562–95; Apel, *Feverish Bodies, Enlightened Minds: Science and the Yellow Fever Controversy in the Early American Republic*.

60   Arner, "Making Yellow Fever American: The Early American Republic, the British Empire and the Geopolitics of Disease in the Atlantic World."

61   Caldwell, *Autobiography of Charles Caldwell, M.D. with a Preface, Notes, and Appendix, by Harriot W. Warner*, 283.

provided an opportunity for the legal-medical connections mentioned above to flourish. In Philadelphia Rush and some of his closest professional allies formed the Philadelphia Academy of Medicine in large part to organize research about the reoccurring ailment and nature of American environments. The academy existed as a rival organization to the College of Physicians of Philadelphia, from which Rush had resigned in 1793. He left the group in protest after they refused to endorse his advice on fever treatment and prevention. This split over yellow fever characterized the new organization far beyond Philadelphia. In 1799, Benjamin Lynde Oliver wrote to Rush about yellow fever from Salem, Massachusetts. Like many letters it contained medical gossip. He noted that "Dr. [Samuel Latham] Mitchill, has informed me that the disease [yellow fever] was not contagious in the City of N York."[62] The fact that Oliver mentioned yellow fever is not especially unusual, but it is worth noting that he connected the opinion to Philadelphia's Academy of Medicine. That same year Mitchill, a New York physician and politician, was elected as a long-distance member of the Academy, strengthening that link.[63]

However, the new group was more than an alternative to the old. The two organizations enshrined different forms of civic outreach into their operation and had different goals as professional organizations. While the College convened to discuss the epidemic and printed recommendations when needed, their main purpose was fostering professional connections and serving as a forum for individual research. The Academy, on the other hand, viewed itself as a potential research organization, which coordinated efforts to shape policy, a think tank or ad hoc public health department as much as a professional organization. From the beginning they actively tried to establish themselves as an advisory body for government officials. This network strategy is again something common in Rush's appeals to correctness and authority. Where one's own experience ended those of a trustworthy source could reasonably pick up the slack.

In the Academy's founding document previsions were made for basic epidemiological research both within and beyond city limits. Caldwell recalled in his autobiography that the organization sent him on a fact-finding mission to inquire into the causes of sporadic cases of yellow fever in New Jersey like that of the Abbots in chapter 6. He concluded that he was "unable to trace

---

62 Benjamin Lynde Oliver to Benjamin Rush (1799) LCP, Rush Family Papers, Series I Benjamin Rush Papers, Subseries I Correspondence, Vol. XII.

63 Samuel Latham Mitchill (1799) LCP, Rush Family Papers, Series I Benjamin Rush Papers, Subseries I Correspondence, Vol. X.

them [the fever's causes] to any source having the slightest connection with a foreign country. Their origin was as clearly domestic as that of intermitting fever or common catarrh."[64] These observations suggested that the excitement produced by organic effluvia was simultaneously harmful and subject to human intervention. This directed research sought out the kind of information that doctors like Rush could only otherwise encounter by chance, such as the Abbot case. In that instance a correspondent in New Jersey effectively gifted Rush information on the fever's spread. Rush did not direct the collection of information the way the Academy was able to direct Caldwell.

In addition to individual missions, the Academy's constitution included several committees with specific duties. One compiled bills of mortality from American cities to decipher patterns of illness throughout the republic. Another was charged with analyzing the chemical composition of the atmosphere in search of correlations between health and the atmospheric environment.[65] This group applied concepts of eudiometry first popularized in Europe and promoted by Rush's international colleagues (as discussed in chapter 2). Priestley, for example, was working with eudiometers by the 1770s and Italian scientist Alessandro Volta (1745–1827) made improvements on the device to detect inflammable air (carbon dioxide) in 1778. In terms of public policy, both Priestley and Pringle supported atmospheric monitoring to better correlate health and environment. After moving to Pennsylvania Priestley measured the air quality of his new home in Northampton and reported approvingly to Rush in 1795.[66] The Academy was likely the first American organization to propose regular measurements in Philadelphia as a means of identifying dangerous spaces and preventing (or at least explaining) epidemics following such recommendations. Academy members noted the temperature, barometric pressure, and air purity with a eudiometer

64   Academy of Medicine of Philadelphia, *Academy of Medicine of Philadelphia Constitution* (Philadelphia, 1798).

65   Assessment of the atmosphere in Philadelphia seems to have followed John Huxham's work in England. Osman, "Alessandro Volta and the Inflammable-Air Eudiometer," 215–42; Weidenhammer, "Patronage and Enlightened Medicine in the Eighteenth-Century British Military: The Rise and Fall of Dr John Pringle, 1707–1787," 41; Schaffer, "Measuring Virtue: Eudiometry, Enlightenment and Pneumatic Medicine," 281–318; Schaffer, "Priestley's Questions: An Historiographic Survey," 151–83; Philadelphia, *Academy of Medicine of Philadelphia Constitution*.

66   Joseph Priestley to Benjamin Rush (1795) LCP, Rush Family Papers, Series I Benjamin Rush Papers, Subseries I Correspondence, Vol. XXX.

and different points within the city to note changes based on population. Most assumed that gasses like carbon dioxide, sulphur, and ammonia (all associated with decomposition) were the key to linking putrid matter with damaged health. Measuring the atmosphere in conjunction with qualitative observations of space lent a sense of scientific certainty to their endeavor.[67]

The goal, however, was not simply to add to the collective knowledge of the scientific community. The Academy (like the College or the American Philosophical Society) was interested in utility. In this case, their observations were designed to influence public policy and individual action. In December 1797 the organization drafted its first public statement, a formal letter to Pennsylvania governor Thomas Mifflin (1744–1800). Mifflin had requested information on the nature of the disease and ideas for how to prevent its annual return following minor outbreaks in 1794 and 1795. The recommendations provided form a concise overview of Rush's theories regarding epidemic prevention and the manner in which they were taking hold in the medical community by the mid-1790s. The Academy authors divided the document into three sections: an introduction, a description of sources of the fever, and means of preventing the fever. In the first and second parts the authors provided a summary of Rush's beliefs with respect to yellow fever's origin and means of propagation. They stated that it stemmed from putrefaction and tended to exert the most damage on the liver, hence the fever's "bilious" nature. To elaborate in section two, several of the authors appealed to their own observations and those of colleagues from other cities and states, like those of Mitchell and Oliver noted earlier.

Finally, they presented an idealized vision of what we would now call public health. The Academy requested regular inspection of urban spaces for filth, which would have taken place in the "streets, gutters, cellars, gardens, yards, stores, vaults, ponds. &c" of Philadelphia and its outlying regions of the Northern Liberties and Southwark.[68] The document also recommended "washing" the city in key areas with pump water, better ventilation in ships, and the unloading of cargo away from the city between June and October. By following strict rules of cleanliness, the authors hoped to make Philadelphia safe from locally generated and imported fevers.[69] As early as the 1770s, the

---

67   Carlson and Wollock, "Benjamin Rush and His Insane Son," 1323.

68   Rush et al, 1797 December- Report to the Governor.

69   Ibid.

healthy park-like port of William Penn's design was a long-lost dream. Blocks were subdivided for denser housing and parks built up over years.[70]

By the 1790s, physicians and city officials faced a serious problem in need of a significant structural overhaul. Even wealthy citizens like Benjamin Franklin drew water from wells dug only feet away from their privies. For the Academy doctors the answer differed little from that of their seventeenth-century colleagues who had advised Penn to build as clean and orderly a city as possible to avoid disease, criminality, and fire. These recommendations took on added emphasis from the application of eighteenth-century science. For example, the Academy called for more space between habitations, which would allow heat and human effluvia to be blown away by healthy prevailing winds. Philadelphia's alleys and backyard tenements as well as the lost downtown squares (now Washington and Franklin squares after restoration) were of particular concern. Add to this the argument by Rush, Jefferson, and others that America's virtue and future lay in pastoral rather than urban landscapes and a patriotic as well as medical reading of the recommendations takes shape.

Most Academy suggestions focused on the city and how to medically police it. In Rush's physiological analogy of society, the medical profession would act as an additional system in concert with the political to maintain the public's health. If the city had followed through with the recommendations it would have granted medical professionals some legal power over the movement of citizens and management of personal property. They planned to identify and eliminate possible sources of putrefying filth in both public and private spaces. The recommendations would have required homeowners to whitewash basements, and the city to wash streets and remove noxious matter left by animal and vegetable waste.[71] Each idea targeted organic sources of putrefaction believed to trigger disease. The authors complained that Philadelphia's water came from contaminated wells, that ships entered the harbor frequently uninspected by physicians, that general organic "filth" accumulated in streets, and that perishable cargo was left on the dockside. This last remark echoes Rush's 1794 argument that rotting coffee and decomposing paper triggered epidemics in Philadelphia and New York City. Laws existed to combat these problems, but according to the physicians, they had

70   Finger, *Contagious City: The Politics of Public Health in Early Philadelphia*, 7–9.

71   Benjamin Rush, et. al. "1797 December–Report to the Governor by Doctor Benj'n Rush and his Associates Physicians of Philadelphia on the Nature and Origin of the late Contagious disease," CPP, Lewis Curio C365.

been poorly enforced.[72] Despite such a comprehensive document and some revised regulations, no true medical policing was authorized in Philadelphia. Individual doctors and professional organizations continued to comment on public policy, but few suggestions were backed up with the power of the law, keeping them in the realm of the American voluntary organization rather than formal governance.

The letter failed to radically change state laws governing waste in the short term, much less make Philadelphia a disease-free city. In 1798 and 1799, yellow fever returned and nearly matched the mortality and terror of 1793. In 1803, Caldwell reviewed municipal-level policies and again publicly called for sanitary reform with physician oversight.[73] He hoped that the pamphlet would help change statutes up for revision that year. However, the political will for medical police (and the means to pay for them) did not exist. Doctors did not gain authority over lay civic leaders and Caldwell felt the city remained dangerously dirty. In many respects he restated the suggestions of the 1797 letter—of which he was a coauthor—in more detail, more demanding terms, and for a wider audience. He wrote "it is literally impossible that yellow fever should ever overrun our city unless it be aided by internal agents. For, whatever be the source from which this disease springs, whether septic exhalation, or secreted contagion, it is known to be an evil that thrives only in a contaminated atmosphere."[74] As much as Rush or Caldwell may have desired a large and powerful medical bureaucracy the city of Philadelphia could neither support nor enforce it without challenging central believes about individual control over persons and property.

Despite continued resistance and limited resources, the medical profession's policing impulse left a lasting mark on Philadelphians' attitudes toward unattended organic substances. Throughout most of the nineteenth century imported goods—especially hides, coffee, and rags—remained a target for

---

72 Health and safety laws for the province and, after independence, commonwealth of Pennsylvania made provisions for ship inspections, set standards for immigrant ship construction, and coordinated medical surveillance between Philadelphia, Southwark, and the Northern Liberties. Their efficacy, however, did not impress the legislature any more than the doctors and they were often revised in the 1780s and 90s. See James T. Mitchell and Henry Flancer, eds., *The Statutes at Large of Pennsylvania, 1680–1809*, www.palrb.us/stlarge/index.php.

73 Caldwell, *Thoughts on the Subject of a Health-Establishment for The City of Philadelphia*, 5.

74 Caldwell, *Thoughts*, 3.

inspection at the lazaretto.[75] Rotting goods and dank ships' holds could brew the required putrefaction for disease spread. Nor did their concern begin and end with yellow fever. Any epidemic could point to the dangers of urban spaces. The very names of some common ailments—ship fever, jail fever, and camp fever—all indicated that poor management of space had deadly consequences.[76] Cities like Philadelphia, crammed at the edge of the Delaware River, fostered some of the same environments as other crowded situations.

Controlling disease during the yellow fever years became a matter of national security. In 1796, the federal government showed support for epidemic prevention by empowering the President to aid in the enforcement of state and local laws. The statute, passed on May 27, specifically stated "[t]hat the President of the United States be, and is hereby authorized [by Congress], to direct the revenue officers and the officers commanding forts and revenue cutters, to aid in the execution of quarantine, and also in the execution of the health laws of the states, respectively, in such manner as may to him appear necessary."[77] Essentially, the statute allowed federal officials to answer to state authorities during a medical emergency and possibly declare a quarantine at the federal level. The statement does not specifically address yellow fever; however, at the time of its passage the tropical epidemic constituted the major cause of quarantine and loomed large in the American imagination. It also hints at the complexity of bringing federal power to bear on matters not directly addressed in the Constitution. What constituted a quarantine, how it would be enforced, and which bodies or goods were prioritized for extra scrutiny were questions left unanswered by the proposed legislation.

Additional attempts at congressional legislation from the same period would have specifically added the setting up of quarantine to the President's executive powers, essentially forming a federal health policy. It failed to pass due to both political resistance to increasing the power of the executive and the practical worry about communicating reliable and timely information

---

75 Barnes, "Cargo, 'Infection,' and the Logic of Quarantine in the Nineteenth Century."

76 This association was clearly and influentially made by military doctors and surgeons, most famously John Pringle. Pringle and Rush, *Observations on the Diseases of the Army.*

77 "Chapter XXXI: An Act relative to Quarantine, May 27, 1796," Fourth Congress, Session 1, 476.

about disease to a President who might be hundreds of miles away.[78] The question of quarantine came before Congress again in 1803 with respect to the District of Columbia. Mitchill, as both a physician and senator for New York, was on the committee to draft the resolution. He wrote in a letter to Rush regarding an enclosed report and hoped Rush would "read it and promulgate it. I have endeavoured to bring the mischief home to the Vessel and Cargo; and to exonerate the ports and their inhabitants between whom the Vessel and Cargo pass.—I made a speech on the subject of Quarantines in the House."[79] On February 5, 1803, Mitchill addressed Congress, stating that the committee he represented "upon the most complete investigation . . . are decidedly of opinion, that the ideas generally entertained concerning quarantine are very erroneous."[80] As he noted to Rush, Mitchill placed the blame for ship sickness not on location and contagion, but the poor living conditions and dangerous cargo within the ships themselves. A lack of cleanliness and purification of spaces on board ship produced pestilential poison the same way a crowded and filthy city created illness.[81] He also was a rare example of a physician who literally took his medical theories into the political arena and consulted with Rush on matters in which medicine and the law crossed paths. As an elite New York City physician and elected representative of his state, Mitchill embodied the association between science and politics in the early republic.

Actions like those of Mitchill in Washington and the physicians of Philadelphia created some small changes. Between large-scale intervention and small-scale changes to personal habit a nation's health, morality, and prosperity could be found. The Philadelphia water system crowns these victories. As if to mark the importance of such a move with an unforgettable symbol, the main hub of the water system, the second pump house, located

---

78 Finger, *Contagious City: The Politics of Public Health in Early Philadelphia*, 141.

79 Samuel Latham Mitchill to Benjamin Rush (1803), LCP, Rush Family Papers, Benjamin Rush Correspondence, Vol. X. Mitctill studied medicine in New York under Samuel Bard and pursued his degree in the mid-1780s at the University of Edinburgh. In addition to his work on changing quarantine laws Mitchill also helped reduce the import duty on rags, a substance often subject to scrutiny according to Barnes. Gross, *Lives of Eminent American Physicians and Surgeons of the Nineteenth Century*, 267–68, 271; Barnes, "Cargo, 'Infection,' and the Logic of Quarantine in the Nineteenth Century."

80 "Legislative Acts/Legal Proceedings." *Morning Chronicle* (New York, New York), April 11, 1803.

81 Ibid.

where Philadelphia City Hall stands now, was also a piece of neoclassical art situated in a designated green space. The system's clean, green setting contrasted with what the architect Benjamin Latrobe (1764–1820) found in the city when he arrived. Upon meeting Latrobe on July 24, 1799, Rush wrote in his commonplace book that the two discussed water and several privies near the river filled with water, presumably mixed with excrement.[82] Such mixing clearly indicated the poor state of Philadelphia's sanitation and was a clear danger to residents. Although the Latrobe system only lasted a decade, Philadelphians' pride in their water endured. The larger Fairmount waterworks replaced Latrobe's original system in 1812 and continued to supply the city for most of the nineteenth century after an upgrade in 1821. By the 1850s, they sat in their own enormous park stretching along both sides of the Schuylkill as a symbol of both health and civic pride.

At the turn of the nineteenth century, an unnamed student recorded Rush claiming, "I am not so sanguine as to suppose that it is possible for man to acquire so much perfection, from science, religion, liberty, & good government as to cease to be mortal; but I am fully persuaded . . . it is possible to produce such a change in his moral character, as shall rise him to a resemblance of angles [sic], nay, more to the likeness of God himself."[83] Such comments certainly fit Rush's style and assumptions about the human body. His optimism about the United States was grounded in his views on medicine, climate, and culture as governed by regular motion. The healthy and republican vision he had for his country rested on scientifically grounded institutions. Those institutions in turn were designed to shape human bodies and minds to become fit republican instruments over decades. Most of his dreams proved too big for implementation. Pennsylvania did not adopt his education policy. Rush's plans for the hospital went forward in a haphazard manner and the city never fully adopted his yellow fever prevention scheme.

Nevertheless, by 1801 Philadelphia boasted the most advanced water works in the country with the Schuylkill River rather than shallow ground water as its source. Pumps and fountains not only provided increased access to clean drinking water, but also water for "washing" the streets of organic detritus. Ships attempting to enter the port during the dangerous summer months first stopped at the new lazaretto several miles downstream for inspection, disinfection, and quarantine of goods (and people if they appeared ill),

---

82   Rush, Commonplace Book (July 24, 1799), APS.
83   Unknown, KCRBM, Mss. Coll 225, Item 17.

marking a middle ground between localist and importationist.[84] By the early nineteenth century, the board of health possessed increased health surveillance powers and additional funding, including a temporary property tax hike to cover the operating costs of the Marine and City Hospitals.[85] Finally, the publication of *Diseases of the Mind* in 1812 solidified Rush's legacy as the "Father of American Psychiatry" and shaped psychiatric treatment well into the nineteenth century.

Medical—and by Rush's reckoning republican—institutions like the Pennsylvania Hospital, Philadelphia Dispensary, and sanitary infrastructure form the tangible results of Rush's theoretical discussions of vibrations and excitement. In these spaces theory and technology intersected with political and social willpower to encourage a particularly American view of "improvement." John Duffy notes the remarkable manner in which Americans responded to yellow fever with public works projects, stating that "[m]uch of what was done probably reflects the paternalism of the eighteenth century, but it also shows the beginnings of social consciousness among middle and upper classes."[86] Benjamin Rush exemplifies this transition to social consciousness. Born into colonial Pennsylvania's "middling sort," his vision of reform reflected the values of social cohesion rather than top-down charity. Collective action, sociability, self-discipline, and applied expert knowledge ensured successful reform. His improvement schemes and attempts to understand the social and physical spheres of human existence through a scientific lens were marshalled to craft a new American society.

Rush's views on the connection between knowledge and republicanism were never far from his mind. Despite claiming in a 1796 letter to radical English physician James Currie that though once a republican "residence in a large city and a wife and eight children have degraded me into a mere physician," the same letter includes insight into the importance of knowledge beyond the political sphere. Writing in the wake of revolution in France, a conservative backlash in Britain, and the presumed retirement of George Washington on the horizon, Rush evaluated the credentials of the

---

84   Barnes, "Cargo, 'Infection,' and the Logic of Quarantine in the Nineteenth Century"; Morman, "Guarding Against Alien Impurities: The Philadelphia Lazaretto 1854–1893."

85   Chapter 2007, "An Act to Alter and Amend the Health Laws of this Commonwealth, and to Incorporate a Board of Managers of a Marine and City Hospitals of the Port of Philadelphia, and for Other Purposes Therein Mentioned," *The Statutes at Large of Pennsylvania* (1798).

86   Duffy, *The Sanitarians: A History of American Public Health*, 50.

likely candidates: Thomas Jefferson and John Adams. As friends and correspondents of both he was in a key position to make such observations. Of Jefferson Rush wrote that he was "a pure republican, enlightened at the same time in chemistry, natural history, and medicine. He is, in a word, a Citizen of the world and the friend of universal peace and happiness." Adams, on the other hand was described as having a problematic attraction of monarchy but "is a republican in his manners and a most upright, worthy man. He will govern without a council, for he possesses great knowledge and the most vigorous internal resources of mind."[87]

Politically (and personally) situated between Adams and Jefferson, Rush highlights the key aspects of republican society that he endeavored to cultivate and support. Knowledge and a lack of self-interest or self-importance characterize a true "republican" for Rush. While on the one hand this definition speaks to personal traits and conduct it also represents the goal of the institutions discussed above. Citizens were not born but constructed. Cities and towns required constant supervision and correction analogous to the care required by the bodies that inhabited them. As evidenced by the prevalence of disease—especially diseases of the mind—no society was yet perfectly healthy in the early nineteenth century. In some of his last letters Rush demonstrated his continued dedication to shaping the health and success of the country. Although he claimed to be tired of party politics, a 69-year-old Rush still had plans for the cultivation of healthy citizens. A little over a month before his death Rush told Jefferson that his "next work will be entitled 'Hygiene, or Rules for the preservation of health accommodated to the climate, diet, manners, and habits of the people of the United States."[88] A month later he concluded a postscript to Adams that stated that he was working on a treatise on disease that would "be accommodated to *all* the classes of readers."[89] Between the two letters Rush demonstrated his commitment to health and access to knowledge about health for American citizens until the last.

---

87 Benjamin Rush, "To James Currie (Philadelphia, July 26, 1796)," in *Letters of Benjamin Rush, Vol. III*, ed. L.H. Butterfield (Princeton, NJ: Princeton University Press, 1951), 779.

88 Benjamin Rush, "To Thomas Jefferson (Philadelphia, March 15th, 1813)," in *Letters of Benjamin Rush, Vol. II*, ed. L.H. Butterfield (Princeton, NJ: Princeton University Press, 1951), 1188.

89 Emphasis in original, Benjamin Rush, "To John Adams (Philadelphia, April 10th, 1813)," in *Letters of Benjamin Rush, Vol. II*, ed. L.H. Butterfield (Princeton, NJ: Princeton University Press, 1951), 1192.

Chapter Eight

Prepping the Next Generation of "Republican Machines"

At the beginning of "An account of the influence of the military and political events of the American Revolution on the Human body," Benjamin Rush listed ten "circumstances" that altered the nature of American bodies (and minds) during the 1770s and 1780s. It is a long list, but worth taking a few moments to consider in Rush's language and its relationship to his thoughts on medicine and politics.

1. The revolution interested every inhabitant of the country of both sexes, and of every rank and age that was capable of reflection. An indifferent, or neutral, spectator of the controversy was scarcely to be found in any of the states.

2. The scenes of war and government, which it introduced, were new to the greatest part of the inhabitants of the United States, and operated with all the force of *novelty* upon the human mind.

3. The controversy was conceived to be the most important of any that had ever engaged the attention of mankind. It was generally believed, by the friends of the revolution, that the very existence of *freedom*, upon our globe, was involved in the issue of the contest in favor of the United States.

4. The American revolution, included in it the care of government, as well as the toils and dangers of war. The American mind was, therefore, frequently occupied, at the *same time*, by the difficult and complicated duties of political and military life.

5. The revolution was conducted by men, who, had been born free, and whose sense of the blessings of liberty was of course more exquisite than if they had just emerged from a state of slavery.

6. The greatest part of the soldiers in the armies of the United States, had family connections and property in the country.

7. The war was carried on by Americans against a nation, to whom they had long been tied by the numerous obligations of consanguinity, laws, religion, commerce, language, interest, and a mutual sense of national glory. The resentment of the Americans of course rose, as is usual in all disputes, in proportion to the number and force of these ancient bonds of affection and union.

8. A predilection to a limited monarchy, as an essential part of a free and safe government, and an attachment to the reigning king of Great Britain . . . were universal in every part of the United States.

9. There was at one time a sudden dissolution of civil government in *all*, and of ecclesiastical establishments in several, of the states.

10. The expenses of the war were supported by means of paper currency, which was continually depreciating.

The anxieties and emotions evident in these paragraphs were not abstract by any means to their original author. Even those who favored independence suffered physical and economic hardship during the war. The early years were especially difficult in the mid-Atlantic with active fighting and territory changing hands. Recounting these aspects in full demonstrates how fundamentally Rush felt changed by the Revolution and how political, economic, and social realities were inextricable from medical concerns. War, economic instability, fears of anarchy, and the realization of starting a new civil society from scratch all affected Rush and his contemporaries.[1] They had to become republicans and become Americans in the crucible of revolution and the violence of civil war. As discussed in the previous chapter not all Americans handled the transition well. The physical and mental damage wrought by war could trigger mental disorder. So too could excessive religious or political enthusiasm associated with liberty. Rush and his friends had to become Americans and republicans carefully. But this would not be the case for his nine children or thousands of other American children of the next generation, sometimes called the "inheriting generation."

Over the course of his career Rush had his eye on the future of republicanism in the United States. Moreover, health required republicanism on a biological as well as social level according to Rush's physiology. Recall, the sympathetic function of organ systems acted as a biological mirror to the shared power he saw in republican families, civil society, and governments. Politics and biology were unavoidably linked. Human bodies were constructed of organ systems that—when working correctly—acted in concert to preserve healthy equilibrium. In Rush's mind, God made human bodies

---

1   Bodle, "The Mid-Atlantic and the American Revolution," 282–99.

in the form of mini-republics and humans should follow that instruction when forming their own societies for political and biological benefits. The survival of self-governance in the United States depended upon the social and biological shaping of the next generation of Americans. Freedom, by Rush's definition, was a state that brought with it enormous responsibility to the community. A republican was free from the tyranny of inherited monarchy and aristocracy, but he was not free from his duties toward fellow citizens. Good citizens were active in politics and voluntary organizations, and interested in family life. The best contributed to the growth of scientific knowledge, reformed religion, and financial improvement of their society. As well-educated, scientifically minded men, physicians were in an excellent position to be the best republicans and instruct their families, colleagues, and patients in the systems of social and physical health.

Rush's views went beyond the more general eighteenth-century assumption that republics required health, at least mental health in the Montesquieu tradition. Rather, he suggested that the republic itself would make health more easily attainable. The relationship was reciprocal rather than linear. Rush placed himself in conversation with other republican scientists of the period who viewed their role as an inherently social one. American thinkers like Franklin, Jefferson, and Noah Webster contemplated the "science" of politics as well as the useful knowledge produced by learned men that could improve the nation's health, culture, and economy.[2] This stance was optimistic, but not without external threats from events across the Atlantic. In Britain and Ireland, the political climate of the 1790s threatened to break the intellectual connections between science, religion, and political identity cultivated by men like Joseph Priestley. The Scotland and England that fostered Rush's intellectual independence and development of republican ideals in the 1760s were slipping away in the 1790s during the conservative backlash to the French Revolution. This was only emphasized by the migration of British radicals in the mid-1790s to the United States. One correspondent in Birmingham explicitly referred to the United States as a political refuge and

---

2   Vinson, "The Society for Political Inquiries: The Limits of Republican Discourse in Philadelphia on the Eve of the Constitutional Convention"; Greene, *American Science in the Age of Jefferson*; Spurlin, *The French Enlightenment in America: Essays on the Times of the Founding Fathers*; Stoll, *Protestantism, Capitalism, and Nature in America*; Jefferson, *Notes on the State of Virginia*; Webster, *Collection of Papers On the Subject of Bilious Fevers, Prevalent in the United States for a Few Years Past*; Park, "The Bonds of Union: Benjamin Rush, Noah Webster, and Defining the Nation in the Early Republic."

sent at least two of his immigrating friends to Rush.[3] From Rush's perspective, the United States looked like the lone place where these associations could flourish and shape society, and that future was far from certain.[4] Writing from Scotland in 1795 one former student Edward Fisher noted that while most in his circle supported the new nation, the government in Britain openly suggested that the United States would not survive if Washington died.[5]

Nevertheless, with proper research and social structures, Rush believed that the United States could prove that republics could succeed and even thrive. In a short note to the Earl of Buchan (David Steuart Erskine) during the unstable 1790s he boasted that "The United States continue to demonstrate by their internal order and external prosperity the practicability, safety, and happiness of republican forms of government and among a people too educated for monarchical principles and habits."[6] Despite—or perhaps because of—anxiety surrounding the future of republics beyond the United States, Rush boldly pronounced his views in classrooms, conversation, and in print. The feedback between health and society could spiral up toward greater harmony between body and society or down toward illness and corruption. As noted in previous chapters, Rush believed that unlearned, unstable, and unhealthy citizens would not work for the good of the state and would in turn prove unfit for self-governance. Meanwhile, the disorganized spaces and institutions they created in their wake would lead to illness and prove unprepared in a crisis. In order to have a strong republic a country first needed republicans; men and women who would automatically and naturally behave moderately, healthfully, and for the good of the populace. Rush used the term "republican machine" to describe this transformation of Americans into natural republicans who would promote social and physical

---

3   D. Milne to Benjamin Rush (1795), LPS Rush Family Papers.

4   Kramnick, "Eighteenth-Century Science and Radical Social Theory: The Case of Joseph Priestley's Scientific Liberalism"; Schaffer, "Measuring Virtue: Eudiometry, Enlightenment and Pneumatic Medicine," 281–318; Haakonssen, *Medicine and Morals in the Enlightenment: John Gregory, Thomas Percival, and Benjamin Rush*; Dolan, "Conservative Politicians, Radical Philosophers and the Aerial Remedy for the Diseases of Civilization," 35–54; Graham, "Revolutionary in Exile: The Emigration of Joseph Priestley to America 1794–1804," 1–213.

5   Edward Fisher to Benjamin Rush (1795), LPS, Rush Family Papers.

6   Benjamin Rush to The Earl of Buchan (June 25, 1795), *Letters of Benjamin Rush, Vol. II*, 761.

health amongst themselves and future generations. Children were the obvious targets for this kind of republican molding.

Medicine was Rush's profession. He worked for decades to improve American health and build institutions to continue that work after his death. The ultimate example of his system, however, appears in his discussions of education and the physical development of children: the future republican machines. This chapter discusses Rush's theories on education, how they used his medical ideas, and how they shaped the republican system of medicine as he understood it by the 1790s. Informed by physiology and in conversation with social theorists, Rush's writing on education highlights the manner in which his politics and projects of improvement had medical science as their foundation.

Republican Children, Republican Machines

Rush's interest in education began in earnest during the 1780s, an era when his writing on social and political institutions in general reached a fever pitch. The country was young and in need of clear direction for its future. At the beginning of his essay "A plan for establishing public schools in Pennsylvania, and for conducting education agreeably to a republican form of government" Rush explicitly stated that, "[f]reedom can exist only in the society of knowledge. Without learning, men are incapable of knowing their rights, and where learning is confined to a few people, liberty can be neither equal nor universal."[7] Without proper education citizens might fall under the influence of demagogues and lose what freedoms they had without fully realizing their mistake. With education Rush believed citizens could become "republican machines," healthy and naturally oriented to enjoy freedom and contribute to the improvement of their country.[8]

These new republican machines were not an abstraction in the Rush household. In 1786 (the year he published "A Plan for Establishing Public Schools") Benjamin and Julia Rush were parents to five children: nine-year-old John, seven-year-old Emily, six-year-old Richard, two-year-old Mary, and infant James. Unlike Rush, his children grew up understanding themselves

---

7   Rush, "A Plan for Establishing Public Schools in Pennsylvania, and for
     Conducting Education Agreeably to a Republican Form of Government.
     Addressed to the Legislature and Citizens of Pennsylvania, in the Year 1786," 1.
8   Rush, "A Plan for Establishing," 14.

to be American citizens not British subjects.[9] They had no king to reject or Parliament to revolt against. The challenges of the "inheriting generation" differed from their parents, something of which their parents were well aware. As inheritors they were tasked with the fulfilment of the republican promise. The transition from subject to citizen was difficult for parents, but Rush believed citizenship and the perfection of the republic could be rendered natural for children in body and mind through strict upbringing and widespread education designed to cultivate the moral faculty. A keen interest in mental health and early childhood development grounded Rush's plans marking them out as a key part of his medical theory. He also practiced these ideas on his own growing family.

Between 1777 and 1801 Julia Stockton Rush gave birth to thirteen children. Nine lived to adulthood; six boys and three girls. Benjamin and Julia were strict parents and concerned with the moral, physical, and intellectual development of their children. This was all the more pressing in early years. Student lecture notes from the 1790s show that Rush, following both John Gregory and Scottish professor of midwifery George Young, believed that early childhood development was a pivotal period for physical and moral health. He argued that "we learn more in the 1st three years of our lives, than in any 30 afterwards," and that "the Treatment of Children during the first Month at least I trust deserves your particular attention."[10] The interconnected systems of mind, nerves, blood vessels, and lymph (introduced in chapter 3) were most malleable early in childhood. The impressions and actions pressed upon not-quite-formed infants could literally direct and shape their future physical and mental health. Structural irregularities caused by a lax upbringing encouraged illness and formed a weak constitution. Meanwhile a lack of mental and physical engagement—through walking, early talking, and learning the nature of different objects—would lead to an underdeveloped and unexercised mind and brain. Small children, according to Rush, needed to be encouraged to exercise their bodies, learn simple works and concepts, and consume a wholesome diet.

In older children, Rush noted the health benefits of fresh air and exercise and argued miasmata and dangerous effluvia were known to build up

---

9   For more on the generational differences between "founders" and "inheritors", see Appleby, *Inheriting the Revolution: The First Generation of Americans*; Yokota, *Unbecoming British: How Revolutionary America Became a Postcolonial Nation*.

10 John Spangler, "Acute and Chronic Diss [sic] taken from the Lectrs [sic] of Doctor Rush Professor of the Theory & Practice of Medicine in the College of Philadelphia 1790 & 91," KCRBM, Ms. Coll 225, Item 4, Vol. 1–2.

in classrooms stuffed with children. While education was important, poorly designed curriculums and classroom spaces could be dangerous. Sedentary lives operated against the natural needs of young bodies, as Rush argued in his work on amusements and punishments.

> I have been called to many hundred children who have been seized with indispositions in school, which evidently arose from the action of morbid effluvia, produced by the confined breath and perspiration of too great a number of children in one room. To obviate these evils, children should be permitted, after they have said their lessons, to amuse themselves in the open air. . . . Their minds will be strengthened, as well as their bodies relieved by them. To oblige a sprightly boy to sit *seven* hours in a day, with his little arms pinioned to his sides and his neck unnaturally bent toward his book; and for *no crime!*—what cruelty and folly are manifested, by such an absurd mode of instructing or governing young people![11]

The physical and academic worked together in Rush's view of childrearing and school design. Schools too often produced sickness and lackluster students rather than the excited and thoughtful pupils the Republic required. Rush took a special interest in the early development of his own children marking the passage of developmental milestones and tinkering with their education and play. Even in moments of external crisis he paid close attention to the education, health, and growth of his large family. When recovering from yellow fever in October 1793 he wrote to Julia inquiring after each of their seven children at the time, despite his weakened state. Lying in bed and fearing the worst—he later wrote "I could hardly expect to survive so violent an attach of the fever"—his thoughts turned to his family, safely ensconced at Julia's childhood home in Princeton.[12] He paid special attention to developmental milestones for their youngest. Little Julia Rush was less than a year old when her father wrote asking about her teeth and if she knew any words and mother responded by proudly noting her attempts to walk and ability to identify articles of clothing.[13] Despite suffering from a bad cold and teething the baby continued satisfactory physical and mental development. Her mother wrote that "she [baby Julia] does not go alone—but can walk all around the room by chairs—and can point out all her articles of dress—and

---

11   Rush, "Thoughts upon the Amusements and Punishments Which Are Proper for Schools. Addressed to George Clymer, Esq.," 62–63.

12   Rush, *An Account of the Bilious Remitting Yellow Fever as It Appeared in the City of Philadelphia in the Year 1793*, 361.

13   Benjamin Rush "To Mrs. Rush" (713).

all her features upon being asked."[14] These activities introduced new concepts to the baby's mind and stimulated physical and psychological growth.

Little Julia's siblings were also carefully monitored during the epidemic. Long-distance parenting meant that Julia Rush relayed regular information about the children to Benjamin, alternately responding to his questions and encouraging him to take an active, if virtual role in their upbringing. Physical development remained central for the youngest children Julia and Benjamin (about 18 months old) while academic pursuits were prescribed for the older children. Anne Emily (14) and Mary (nine) attended a boarding school in Trenton. In Princeton James (seven) attended a local day school while his elder brothers John (16) and Richard (12) undertook independent study supervised by their mother and occasionally directed by their father by post.[15] Formal education was not an artifact of being away from home during the epidemic for the boys or girls. Between 1798 and 1800 James Rush attended boarding school in Maryland run by one of his father's Hall cousins.[16] Meanwhile, Julia stayed closer to home and graduated from Madame Rivardi's intellectually rigorous female seminary in Philadelphia in 1808. Benjamin Rush was a trustee.[17]

In addition to observing his children, Rush tested his theories on them. For example, he tried new forms of corrective punishment designed to change behavior by manipulating the faculties of the mind. Unusually for the era, Rush did not use corporal punishment on children. He argued that it was unlikely to result in positive permanent change and likely to damage the moral sense of children (not to mention their bodies). Instead, he used psychology to try and reform their behaviors, bodies, and minds for good.[18] As a father, Rush punished bad behavior by isolating the child from his or her siblings. In some instances, a child might be left alone without amusement or contact with others for a whole day. Such isolation was supposed to calm the mind as well as frustrate the child (it was after all a punishment). This approach mimicked tactics Rush used on "insane" patients at

---

14   Julia Rush to Benjamin Rush (October 18, 1793), APS, Julia Stockton Rush Collection of 20 Letters, Mss.B.R.894.

15   Julia Rush to Benjamin Rush, Mss.B.R.894.

16   Letters to Benjamin Rush detail his son's progress and education. J. Hall to Benjamin Rush (1798–1800), LCP, Rush Family Papers, Benjamin Rush Correspondence, Vol. XXII and XXIV.

17   Johnson, "Madame Rivardi's Seminary in the Gothic Mansion," 5, 23.

18   Rush, "Thoughts upon the Amusements and Punishments," 65–66.

the Pennsylvania Hospital and recommended for convicts to reform adult criminal behavior.[19]

Boredom, Rush felt, forced children (and adults) into a mode of self-reflection and calmed the irregular motions of nervous tissue excited by bad behavior. Corporal punishment, on the other hand, created the irregular motions that defined disease and could even desensitize the child to such actions. A loss of physical sensitivity could ultimately reduce a person's ability to be affected emotionally by others, eventually dehumanizing both the punished and the punisher. In extreme cases permanent physical damage could destroy a child and their chances to be a healthy and productive member of society. Rush noted that "the effects of thumping the head, boxing the ears, and pulling the hair, in impairing the intellects, by means of injuries done to the brain, are too obvious to be mentioned." At one point in his essay "Thoughts upon the Amusements and Punishments Which Are Proper for Schools," Rush went so far as to associate corporal punishments with the work of the Devil—"who knows how great an enemy knowledge is to his kingdom"—who was trying to subvert the better nature of humans and halt the evolution of society. In place of physical punishment Rush recommended—and utilized—isolation and shame to alter behavior and hopefully enforce republican virtues of selflessness and moderation.[20]

As demonstrated here, education in a republic was, above all, designed to create good citizens, with an emphasis on the word *good*. The "moral faculty" Rush spoke of operated like other innate faculties or abilities of the mind. In his *Medical Inquiries and Observations Upon Diseases of the Mind* from 1812, Rush enumerated nine such faculties: understanding, memory, imagination, passions, principle of faith, will, moral faculty, conscience, and "sense of Deity."[21] The general concept grew in popularity during the eighteenth century, especially in the Scottish Enlightenment circles Rush emulated as a

---

19 Carlson and Wollock, "Benjamin Rush and His Insane Son," 1319–20; Rush, "Thoughts upon the Amusements and Punishments," 69–70; Manion, *Liberty's Prisoners: Carceral Culture in Early America*; Rush, "An Enquiry into the Effects of Public Punishments upon Criminals, and upon Society. Read in the Society for Promoting Political Enquiries, Convened at the Hosue of Benjamin Franklin, Esq. in Philadelphia, March 9th, 1787," 136–63.

20 Rush, "Thoughts upon the Amusements and Punishments Which Are Proper for Schools. Addressed to George Clymer, Esq.," 64–68.

21 Rush, *Medical Inquiries and Observations Upon the Diseases of the Mind*, 2.

young man.[22] The theory of faculties provided a framework for early psychology to build from. The exact nature and number of faculties varied between thinkers, including Francis Hutcheson, Joseph Priestley, William Cullen, and David Hartley. Despite variation, however, each system agreed that certain mental abilities were inherent to the mind and could be cultivated or left unimproved depending on education.

That sense of right and wrong required careful cultivation if the republic were to be protected from corruption and self-interest. In a 1786 oration to the American Philosophical Society Rush defined the moral faculty as "a power in the human mind of distinguishing and chusing [sic] good and evil; or, in other words, virtue and vice. It is a native principle, and though it is capable of improvement by experience and reflection, it is not derived from either of them."[23] That improvement of the moral faculty on a national scale was required, in Rush's opinion. He and like-minded thinkers agreed that universal education for American boys (and possibly girls) was the ideal mechanism to shape the faculties from an early age. Schools would have the ability not only to promote the spread of factual information, but also to instill a sense of public duty and private morality. These ideas surrounding education, meanwhile, are directly related to Rush's professional interests in mental and physical development in childhood and "diseases of the mind" in adults. Education had the potential to end or exacerbate social problems in the republic.

A peculiar example of this is found in Rush's views on Greek and Latin language instruction. Above all, Rush despised the manner in which Greek and Latin dominated boys' early education. At the time, classical education dominated elite education and continued to do so for a century more.[24] The texts, he argued, taxed their brains in unnatural ways. Stories and myths also exposed them to immoral concepts. Rush wrote in an essay on Greek and Latin that "[t]he study of some . . . classics is unfavourable [sic] to morals

---

22   Rush specifically cited Lord Kames as the originator of the concept of an innate sense of the Deity; Rush, 355; McCosh, *The Scottish Philosophy, Biographical, Expository, Critical, From Hutcheson to Hamilton*, 175.

23   Rush, *An Oration, Delivered before the American Philosophical Society: Held in Philadelphia on the 27th of February, 1786; Containing an Enquiry into the Influence of Physical Causes upon the Moral Faculty* ..., 1.

24   For a discussion of American uses of classical texts and education, see Caroline Winterer, *The Culture of Classicism: Ancient Greece and Rome in American Intellectual Life, 1780–1910* (Baltimore: The Johns Hopkins University Press, 2002).

and religions. Indelicate amours, and shocking vices both of gods and men, fill many parts of them. Hence an early and dangerous acquaintance with vice; and hence . . . a diminished respect for the unity and perfections of the true God."[25]

Rush feared that by stuffing the minds of young boys (four or five years old) with knowledge of Greek and Latin words rather than ideas about physical objects they would not develop a sufficient understanding of the world around them. This difficulty explained why boys disliked their lessons in Latin and only enjoyed them for stories (of dubious morality) or for the honor of competition with classmates. Small children were simply not ready for the abstract principles introduced in language lessons. Nor would many of them actually need Latin or Greek in their future careers. The true joy of language acquisition, Rush argued, belonged to a more mature brain.[26] In extreme circumstances, he wrote, "sprightly boys of excellent capacities for useful knowledge, have been so disgusted with the dead languages, as to retreat from the drudgery of schools, to low company, whereby they have become bad members of society."[27] For a country whose future relied upon an upright citizenry and innovation in the fields of "useful knowledge" even the theoretical possibility of a "Latin to crime" pipeline was viewed by Rush as an existential threat.

Rather than study the classics, Rush argued that natural history and geography were subjects better suited to the minds of children. The active learning and inquisitive nature of science matched a young child's inclination to acquire new ideas. They picked up new words, images, and simple ideas. In later childhood and early adulthood those simple ideas could compound and lead to an appreciation of philosophy, theology, and linguistics. For Rush, the basic principles of childrearing and the techniques of active lecturing were designed to produce well-educated republicans as discussed below. Healthy mental and physical development were prerequisites for healthy moral development. Behavioral management remained a key concern for Rush with respect to education.

---

25 Rush, "Observations upon the Study of the Latin and Greek Languages, as a Branch of Liberal Education, with Hints of a Plan of Liberal Instruction, without Them, Accommodated to the Present State of Society, Manners, and Government in the United States," 24.

26 Rush, "Observations," 22–23. Rush worried that the content of the classics were largely amoral or too violent for children and would provide bad lessons for life and public service, Rush, 24.

27 Rush, "Observations," 23–24.

Even beyond the confines of the home he tried to control his growing children's behavior by shaping their environments. When his eldest son John enrolled at the College of New Jersey (Princeton) Rush refused to allow his son to board with other students who might encourage poor behavior or slacking off. This fear seems to have originated from Rush's own self-reflection on his teen years, which he considered ill-used. Perhaps, like many first-time parents, Rush was overanxious about John's future. To prevent what the father considered time-wasting, the son lived with a faculty member and friend of his parents, Walter Minto. Nevertheless, John managed to misbehave and was caught playing cards on a Sunday, a serious transgression at Presbyterian Princeton. Rush pulled his son out of school permanently (rather than re-enroll after a school-mandated suspension) and educated him at home fearing that the boy was falling into moral corruption through contact with his classmates. At the end of a letter to Minto the distressed father wrote, "I conceive, after what has past, he [John] can never recover his character so as to appear to advantage either with his masters or among his fellow students" and "[w]e shall always retain a grateful sense of your kindness to our poor deluded boy."[28] Moral education, according to Rush's republican ideology needed to go hand in hand with academics. In John's case than meant a medical education carried out at home under the careful supervision of his worried and disappointed father. That anxiety only continued in the case of John Rush ultimately leading to his ill-fated naval career and incarceration in the Pennsylvania Hospital for psychosis detailed in the previous chapter.

Republican Education

In 1801, Benjamin and Julia Rush's third son James was studying at Princeton. Unlike his oldest brother John with his checkered educational history, James appeared to be the ideal student. Never in trouble for card-playing like John, James had roommates of whom his parents approved and did not participate in a college "insurrection" in early 1802. Throughout this period, Benjamin's letters to his son were full of advice and instructions both large and small. He praised his son's letter writing, noting and correcting

---

28   Benjamin Rush to Walter Minto (Philadelphia, September 19, 1792), Rush, *Letters of Benjamin Rush*, 622. despite the initial expulsion John's fellow students were readmitted the next year Carlson and Wollock, "Benjamin Rush and His Insane Son," 1320–21.

spelling and grammar.[29] On the other hand, he also pressured James to be more productive in a letter from May 1802.

> Recollect, my dear boy, your age and the years you have lost. Improve every moment you can spare from your recitations in reading useful books. Your uncle's [Richard Stockton's] library I presume will always be open to you, where you will find history, poetry, and probably other books suited to your age. . . . Remember the profession for which you are destined. Without an extensive and correct education, you cannot expect to succeed in it. Do not, my dear son, disappoint my expectations and wishes of bequeathing my patients to an enlightened and philosophical physician. If you discover a relish for knowledge, your wishes shall be gratified to the utmost of my power. . . . You shall visit Europe, if my life be spared, and draw from foreign universities all that you require to enable you to settle with advantage in Philadelphia.[30]

At the time Rush wrote this letter, the boy who had "lost" so many years was only 16. However, he represented the only Rush son with a clear medical future after the disappointment of John and of the second son, Richard Rush, who chose to study law and entered politics. Younger sons Benjamin (10), Samuel (5), and infant William were still too small for such specific scrutiny. Being Benjamin Rush's son was not easy. The expectations placed on James were intense and those on his siblings only slightly less so. While not all took a medical path, the call for enlightened—that is rational, informed, and scientifically minded—citizens crossed professional boundaries.

What Rush wrote to James he could just as easily have addressed to this next generation: Work hard, keep regular habits, and don't waste time. These virtues permeate Rush's educational and medical thinking. Intellectual engagement, thoughtfulness, and the fight against boredom also came to bear on educational instruction and training young memories. Although Rush mainly published on the question of how children were best instructed, he used similar techniques in the medical lecture hall to engage the minds and faculties of adult men. The only difference was that in the case of medical students he openly explained his tactics.

Medical lectures were long and for many students a repetition of previous years' study. Discipline may not have been a concern but knowledge retention

---

29   Butterfield, 839, 843; Benjamin Rush "To James Rush (Philadelphia, November 23rd 1801)," *Letters of Benjamin Rush*, Vol. II, 839; Benjamin Rush "To James Rush (Philadelphia, January 25, 1802)," *Letters of Benjamin Rush*, Vol. II, 842.

30   Benjamin Rush "To James Rush (Philadelphia, May 25, 1802)," *Letters of Benjamin Rush*, Vol. II, 849–50.

and fighting boredom remained important for the instructor. In the class-room, Rush demonstrated the importance of engaging multiple senses for the sake of memory. His techniques seemed to work. Many years after Rush's death former students discussed the impressive nature of his lecture style. Thomas D. Mitchell (1791–1865), opened his series of medical lectures for the year 1848 at the University of Pennsylvania with a talk on Rush's character as a physician, teacher, patriot, and friend. Under the heading of "teacher" Mitchell claimed that Rush possessed a unique manner of oratory.

> Of Dr. Rush's manner of lecturing, it is impossible to convey an adequate idea. His voice was one of sweetest euphony, adapting itself most easily to the *variety of sentiment and presented, an eminently calculated to riven the attention of his class.* Although he read almost every word, and occupied the sitting posture through-out his course, with only now and then an exception, he was unquestionably the most *eloquent and instructive* teacher I have ever heard. When he desired to give peculiar and unwonted emphasis and power to something he regarded as specially [sic] important, he *rose from his chair, and with inexpressible dignity, pronounced the sentiment.*[31]

Strong oratory and engagement of the senses by changing his physical posi-tion to add emphasis helped Rush's students remember and engage with material. That same year, another former student, Charles Meigs (1792–1869) wrote that when Rush "arose and stood up . . . casting his eyes over the large hall, looking to the left, and then to the right, and then to those in front of him." This movement and pause were followed by the phrase, "obsta principiis," that he wished them to remember.[32] Rush stood and engaged the sense of sight, paused to break the rhythm of the lecture, and spoke loudly and clearly to address the sense of hearing. A firm memory resulted. Presumably a monotone and unmoving lecture was easily forgotten due to lack of stimulation. Simple reading, meanwhile, did not aid memory and was easily forgotten because it stimulated only one sense, that of sight. Rush even went so far as to claim that sight was not necessarily the strongest sense humans possessed, recalling that Benjamin Franklin "could never recollect

---

31 Emphasis added, Mitchell, *The Character of Rush, an Introductory to the Course on the Theory and Practice of Medicine in the Philadelphia College of Medicine*, 13.

32 Meigs, *Females and Their Diseases: A Series of Letters to His Class*, 372–73. The phrase "obsta principiis" seems to be a quote from Ovid's "Remedia Amoris" and indicate the association between emotion and health and the need to stave off disease from the very start. Ovid, "Remedia Amoris," 320–52; Kruschwitz, "Principiis Obsta: Resist Beginnings!" 2017.

his old acquaintances until they spoke," suggesting the power of auditory learning.[33] Meigs may have subconsciously applied the same logic—engagement of the senses and alteration of expectations to aid memory—to his own work. *Females and Their Diseases*—the book that included the above anecdote—is an epistolary textbook with short chapters written in an easy and memorable style. By mixing styles and writing clearly, Meigs captured the imagination, and memory, of his readers as his preceptor may have done.

The lecture Meigs described took place at the very end of Rush's life and career in 1813, by which time the senior physician was an experienced teacher and convinced of the value of education.[34] Numerous lecture notes (Rush's and those of his students) include records of emphatic language, including repetition of key concepts, statements in "all caps," underlining, and exclamation points that may echo in writing the dynamism of the lecture itself. Mitchell also hinted at Rush's style of examination and questioning. He claimed that "[p]upils were compelled to meditate, reason and judge for themselves, and the habit thus formed by daily practice . . . may serve to explain the fact, that in no similar portion of our country's history was so much useful and original matter issued from the press, as during the last twenty years of the life of Dr. Rush."[35] Student meditation and questions formed the basis for original medical work and empowered learners. Rush encouraged students to continue their learning outside of the classroom. He told Henry Powell's class to "[m]ake it a constant practice to think & talk over the Lectures which you have heard when you return home, this will serve as a test to discover whether you understand them."[36]

As an instructor, Rush provided biological reasons for the improvement of understanding through discussion. He argued that proper study invigorated the mind and better trained it to analyze local situations and remember content introduced in medical school and hospital practice. In this manner Rush medicalized a common practice, that of exchanging and editing classroom notes as a group.[37] This was all the more urgent, as Rush noted in his "American Editions" of British medical texts as well as in

---

33 Hare (1796), KCRBM, Ms. Coll. 225, Box 6, Item 9.

34 According to Rush's records Meigs attended lectures in the winter of 1812–1813, the last year Rush taught before his death in April 1813. LCP, Rush Family Papers, Benjamin Rush Papers, Vol. 106, Yi2 7270.

35 Mitchell, *The Character of Rush*, 17–18.

36 Powell, UPenn, Ms. Coll. 225, Box 3, Item 7, Vol. I, 1809.

37 Taylor, "Plummer to Cullen: Novelty in William Cullen's Chemical Pedagogy," 68–69.

correspondence, because American doctors were more likely to encounter unexpected environments, diseases, and social situations than those of their European counterparts. The twin characteristics of republics—their promise and instability—are never far from Rush's mind here. Nor the instability of the American climate.[38]

Rush believed that proper medical education and the resulting profession of gentlemen best served the interests of the country. He worried that dependence on education and books alone would not be enough. Journals and professional organizations could go a long way in ensuring that such an education continued beyond the lecture hall. In 1812, Samuel Bard similarly proposed to the medical students of New York that: "[i]t is . . . in the constitution of our frame, and in the natural structure of our minds, that we discover the reason and truth of the maxim, that peace of society and the stability of government, especially of free governments, depend upon the instruction, information, and correct habits of the people."[39] Good government for these men literally required educated minds and healthy bodies. Moreover, nature required health and education to function properly in accordance with her own natural laws. For the United States to function, therefore, the bodies that made up the body politic had to function. The future of the country could very literally be in the hands of the young men gathered to hear Rush speak.

Of course, not all of Rush's "republican machines" were identical. Republican educational roles broke down along gendered lines. Rush believed men and women fundamentally differed on a physical and mental level from birth. In the case of education and republican society, this belief led directly to Rush's advocacy for single-sex education with curricular differences based on age and sex. Education in general would cultivate the faculties in both boys and girls but to different degrees and with different aims. It would also introduce gendered forms of labor. Rush considered idleness dangerous to both moral and physical development and appropriate work necessary to children's development, writing in 1786 that "[t]he effects of steady labour [sic] in early life, in creating virtuous habits is . . . remarkable."[40]

---

38 Taylor, 68–69.

39 Bard, "A Discourse on the Importance of Medical Education; Delivered on the 4th of November, 1811, at the Opening of the Present Session of the Medical School of the College of Physicians and Surgeons. By Samuel Bard, M.D. President of the College of Physicians," 371.

40 Rush, *An Inquiry Into the Influence of Physical Causes Upon the Moral Faculty: Delivered Before a Meeting of the American Philosophical Society, Held at*

Boys, in a republican system, were encouraged to be active and self-sufficient. An educated male population, Rush specifically argued, would be less of a burden on the state's resources and have the ability to work toward the greater good. Moral and educated men would commit fewer crimes and contribute more to the agricultural, industrial, and internal improvements required of a growing, independent economy. Educated women, meanwhile, would act as moral compasses for their fathers, brothers, husbands, and male friends. Within the home, Rush expected women to uphold the republican virtues of moderation and rationality by managing efficient homes without extravagance or waste. Furthermore, he frequently remarked on the natural morality of women and their greater sense of the deity. Although these faculties could be corrupted, with proper education women would check men's ambitions and self-interestedness with examples of domestic morality. Like the system of republican government with its various parts checking each other, the domestic balance of morality and power would set the tone for society as a whole. Republican homes modeled greater social values. Marriages formed partnerships and children were expected to grow up in safety, punished when necessary for correction but never arbitrarily or capriciously. Schools could further reinforce these ideals making them universal in the next generation of Americans. From carful parental guidance and correct institutions, the minds (and ultimately bodies) of young Americans would be shaped to fit their society. In the end, Rush argued that education more than paid for itself.[41]

For boys, Rush viewed formal education as the best way to shape "republican machines." In terms of a theoretical structure, Rush's ideas appear most clearly in a 1786 essay for the establishment of public schools in Pennsylvania where he set out his plan for all levels of male education. In the text he used medical and psychological theory to support changes to the traditional systems that dominated eighteenth-century schoolrooms. In its most basic format, the plan recommended that all boys receive as much education as society required and their personal talents allowed. Each town of 100 families or more would be required to provide a primary school. Students who excelled could continue their education and take advantage of county-wide college preparatory academies, regional colleges (in Philadelphia, Pittsburgh, Lancaster, and Carlisle), and the University of Pennsylvania for post-graduate professional training in law, medicine, politics, and the sciences.[42]

Philadelphia, on the Twenty-Seventh of February, 1786, 14.

41 Rush, "Of the Mode of Education Proper in a Republic," 7–20.

42 Rush, "A Plan for Establishing," 1–5.

This hypothetical public system would have allowed those of modest means but extraordinary talent to pursue higher education, which in turn they (as good citizens) would use for the improvement of their whole country. One can imagine how such a system would have benefited a young Benjamin Rush—especially a version of Benjamin Rush who lacked the family support and commitment of his mother. In this respect, Rush was like his friend Thomas Jefferson, who proposed a public system for Virginia around the same time. They differed, however, in terms of local control, with Jefferson favoring a secular centralized system and Rush promoting a more flexible system. Rush, in his quest for promoting morality along with knowledge, argued that religious groups should run local schools and that the Bible should be taught alongside modern subjects. He was also open to schools in which the language of instruction was German rather than English, based on local populations.[43] Although Rush's plan was not adopted neither were the grand schemes of contemporaries championing public education, such as Noah Webster, despite attention from the press.[44] Nevertheless, Rush celebrated what he viewed as steps in the right direction, like Pennsylvania's 1792 decision to fund public schools for boys.[45] He also appeared to influence the views of his students. The historian Benjamin Justice notes that two anonymous submissions to the American Philosophical Society's 1797 contest to propose a new educational system had a medical background and followed many of Rush's suggestions although not written by Rush himself.[46] He implies that such submissions are a reasonable approximation of Rush's ideas and the appeal of such ideas among medical men.

Beyond access to education, Rush had clear opinions about what boys needed to learn in school. Unsurprisingly, Rush also promoted wide knowledge of science among the population. This shaped his second major objection to the instruction of Latin and opposition to writing in Latin. Keeping the sciences cloaked in dead languages kept the pool of potential American

---

43 Justice, "'The Great Contest': The American Philosophical Society Education Prize of 1795 and the Problem of American Education," 199; Rush, "'A Defense of the Use of the Bible as a School Book. Addressed to the Rev. Jeremy Belknap of Boston,'" 92–113.

44 Justice, *Founding Fathers, Education, and "the Great Contest": The American Philosophical Society Prize of 1797*, 2–3.

45 Rush and Biddle, *A Memorial Containing Travels Through Life Or Sundry Incidents in the Life of Dr. Benjamin Rush, Born Dec. 24, 1745 (Old Style) Died April 19, 1813*, 133.

46 Justice, "Introduction," 12.

men of science too small for a new republic. Rush argued that as long as "Greek and Latin are the only avenues of science, education will always be confined to a few people. It is only by rendering knowledge universal, that a republican form of government can be preserved in our country."[47] To thrive as a republic, or simply as an independent nation, the United States needed to produce knowledge, agricultural products, and manufactures in the most efficient manner possible. Similarly, for individuals, the assumption that intelligence could be measured only by competence in dead languages ignored other types of brilliance that Rush wanted to cultivate.

On the other hand, he thought modern languages were far more appropriate for republicans to study. Rush argued that boys could begin lessons in French and German, by their early teen years. German in particular loomed large in Pennsylvania, which Rush thought of as a potentially bilingual state in the 1780s. Contrary to his friend and mentor Benjamin Franklin, who worried about the increasing numbers of German-speaking immigrants in the mid-eighteenth century, Benjamin Rush had little issue with linguistic or cultural diversity as long as it did not act as an impediment for higher education. Such an outlook may have seemed all the more practical in a United States where one in four people spoke something other than English as their first language.[48] In his plan for a Pennsylvanian educational system, Rush recommended that public schools be conducted in *either* English or German, depending on the local population. He also became deeply involved with the establishment of Franklin College (now Franklin and Marshall College) in Lancaster as an ecumenical and bilingual institution to bring German-Pennsylvanians into the learned professions from both Lutheran and Reformed families. A degree from Franklin, he hoped when writing to his mother-in-law Annis Boudinot Stockton, would allow German-American men to attend the University of Pennsylvania and serve their communities as educated ministers, lawyers, and physicians.[49]

---

47 Rush, "Observations upon the Study of the Latin and Greek Languages, as a Branch of Liberal Education, with Hints of a Plan of Liberal Instruction, without Them, Accommodated to the Present State of Society, Manners, and Government in the United States," 25.

48 Lepore, *A Is for American: Letters and Other Characters in the Newly United States*, 28.

49 Rush, *A Letter by Dr. Benjamin Rush Describing the Consecration of the German College at Lancaster in June, 1787: Printed, with an Introduction, from a Newly Discovered Manuscript, Now in the Fackenthal Library at Franklin and Marshall College.*

Despite Rush's intentions, reform of American language education remained in the future. Even his sons largely conformed to expected educational practice. Letters from J. Hall (a schoolmaster and cousin of Rush on his mother's side) between 1798 and 1800 detail the academy education of James Rush (1786–1869). Hall wrote about James's language study, claiming, "[w]ithout your knowledge, no doubt, he [James] has been studying a foreign language [Latin], before he learned ye Rudiments of his own."[50] A year later, he wrote that James was making good progress in both Latin and French.[51] However, Hall agreed with Rush with respect to the importance of science education. In the same letter in which he discussed James's progress in foreign languages, he noted the arrival from London of "Terrestrial & Celestial Globes; . . . a Medical Electrical Machine, a Theodolite for surveying Land with an apparatus for levelling water courses, taking angles of Elevation &ct. . . . Besides the use of these Instruments . . . pupils will have the benefit of seeing ye practice of extensively carried on."[52] Practical skills, especially geography and surveying, certainly appealed to those Americans focused on the physical improvement and western expansion of their republic. Electricity too, was increasingly viewed as a skill with practical and perhaps medical uses during this period . . . an appropriate subject for a future physician.[53]

By stressing the practical as well as the social and moral advantages of education, Rush hoped that the country would contribute more than its fair share to commerce, manufacture, and especially agriculture and medicine. A letter to Rush from his New York colleague David Hosack praised the republican virtues of medical education and the role Rush played in encouraging American practitioners to make this connection. Hosack wrote: "America has already shewn the predicability (sic) of a republican form of government I have no doubt she is also destined to give the world many important productive lessons in science and medicine—you have done much for the formation of medical literature and in elevating the character of our country."[54]

---

50 J. Hall (1798), LCP, Rush Family Papers, Benjamin Rush Correspondence, Vol. XXII.

51 J. Hall (1799), Vol. XXIV.

52 J. Hall (1798), Vol. XXII.

53 Delbourgo, *A Most Amazing Scene of Wonders: Electricity and Enlightenment in Early America.*

54 David Hosack to Benjamin Rush, Vol. XXVII, Benjamin Rush Correspondence, Rush Family Papers, LCP.

Science, in this instance, benefited from the republic and vice versa due, in part, to Rush's promotional work.

Despite their democratic flavor, the educational opportunities outlined above were nearly all designed for the benefit of boys, not girls. Calls to correct the perceived deficiency of female education in the United States started to gain traction in the late 1780s through the 1790s. This accompanied the growing popularity of reforming writers like British proto-feminist Mary Wollstonecraft, who argued that any perceived inferiority of women's minds was the result of neglecting the education of girls.[55] In part this reflects the general assumption that a successful society required a standard level of knowledge—reading, writing, grammar, and basic mathematics— as intimated by Philadelphia clergyman and vice-provost of the University of Pennsylvania Samuel Magaw in his 1787 address to the Young Ladies' Academy.[56] In the past historians have characterized Rush as a champion for improved education for girls based on his involvement with the Young Ladies' Academy and his educational writings.[57] It is true that he promoted improved education for girls in general and oversaw the education of his own daughters. But that does not mean that he shared the ideas of a contemporary like Mary Wollstonecraft and endorsed real equality of the sexes.

Nevertheless, his writings do point to a shift in the perceived role of women in the United States, acknowledging the considerable intellectual work done by women and girls in educating children, supporting family members, managing households, and working in family businesses. A 1776 letter from Benjamin to Julia Rush hints at the role of women in business. Although the document comes from only their first year of marriage, it is clear that Julia Rush was already a necessary part of the household. After spending several weeks with her parents in New Jersey her husband wrote that "business suffers from the want of you. My pretices [sic] are young,

---

55 Wollstonecraft, *Thoughts on the Education of Daughters: With Reflections on Female Conduct, in the More Important Duties of Life.*

56 Magaw, "Address Delivered in the Young Ladies' Academy, at Philadelphia, on February 8th, 1787, at the Close of a Public Examination," 25–28.

57 For more on Rush's work and ideas on the Academy, see McMahon, *Mere Equals: The Paradox of Educated Women in the Early American Republic*; Nash, "Rethinking Republican Motherhood: Benjamin Rush and the Young Ladies' Academy of Philadelphia"; Branson, *These Fiery* Frenchified *Dames: Women and Political Culture in Early National Philadelphia*; Knott, "Benjamin Rush's Ferment: Enlightenment Medicine and Female Citizenship in Revolutionary America," 649–66.

and Betsey too much out of the way to give answers. Do come home as soon as possible, or I tremble at the consequences. I languish for want of company . . . How I long to tell you how much I love you!" While in part the pleas of a love-struck young spouse, the note argues that Julia was required at home to watch after students, provide clear domestic directions, and act as an intellectual companion to her husband. Further down the page more practical matters appear as well. Benjamin discusses the finances associated with a new apprentice that Julia may have recruited, adding 100 guineas to their name as well as his modest income as a member of the Continental Congress. All this goes to show that his concerns about the education of girls were not abstract. At sixteen Julia Rush was expected to be an active player in all parts of household management.[58]

In 1797, Rush reflected his feelings from two decades prior as he addressed visitors to the Young Ladies' Academy on the proper education for girls "accommodated to the present state of society, manners, and government, in the United States of America."[59] Like boys, American girls needed a new educational system suited to a republic; however, that did not mean they would study the same curriculum as their brothers. This gender division in terms of education (and the increased availability of formal schooling for girls) provides one of the best windows into the intersection between medicine, republicanism, and education in the Early Republic. Education for girls needed to be crafted from scratch, defended, and explained to the public leaving a substantial paper trail. Donald Fraser, a writer from New York, praised Rush in a letter, stating, "[y]our very laudable & able exertions to promote the best interest of the Female-Sex, in particular, induces me to think that you will be inclined to view in a favorable light, every attempt, however feeble, to promote the mental improvement of the same Daughters of Columbia."[60]

Rush articulated an ideal curriculum for girls' schools in that 1797 speech. For example, he argued that girls should learn chemistry and other natural

58 Benjamin Rush "To Mrs. Rush (Tuesday night [23 July 1776])," *Letters of Benjamin Rush,* Vol. I, 106.

59 Rush, "Thoughts upon Female Education, Accomodated to the Present State of Society, Manners, and Government, in the United States of America. Addressed to the Visitors of the Young Ladies' Academy in Philadelphia, 28th July, 1787, at the Close of the Quarterly E," 75.

60 Donald Fraser (1800), LCP, Rush Family Papers, Benjamin Rush Correspondence, Vol. V.

sciences as well as mathematics for bookkeeping.[61] The rational nature of the sciences was supposed to counter feminine propensities for irrationality and enthusiasm by providing an explanation for everyday tasks. For example, chemistry for women could demystify the processes of cooking, baking, brewing, and making cleaning products, all common household duties.[62] Mathematics and bookkeeping, meanwhile, had the additional benefit of being practical for women who might act as their husband's clerks or find themselves widowed (or single) and running a business much like Rush's mother who ran two stores during her widowhood.[63] This was certainly a change from previous generations in which American female literacy and writing ability lagged behind that of men.[64]

For girls, education centered around what it could do for the family just as boys were educated with regard to their economic and social utility to the republic. The literature on republican motherhood and womanhood is too extensive to fully treat here.[65] The most important facet for the current discussion of education is the concept that women were supposed to act as partners in their marriages (which at this point still included family businesses), stemming from their physiological distinctness. Although the late-eighteenth and early-nineteenth centuries are notable for the shift toward a disembodied sentimental version of motherhood they remained transitory, especially

---

61   Rush, "Thoughts upon Female Education," 79; Nash, "Rethinking Republican Motherhood: Benjamin Rush and the Young Ladies' Academy of Philadelphia," 177.

62   Rush, "Thoughts upon Female Education," 79–80.

63   For more on women in business, see Wulf, *Not All Wives: Women of Colonial Philadelphia.*

64   Branson, *These Fiery Frenchified Dames: Women and Political Culture in Early National Philadelphia,* 21–22.

65   For more on republican motherhood/womanhood and its limits see: Norton, *Liberty's Daughters: The Revolutionary Experience of American Women, 1750–1800*; Norton, *Separated by Their Sex: Women in Public and Private in the Colonial Atlantic World*; Zagarri, "Morals, Manners, and the Republican Mother"; Zagarri, "The Rights of Man and Woman in Post-Revolutionary America," 203–30; Nash, "Rethinking Republican Motherhood: Benjamin Rush and the Young Ladies' Academy of Philadelphia"; Knott, "Sensibility and the American War for Independence," 19–40; Knott, "Benjamin Rush's Ferment: Enlightenment Medicine and Female Citizenship in Revolutionary America."

in the medical profession.[66] For someone like Rush, the innate differences between men and women made them complementary parts of a whole. Recall from chapter 4 that, in a physiological sense, women were thought to be shaped by their lymphatics and the abstraction of stimulus while men required stimulation and were therefore more subject to the power of the blood vessels. This basic physiological difference in turn governed social and emotional behavior. Rush considered women naturally more sensitive to their surroundings, more religious, and a moral center for the household (and by extension the nation). Education, therefore, would enhance important feminine qualities while also directing girls away from "natural" foibles. For example, Rush promoted the study of geography, history, and chemistry as a means of combatting superstition, especially religious superstition.[67]

Rush certainly believed that gender roles were firm and founded in nature. In his medical lectures, he specifically challenged Wollstonecraft's idea that difference in education accounted for observed gender differences and claimed, "[t]here is no girl fond of riding a stick; nor boy of playing with a doll. Their minds & bodies are originally different the celebrated [Wollstonecraft] is hypothetically absurd. . . . Tis necessary to social as well as to domestic happiness that this inferiority should exist. My opinion is supported not only by reason & observation but by divine revelation."[68] He used the presumed independence of play to show innateness of gendered behaviors. Boys anticipated becoming men—who rode horses—and girls anticipated becoming women—who cared for children—based on their play. There is no evidence that Rush considered the possibility that these forms of play were a form of mimicry, in which children were told by their parents, siblings, and peers which group they belonged to and copied that behavior. This contrasts with Wollstonecraft's descriptions of early childhood in *Thoughts on the Education of Daughters*, in which she argues that children of both sexes copied the behavior of those around them.[69] Like the faculties, gender was for Rush an innate state of being that acted as a lens through which bodies perceived and interacted with their world.

---

66   For a discussion of this shift and the embodied nature of motherhood in the United States, see Doyle, *Maternal Bodies: Redefining Motherhood in Early America*.

67   Rush, "Thoughts upon Female Education," 79.

68   Hare (1796), KCRBM, Ms. Coll. 225, Box 5, Item 9, Vol. I.

69   Wollstonecraft, *Thoughts*, 5.

Women might learn chemistry, for example, and even publish on it in exceptional cases like French chemist Marie-Genevieve-Charlotte Thiroux d'Arconville (1720–1805), who Rush read and citied in his own work. However, women were not supposed to use their skills in public or for profit. At least not the European-descended middling women on whom Rush focused his attention.[70] In another example from his own life Benjamin wrote to Julia how much he looked forward to reading with her. On August 16, 1787, while Julia and the children visited her family in Princeton he wrote "to a mind like mine, which so soon (perhaps from its slender size) becomes plethoric with ideas and which delights so much in communicating them, it is a new and peculiar hardship to lose at once a domestic friend, and wife, and five children. . . . Had I married a fool, I never should have disturbed a single sleeping prejudice upon any subject."[71] A few days later he noted in another letter that he longed to discuss William Paley's *Moral Philosophy* with Julia, noting, "it will qualify you above all things to educate our children properly."[72] In both instances Benjamin simultaneously acknowledged Julia's intelligence and influence while making clear her prescribed role in the nuclear family. Susan Branson notes, however, that despite the intentions of men like Rush, Philadelphia's educated women had their own ideas about their abilities. Women participated in political activities, including parades; girls at the Young Ladies Academy argued that they should have a public role; and Mary Wollstonecraft's books were popular reading for young women and men in American cities.[73]

Nevertheless, Rush's essentialist views found considerable support, most evidently among his educated, male peers. Samuel Stanhope Smith wrote to Rush congratulating him on his work on female education in 1787, stating, "[h]appy in a sensible & amiable woman yourself, you will desire well of your country men if you can contribute to make such wives common. . . . I

---

70 Rush owned a copy of Thiroux d'Arconville's treatise on putrefaction and cited it in his description of Pennsylvania mineral waters. Thiroux d'Arconville, *Essai Pour Servier a l'histoire de La Putréfaction*; Rush, *Experiments and Observations on the Mineral Waters of Philadelphia, Abington, and Bristol, in the Province of Pennsylvania*.

71 Benjamin Rush to Julia Rush (August 16, 1787), *Letters of Benjamin Rush*, Vol. I, 435–36.

72 Benjamin Rush to Julia Rush, *Letters*, 436.

73 Branson, *These Fiery Frenchified Dames: Women and Political Culture in Early National Philadelphia*; Zagarri, "Morals, Manners, and the Republican Mother," 207.

do not know whether you can do a greater service to mankind than by assisting & directing female education."[74] Women like his wife, Julia Stockton Rush, were educated for the benefit of their husbands and families, not for any sense of individual fulfillment.

The exact extent of Julia Stockton Rush's education is unclear; however, her reading knowledge, journal-keeping, and musicality suggest that she was taught at home to a fairly high level. Her mother, Annis Boudinot Stockton, was certainly well-educated for her time and was one of the country's first published poets. She also publicly critiqued the poor education of girls and men's assumptions of women's intellectual inferiority, so it is unlikely that she would have neglected her own daughter.[75] After marriage, Julia had access to her husband's growing library and possessed a great deal of medical knowledge herself. A generation later, Julia's daughters received a formal education at school that included serious academic study. In 1804, while visiting family in Princeton, she wrote to say that she had visited their youngest daughter Julia along the way, who was at boarding school in Burlington, New Jersey. The younger Julia was learning French, an increasingly common accomplishment for girls at the turn of the nineteenth century.[76]

Despite the enduring image of the painting that keeps Julia as an eternal teenager (in chapter 2), most mentions of her come from later in her marriage as a self-confident woman raising a large family and looking after a home that included an average of four private medical students at a time. Charles Caldwell described an encounter with Julia Rush in his autobiography that presents her in this manner. Their conversation demonstrates her general sociability and a knowledge of Philadelphia's medical world and society that rivaled her husband's. Caldwell wrote:

> I discovered, to my surprise . . . that she knew more of my history than I had believed to be known by all the inhabitants of Philadelphia. She even spoke of events connected with me which I myself had almost forgotten. . . . I begged her to inform me through what channel she had become possessed of it. "For, cer-

---

74 Samuel Stanhope Smith (1787) LCP, Rush Family Papers, Benjamin Rush Correspondence, Vol. XXII.

75 Branson, *These Fiery Frenchified Dames*, 44.

76 Julia Stockton Rush to Benjamin Rush (August 11, 1804), APS, Julia Stockton Rush Collection of 20 Letters, Mss.B.R894. Johnson, "Madame Rivardi's Seminary in the Gothic Mansion," 7, 10; Kilbride, "Southern Medical Students in Philadelphia, 1800–1861: Science and Sociability in the 'Republic of Medicine,'" 731.

tainly," said I, "Dr. Rush cannot have informed you of all this." "Oh! no," she said; "though the doctor has often spoken of you he did not tell me that; I learned if from Mr. N___w___n, who knew you in Salisbury. He has called here several times since the commencement of the lectures . . . he always speaks of you in the highest terms.[77]

The version of Julia Rush presented by Caldwell is that of a woman acutely aware of her surroundings and likely keeping track of the myriad of personal and professional relationships that surrounded her family. It also suggests that though uncommented upon by Benjamin in his commonplace book, Julia was present for many of his meetings with out-of-town visitors and participated in those conversations. In a professional landscape shaped by personal connections such information was part of the medical business, part of the family business, and thus Julia's business. Letters to Benjamin Rush from then Professor Samuel Stanhope Smith in 1790 present a similar image of a woman valued in heterosocial circles in Princeton for her conversational skills and intelligence. Smith wrote that he must "thank you, for your consent that she should stay so long to enliven our society here. If you will allow another gentleman to say it, she charms wherever she goes. And I cannot refrain from congratulating you, that at your time of life & hers, you have so much elegance, & beauty & good sense, visited in the mother of an amiable group of children, & the wife of a man who has taste & sentiment enough to relish them."[78] Like Rush, Smith emphasized sociability as feminine and the traditional roles of wife and mother that Julia Stockton Rush carried out. Her power was her private influence over family and friends rather than public, political action. This matched the republican worldview Rush imagined, as well as the virtuous society proposed by Catherine Macaulay, in which women and men were partners: one in the public eye and one acting as the critic away from the spotlight.[79]

Nevertheless, as evidenced by her own hand, Julia Stockton Rush could navigate even the "masculine" world of medicine. Not only did she hold her own in conversation, but she also had some theoretical knowledge. In a letter to her husband during the yellow fever epidemic she noted that his treatment

---

77 Caldwell, *Autobiography of Charles Caldwell, M.D. with a Preface, Notes, and Appendix, by Harriot W. Warner*, 145–46.

78 Samuel Stanhope Smith to Benjamin Rush (1790), LCP, Rush Family Papers, Benjamin Rush Correspondence, Vol. XXII.

79 Gunther-Canada, "Cultivating Virtue: Catherine Macaulay and Mary Wollstonecraft on Civic Education," 56.

seemed akin to that of British physician Benjamin Moseley.[80] Additional evidence comes from her correspondence immediately after Rush's death in 1813. Following the initial news of his demise Abigail Adams requested information on the doctor's last days, which Julia Rush responded to in detail. The winter before his death, she noted, Rush suffered from a cough when damp (which was in accordance with his constitution). She went on to explain his treatment for it: water with warm molasses, occasionally with the addition of brandy, lime, or laudanum, and the total abstinence from wine. Here, apparently, they disagreed; Julia wrote "I remonstrated against this plan and said that I thought his labours and his advancing years required more generous living."[81] Despite her evident ability and keen eye for observation, gender prevented Julia Rush from being anything beyond a doctor's wife.

In the end, for Rush, the education of both boys and girls was aimed at producing future republican men and women. That is, civic minded and industrious voting men and moral, rational, and sensible women. Schools would help the country get off on the right foot with respect to health. When health failed, however, other institutions were required to restore republican order. In his own family many of his children followed their pre-designed path. Richard engaged in a successful legal and political career and James followed his father into the medical profession. Meanwhile, by the early 1800s both of the elder Rush daughters, Mary and Emily, were married to respectable men (although not American citizens) and starting families of their own. For the most part the plan seemed to work. Republican machines could be constructed.

Rush's essays on education provide an important opportunity to address his ideas about childhood and children's mental development as well as the role of schools in supporting good government and good health. His contemporaries in other parts of the world also increasingly looked to education and schools as a national resource and necessity for producing a successful generation of young people. In Ireland, physician William Drennan (like Rush, educated in Enlightenment Scotland and a republican) highlighted the need for improved education in his own country in 1795. He echoed ideas that would have been at home in American discussions of public education

---

80 Julia Stockton Rush to Benjamin Rush (October 1, 1793), APS, Julia Stockton Rush Collection of 20 Letters, Mss.B.R894.

81 "From Julia Stockton Rush to Abigail Smith Adams, 23 June 1813," Founders Online, National Archives, last modified February 1, 2018, http://founders.archives.gov/documents/Adams/99-03-02-2314.

in the 1780s. In a published letter to the new lord lieutenant of Ireland, Drennan foregrounded educational reform, stating, "the most pernicious error that ever poisoned the happiness of mankind, has been the prejudice, that there is one sort of knowledge fit for the learned, and another adapted to the vulgar."[82] Drennan feared future instability as well as a waste of talent among the "vulgar," citing Benjamin Franklin as an example of scientific genius from a humble background. He might also have cited Benjamin Rush, a man very aware of the manner in which education took the son of a farmer and blacksmith and turned him into a leading physician. Although less concerned about an entrenched class system than Drennan, Rush shared his contemporary's view that the social order benefited from an educated public and feared wasted natural talent. Both men espoused a type of social republicanism, pointing to the broad benefit that equality of educational opportunity could have on a population and doing so from the perspective of the medical profession.

---

82   Drennan, *A Letter to His Excellency Earl Fitzwilliam Lord Lieutenant, &c. of Ireland*, 5.

Epilogue

> In this frontier of the Republic of Letters, in the 'ultima Thule' of
> Literature your writings have brought with them some of the purest
> rays of truth that have yet enlightened our horizon. Remote from the
> authority of Colleges & unawed by any unbounded admiration for old
> systems, it is not impossible that Kentucky may, before many years,
> make considerable additions to our stock of Medical knowledge.[1]

Writing from Lexington, Kentucky, on behalf of their newly formed medical society, Dr. Samuel Brown turned his eyes eastward for a moment to congratulate Benjamin Rush on his inclusion to their number as an honorary member. Historians, with their gaze focused on established universities, have remembered Rush as the last of the great system builders of the eighteenth century, but that is only half the story. He may equally be viewed as the beginning and inspiration for American regional medicine in the South and Midwest. The American system may not have turned out exactly how Rush planned, but his inspiration, focus on location, and model of physician behavior lasted well into the nineteenth century.

Like so many things, Brown's address was exaggerated. Lexington in 1799 was a western settlement, but not beyond the known world. Beyond the hyperbole, however, Brown's letter hints at the future of Rush's American medicine and his value to the profession at the dawn of the nineteenth century. The flexibility and independence Rush built into his medical and educational philosophy opened the door for regional variation and adaptation to new regions annexed to the United States. To men like Brown, Rush showed that American medicine could be truly American. He helped Britons in the American colonies see themselves as inhabiting a biologically distinct nation with its own character, institutions, and diseases. Together these parameters shaped a new bodily constitution within a new continent, a concept that remained in flux as the country grew, both demographically and geographically. Rush argued that the country required its own distinctive educational

---

1   Samuel Brown to Benjamin Rush (1799), LCP, Rush Family Papers, Benjamin Rush Correspondence, Vol. XXI.

system in order for the profession and the nation to succeed as an equal part-ner in the world of science. This tension between independence and connec-tion continued to play out within the United States. The challenges faced by American bodies, minds, and institutions were unique and required a clear and concise approach to medicine. Rush's system, which focused on general terms of excitement and excitability could readily move from one region to another and interpret the different physical and social environments. That environmental approach evolved into the medical geography that drove men like Rush's student, Daniel Drake,[2] later in the century.

From the heady optimism of Enlightenment and a world turned upside down to the despair of epidemics and political infighting, Benjamin Rush clutched ever more tightly to the dream of explaining the human condi-tion and reshaping the world in God's image—revelation not in theology, but in physiology. The human body and mind, if properly managed could bring men close to angels and the American republic closer to the kingdom of heaven. In hindsight, his quest appears quixotic and hopelessly utopian. The end of Rush's road produced no appendectomy, penicillin, or germ theory. The nineteenth-century prizes for great insight and understand-ing have been bestowed upon French pathologists, British sanitarians, and German biochemists. From one perspective Rush looks like the last gasp of an eighteenth-century tradition of medical systematizing. Meanwhile, latter-day system-builders cast as irregulars and quacks looked down their noses at the thoroughly "regular" Rush.[3]

Nevertheless, Benjamin Rush stubbornly remained a fixture of the American medical landscape. His influence and work as an educator and prolific writer have never fully disappeared. As John Duffy puts it, "[n]ineteenth-century medicine took its unique character in America from the dialectic between professionalism and the nation's democratic culture."[4] This book has argued that Benjamin Rush first sketched the parameters of that dialectic. He both relied upon insights and theories from Europe and rejected them in the name of a more republican version of theory and a

---

2   Frank A. Barrett, "Daniel Drake's Medical Geography," *Social Science and Medicine,* 42.6 (1996): 792.

3   Duffy, *A History of Public Health in New York City, 1625–1866,* 54–55; Shryock, *Medicine in America: Historical Essays,* 206–7; Warner, *The Therapeutic Perspective: Medical Practice, Knowledge, and Identity in America, 1820–1885,* 37–41; Burnham, *Health Care in America: A History,* 90.

4   Duffy, *A History of Public Health,* 54.

practice designed to promote and heal republican bodies. He frequently wrote for public audiences and believed in spreading knowledge about the public's health. At the same time, he remained dedicated not only to upholding medicine as one of the learned professions, but indeed expanding the power and privilege of regularly trained physicians. His hopes for a state university system, encouragement of young trainees, and publication of the "American Editions" all served to discipline the boundaries of the medical profession.

The American system Rush built relied on a strong tradition of practice interested in the social applications of medicine borrowed from Scotland. At the same time questions of the physical and political health of the republic fundamentally shaped the manner in which American medicine developed. Independence became a lasting rallying cry for the profession well into the nineteenth century. This patriotism informed Thomas Mitchell's choice of Rush as the subject of his introductory essay for the year 1848. He praised Rush's memory as a man committed to the improvement of his country, stating that Rush "more than any who had preceded him, felt and acted under the inspiration of the spirit of improvement. He was not one of your *in statu quo* men, but in the phraseology of the West, he *believed in going ahead*."[5] Mitchell's summation of Rush helps put his life and legacy in context. The constant motion and desire for improvement is evident in all of Rush's writings. Even when recounting something as devastating as yellow fever, he preserved a kernel of optimism.

That Rush believed in improvement is evident. His quest for perfection of bodies, minds, and society drove what might be called his research project. However, this book also argues that Rush's social and political agendas are not sufficient to explain the system he arrived at or his professional appeal. Like many of his generation, Rush mixed areas of inquiry that are now separate disciplines. This work elucidates the framework of Rush's thinking and some of its consequences for the early nineteenth century. It cannot recover everything that Rush's work touched. His thousands of students and correspondents left important marks on the medical and social framework of the United States far beyond the scope of a single project. What it can demonstrate is the way one figure of the Revolutionary era gathered information, made sense of a world turned upside down, and struggled to impose a rational framework on the messiness that is social and biological life.

---

5   Mitchell, *The Character of Rush, an Introductory to the Course on the Theory and Practice of Medicine in the Philadelphia College of Medicine*, 15.

Benjamin Rush died on April 19, 1813, with a country redefining its independence once again in the crucible, of the War of 1812. His final illness carried him off fairly suddenly. He suffered from a "low" fever for a few days—possibly typhoid or typhus—and then faded away. Rush left the country at a moment of transition. The ongoing War of 1812 was interpreted by some Americans as their second great reckoning with the British Empire, a chance to prove their independence once more. It also foreshadowed a change in the cast of characters who dominated the next quarter century of American public life. Washington, Hamilton, and Franklin were already gone. Adams and Jefferson sat at home in retirement and reconciliation (in part credited to Rush). In politics, the First Party System of Federalists and Democratic-Republicans faded, replaced eventually by the Democrats and Whigs of the 1830s. Democratic principles and virtues started to dominate over the republican ones championed by Rush. The individualist spirit and celebration of equality (among white men) arguably eroded the power of medical professionals by the 1840s. Irregular systems popped up to move against the now entrenched elites of Philadelphia, New York, and Boston. Even among the "regular" physicians, the descendants of Rush and his institutions no longer held on to his American system. Mitchell would praise Rush's teaching style, citizenship, and patriotism, but not his therapeutics, which were dated. Bloodletting aside, however, the fact that there was an American medical profession, that for good and ill its practitioners spread across the country providing healthcare and facilitating settlers, is in large part due to Rush. During his lifetime he forced himself into international conversations and pushed himself to the top of his profession. He always believed in getting ahead.

Bibliography

(1887), Transactions of the College of Physicians of Philadelphia. "Currie, William (1754–1828)." In *A Cyclopedia of American Medical Biography, Comprising the Lives of Eminent Deceased Physicians and Surgeons from 1610 to 1910*, 267. W.B. Saunders Company, 1912.

Academy of Medicine of Philadelphia. *Academy of Medicine of Philadelphia Constitution*. Philadelphia, 1798.

Ackerknecht, Erwin H. "Anticontagionism Between 1821 and 1867." *Bulletin of the History of Medicine* 22 (1948): 562–95.

Adamson, George C.D. "'The Languor of the Hot Weather': Everyday Perspectives on Weather and Climate in Colonial Bombay, 1819–1828." *Journal of Historical Geography* 38, no. 2 (2012): 143–54.

Altschuler, Sari. "From Blood Vessels to Global Networks of Exchange: The Physiology of Benjamin Rush's Early Republic From Blood Vessels to Global Networks of Exchange." *Journal of the Early Republic* 32, no. 2 (2012): 207–31.

———. *The Medical Imagination: Literature and Health in the Early United States.* Philadelphia: University of Pennsylvania Press, 2018.

Altschuler, Sari, and Christopher J. Bilodeau. "Ecce Homo!: The Figure of Benjamin Rush." *Early American Studies*, no. Spring (2017): 233–45.

Ambrose, Charles T. "The Priority Dispute over the Function of the Lymphatic System and Glisson's Ghost (the 18th-Century Hunter-Monro Feud)." *Cellular Immunology* 245, no. 1 (2007): 7–15.

Apel, Thomas. *Feverish Bodies, Enlightened Minds: Science and the Yellow Fever Controversy in the Early American Republic.* Stanford University Press, 2016.

———. "The Thucydidean Moment: History, Science, and the Yellow-Fever Controversy, 1793–1805." *Journal of the Early Republic* 34, no. 3 (2014): 315–47.

Appleby, Joyce. *Inheriting the Revolution: The First Generation of Americans.* Cambridge and London: The Belknap Press of Harvard University Press, 2000.

Arner, Katherine. "Making Yellow Fever American: The Early American Republic, the British Empire and the Geopolitics of Disease in the Atlantic World." *Atlantic Studies* 7, no. 4 (2010): 447–71.

Bard, Samuel. "A Discourse on the Importance of Medical Education; Delivered on the 4th of November, 1811, at the Opening of the Present Session of the Medical School of the College of Physicians and Surgeons. By Samuel Bard, M.D. President of the College of Physicians." *American Medical and Philosophical Register, or, Annals of Medicine, Natural History, Agriculture and the Arts* 2 (1812): 369–82.

Barfoot, Michael. "Brunonianism under the Bed: An Alternative to University Medicine in Edinburgh in the 1780s." *Medical History*, no. 8 (1988): 22–45.

———. "James Gregory (1753–1821) and Scottish Scientific Metaphysics, 1750–1800." University of Edinburgh, 1983. https://core.ac.uk/download/pdf/12812852.pdf.

Barnes, David S. "Cargo, 'Infection,' and the Logic of Quarantine in the Nineteenth Century." *Bulletin of the History of Medicine* 88, no. 1 (2014): 75–101.

———. *The Great Stink of Paris and the Nineteenth-Century Struggle against Filth and Germs*. Baltimore: The Johns Hopkins University Press, 2006.

Baron De Montesquieu, Charles de Secondat, Jean le Rond D'Almbert, Thomas Nugent, trans, and Frederic R. Coudert. *The Spirit of Laws, Vol. I*. New York: P.F. Collier & Son, 1900.

Barrett, Frank A. "Daniel Drake's Medical Geography." *Social Science and Medicine*, 42.6 (1996): XX–XX.

Barton, Benjamin Smith. *A Memoir Concerning the Disease of Goitre as It Prevails in Different Parts of North-America*. Philadelphia: Printed for the author by Way & Groff, 1800.

Bassiri, Nima. "The Brain and the Unconscious Soul in Eighteenth-Century Nervous Physiology: Robert Whytt's Sensorium Commune." *Journal of the History of Ideas* 74, no. 3 (2013): 425–48.

Baynham, William. "An Account of Two Cases of Extra-Uterine Conception; in Each of Which the Foetus Was Extracted by an Operation with Success." *New York Medical and Philosophical Journal and Review* I, no. 2 (1809): 161–70.

Beattie, James. *Elements of Moral Science*. Philadelphia: From the Press of Mathew Carey, 1792.

———. *Essai Sur La Poésie et Sur La Musique*. Paris: H. Tardieu, 1798.

———. *Essays: On Peotry and Music, as They Affect the Mind*. Edinburgh and London: Printed for Edward and Charles Dilly in London; and William Creach, Edinburgh, 1778.

Beatty, Heather R. *Nervous Disease in Late Eighteenth-Century Britain: The Reality of a Fashionable Disorder*. London: Pickering & Chatto, 2012.

Beck, Andrew, Hilda Guzman, Li Li, Brett Ellis, Robert B Tesh, and Alan D T Barrett. "Phylogeographic Reconstruction of African Yellow Fever Virus Isolates Indicates Recent Simultaneous Dispersal into East and West Africa." *PLoS Neglected Tropical Diseases* 7, no. 3 (2013).

Bell, Richard. "The Moral Thermometer: Rush, Republicanism, and Suicide." *Early American Studies*, no. Spring (2017): 308–31.

———. *We Shall Be No More: Suicide and Self-Government in the Newly United States*. Cambridge and London: Harvard University Press, 2012.

Bell, Whitfield. *The College of Physicians of Philadelphia: A Bicentennial History*. Canton, MA: Science History Publications/USA, 1987.

Bell, Whitfield J. "Benjamin Smith Barton, M.D. (Kiel)." *Journal of the History of Medicine*, 1971, 197–203.

Berrios, GE. "'Febrile Anxiety,' by Robert James (1745)." *History of Psychiatry* 25, no. 1 (2014): 112–24.

Berry, Christopher J. "'Climate' in the Eighteenth Century: James Dunbar and the Scottish Case." *Texas Studies in Literature and Language* 16, no. 2 (1974): 281–92.

Binger, Carl. *Revolutionary Doctor: Benjamin Rush, 1746–1813*. New York: Norton, 1966.

Block, Sharon. *Colonial Complexions: Race and Bodies in Eighteenth-Century America*. Philadelphia: University of Pennsylvania Press, 2018.

Bodle, Wayne. "The Mid-Atlantic and the American Revolution." *Pennsylvania History: A Journal of Mid-Atlantic Studies* 82, no. 3 (2015): 282–99.

Boerhaave, Herman. *Boerhaave's Aphorisms*. London: printed for W. Innys and J. Richardson, and C. Hitch and L. Hawes, 1755.

———. *Boerhaave's Medical Correspondence*. London: printed for John Nourse, 1745.

———. *De Viribus Medicamentorum*. London: printed for J. Wilcox, B Creake, and John Sackfield, 1720.

———. *Dr. Boerhaave's Academical Lectures on the Theory of Physic: Being a Genuine Translation of His Institutes and Explanatory Comment, Collated and Adjusted to Each Other, as They Were Dictated to His Students at the University of Leyden . . .* London: W. Inny, 1744.

———. *Dr. Boerhaave's Academical Lectures on the Theory of Physic Being A Genuine Translation of His Institutes and Explanatory Comments, Collated and Adjusted to Each Other, as They Were Dictated to His STUDENTS at the University of Leyden, Vol. II*. London: printed for W. Innys, at the West End of St. Paul's, 1749.

———. *Dr. Boerhaave's Elements of Chymistry*. London: printed for C. Rivington, 1737.

———. *Elemens de Chymie*. Amsterdam: Chez J. Wetstein, 1752.

———. *Elementa Chemiae*. Paris, 1724.

———. *Hermanni Boerhaave Libellus de Materie Medica*. Lugduni Batavorum: apud I. Severinum, 1740.

———. *Institutiones Medicae*. Lugduni Batavorum: Apud Johannem vander Linden, 1713.

Bolton Valencius, Conevery, David I. Spanagel, Emily Pawley, Sara Stidstone Gronim, and Paul Lucier. "Science in Early America: Print Culture and the Sciences of Territoriality." *Journal of the Early Republic* 36, no. 1 (2016): 73–123.

Boott, Francis. *Memoir of the Life and Medical Opinions of John Armstrong . . . : To Which Is Added an Inquiry into the Facts Connected with Those Forms of Fever Attributed to Malaria or Marsh Effluvium, Volume 1*. London: Baldwin and Cradock, 1833.

Bow, Charles Bradford. "Reforming Witherspoon's Legacy at Princeton: John Witherspoon, Samuel Stanhope Smith and James McCosh on Didactic Enlightenment, 1768–1888." *History of European Ideas* 39, no. 5 (2013): 1768–1888.

Bradburn, Douglas. *The Citizenship Revolution: Politics and the Creation of the American Union, 1774–1804.* Charlottsville: University of Virginia Press, 2009.

Brandt, Susan H. *Women Healers: Gender, Authority, and Medicine in Early Philadelphia.* Philadelphia: University of Pennsylvania Press, 2022.

Branson, Susan. *These Fiery Frenchified Dames: Women and Political Culture in Early National Philadelphia.* Philadelphia: University of Pennsylvania, 2001.

Breen, T.H. *American Insurgents, American Patriots: The Revolution of the People.* New York: Hill and Wang, 2010.

Breslaw, Elaine G. *Lotions, Potions, Pills, and Magic.* New York and London: New York University Press, 2012.

Brodsky, Alyn. *Benjamin Rush: Patriot and Physician.* New York: Truman Talley Books, 2004.

Brown, T M. "From Mechanism to Vitalism in Eighteenth Century English Physiology." *Journal of the History of Biology* 7, no. 2 (1974): 179–216.

Brunton, Deborah C. "The Transfer of Medical Education: Teaching at the Edinbrugh and Philadelphia Medical Schools." In *Scotland and America in the Age of Enlightenment*, edited by Richard B. Sher and Jeffrey R. Smitten, 242–58. Princeton, NJ: Princeton University Press, 1990.

Bullough, Vern, and Martha Voght. "Women, Menstruation, and Nineteenth-Century Medicine." *Bulletin of the History of Medicine* 47, no. 1 (1973): 66–82.

Burnham, John C. *Health Care in America: A History.* Baltimore: The Johns Hopkins University Press, 2015.

Burns, John. *Observations on Abortion Containing an Account of the Manner in Which It Is Accomplished, the Causes Whic Prodiced It, and the Method of Preventing or Treating It.* London: Printed for Longman, Hurst, Rees, and Orme, Pater-Noster Row, 1807.

———. *Pracitcal Observations on the Uterine Hemorrhage; With Remarks on the Management of the Placenta.* London: Printed for Longman, Hurst Rees, and Orme Paternoster Row, 1807.

Bynum, William F. "The Nervous Patient in Eighteenth- and Nineteenth-Century Britain: The Psychiatric Origins of British Neurology." In *The Anatomy of Madness: Essays in the History of Psychiatry, Vol. I.*, edited by William F. Bynum, Roy Porter, and Michael Shepherd, 89–102. London and New York: Tavistock Publications, 1985.

Cadogan, William. *Dissertation on the Gout, and All Chronic Diseases, Jointly Considered, As Proceeding from the Same Causes; What Those Causes Are; and A Rational and Natural Method of Cure Proposed.* London and Philadelphia: Reprinted and Sold by William and Thomas Bradford, 1772.

Caldwell, Charles. *Autobiography of Charles Caldwell, M.D. with a Preface, Notes, and Appendix, by Harriot W. Warner*. Edited by Harriot W. Warner. Philadelphia: Lippincott, Grambo and Company, 1855.

———. *Medical & Physical Memoirs, Containing Among Other Subjects a Partiuclar Enquiry into the Origin and Nature of the Late Pestilential Epidemics of the United States*. Philadelphia: Printed by Thomas & William Bradford, 1801.

———. *Thoughts on the Subject of a Health-Establishment for The City of Philadelphia*. Philadelphia, 1803.

Calvi, Giulia. *Histories of a Plague Year: The Social and the Imaginary in Baroque Florence*, Dario Biocca and Bryant T. Ragan Jr., trans, Berkeley: University of California Press, 1989

Cañizares-Esguerra, Jorge. "New World, New Stars : Patriotic Astrology and the Invention of Indian and Creole Bodies in Colonial Spanish America , 1600– 1650." *The American Historical Review* 104, no. 1 (1999): 33–68.

Carlson, Eric T., and Jeffrey L. Wollock. "Benjamin Rush and His Insane Son." *Bulletin of the New York Academy of Medicine* 51, no. 11 (1975).

Carlson, Eric T. "Benjamin Rush on Revolutionary War Hygiene" 55, no. 7 (1979).

Castel, Robert, and W.D. Halls. *The Regulation of Madness: The Origins of Incarceration in France*. Berkeley and Los Angeles: University of California Press, 1988.

Catalogue of the Medical Library, Belonging to the Pennsylvania Hospital: Exhibiting the Names of Authors and Editors, in Alphabetical Order, and an Arrangement of Them Under Distinct Heads. Also, a List of Articles Contained in the Anatomical Museum; A. Philadelphia, 1806.

Chakrabarti, Pratik. "'Neither of Meate nor Drinke, but What the Doctor Alloweth': Medicine amidst War and Commerce in Eighteenth-Century Madras." *Bulletin of the History of Medicine* 80, no. 1 (2006): 1–38.

Chaplin, Joyce E. *Subject Matter: Technology, the Body, and Science on the Anglo-American Frontier, 1500–1676*. Cambridge and London: Harvard University Press, 2009.

———. "Natural Philosophy and an Early Racial Idiom in North America: Comparing English and Indian Bodies." *The William and Mary Quarterly* 54, no. 1 (1997): 229–52.

Chard, Chloe. "Lassitude and Revival in the Warm South: Relaxing and Exciting Travel, 1750–1830." In *Pathologies of Travel*, edited by Richard Wrigley and George Revill, 179–205. Rodopi, 2000.

Chervin, Nicholas. *De L'Opinion Des Médecins Américains Sur La Contagion Ou La Non-Contagion de La Fievre Jaune, Our Réponse Aux Allégations de MM. Les Docteurs Hosack et Townsend de New-York, Publiées, l'an Dernier, Dans La Revue Médicale La Gazette De France et Le New-Yor*. Paris and London: Chez J.-B. Bailliere, Libraire, 1829.

Cheyne, George. *The English Malady: Or, a Treatise of Nervous Diseases of All Kinds; as Spleen, Vapours, Lowness of Spirits, Hypochondrical, and Hysterical Distempers, &c*. 3rd ed. London: Printed for G. Strahan, 1734.

Christie, J. R. R. "Historiography of Chemistry in the Eighteenth Century: Hermann Boerhaave and William Cullen." *Ambix* 41, no. 1 (1994): 4–19.

Churchill, Wendy D. "Bodily Differences?: Gender, Race, and Class in Hans Sloane's Jamican Medical Practice, 1678–1688." *Journal of the History of Medicine and Allied Sciences* 60, no. 4 (2005): 391–443.

Cimino, Guido, François Duchesneau, François Azouvi, Giulio Barsanti, Jacalyn Duffin, Dietrich von Engelhardt, Frederick Gregory, et al. *Vitalisms: From Haller to the Cell Theory.* Firenze: Leo S. Olschki Editore, 1997.

Cipolla, Carlo M. *Fighting the Plague in Seventeenth-Century Italy,* Madison: University of Wisconsin Press, 1981

Clark, George. "Case of Extra-Uterine Gestation." *The Philadelphia Medical Museum* 2 (1806): 292–95.

Cleghorn, George, and Benjamin Rush. *Observations on the Epidemical Diseases of Minorca from the Year 1744 to 1749 to Which Is Prefixed A Short Account of the Climate Productions, Inhabitants, and Endemical Distempers of Minorca.* 2nd ed. Philadelphia: F. Nichols, 1812.

Cogliano, Francis D. *Emperor of Liberty: Thomas Jefferson's Foreign Policy.* New Haven and London: Yale University Press, 2014.

Coleman, William. *Yellow Fever in the North: The Methods of Early Epidemiology.* Madison, WI: University of Wisconsin Press, 1987.

Corvisart des Marets, Jean Nicolas (baron), C.E. Horeau, and Jacob Gates. *An Essay on the Organic Diseases and Lesions of the Heart and Great Vessels From the Clinical Lectures of J.N. Corvisart.* Boston: Bradford & Read, 1812.

Cowan, Charles F. "Horsfield, Moore, and the Catalogues of the East India Company Museum." *The Journal of the Society for the Bibliography of Natural History* 7, no. 3 (1975): 273–84.

Coxe, William. *Travels in Switzerland. In a Series of Letters to William Melmoth, Esq. from William Coxe, M.A. F.R.S.F.A.S. . . .* London: printed for T. Cadell, 1789.

Crenson, Matthew A. *Baltimore: A Political History.* Baltimore: Johns Hopkins University Press, 2017.

Crichton, Alexander. *An Inquiry into the Nature and Origin of Mental Derangement Comprehending a Concise System of the Physiology and Pathology of the Human Mind and a History of the Passions and Their Effects, Vol. I.* London: Printed for T. Cadell, Junior, and W. Davies. in the Strand, 1798.

Cullen, William. *First Lines of the Practice of Physic, Vol. I.* Edited by John Rotheram. Edinburgh: Bell & Bradfutte, and William Creech, 1791.

Cullen, William, and Benjamin Rush. *First Lines of the Practice of Physic, for the Use of Students, in the University of Edinburgh, Vol. I.* Philadelphia: Printed by Steiner and Cist., 1781.

Currie, William. *An Historical Account of the Climates and Diseases of the United States of America and of the Remedies and Methods of Treatment . . .* Philadelphia: Thomas Dobson, 1792.

———. "Facts and Arguments in Favour of the Foreign Origin and Contagious Nature of the Pestilential or Malignant Yellow Fever, Which Has Prevailed in Different Commercial Cities and Seaport Towns of the United States, More Particularly since the Summer of 1793." *American Medical and Philosophical Register, or Annals of Medicine, Natural History, Agriculture and the Arts* 1, no. 1 (1811): 181–96.

D'Elia, Donald J. "Benjamin Rush, David Hartley, and the Revolutionary Uses of Psychology." *Proceedings of the American Philosophical Society* 114, no. 2 (1970): 109–18.

Darwin, Erasmus. *Zoonomia; Or, The Laws of Organic Life, Vol. 1.* Dublin: Byrne, 1800.

Daston, Lorraine. "Baconian Facts, Academic Civility, and the Prehistory of Objectivity." *Annals of Scholarship* 8 (1991): 337–63.

Deacon, Harriet. "The Politics of Medical Topograhy: Seeking Healthiness at the Cape during the Nineteenth Century." In *Pathologies of Travel*, edited by Richard Wrigley and George Revill, 279–97. Rodopi, 2000.

Dear, Peter. "The Meanings of Experience." In *The Cambridge History of Science*, edited by Katherine Park and Lorraine Daston, 3:106–31. Cambridge: Cambridge University Press, 2006.

Delbourgo, James. *A Most Amazing Scene of Wonders: Electricity and Enlightenment in Early America.* Cambridge and London: Harvard University Press, 2006.

———. "The Newtonian Slave Body: Racial Enlightenment in the Atlantic World." *Atlantic Studies* 9, no. 2 (2012): 185–207.

Demos, John. *The Unredeemed Captive: A Family Story from Early America.* New York: Vintage Books, 1994.

Digby, Anne. *Madness, Morality, and Medicine: A Study of the York Retreat, 1796–1914.* Cambridge and New York: Cambridge University Press, 1985.

Dingwall, Helen M. *A History of Scottish Medicine: Themes and Influences.* Edinburgh: Edinburgh University Press, 2003.

Doig, A., J.P.S. Ferguson, I.A. Milne, and R. Passmore. *William Cullen and the 18th Century Medical World: A Bicentenary Exhibition and Symposium Arranged by the Royal College of Physicians of Edinburgh in 1990.* Edited by A. Doig, J. P. S. Ferguson, I.A. Milne, and R. Passmore. Edinburgh: Edinburgh University Press, 1993.

Dolan, Brian. "Conservative Politicians, Radical Philosophers and the Aerial Remedy for the Diseases of Civilization." *History of the Human Sciences* 15, no. 2 (2002): 35–54.

Dorr, Jonathan. "Facts Concerning Goitre, as It Occurs in the Towns of Camden, Sandgate, and Chester, within the States of New-York and Vermont; and Conjectures Concerning Its Cause." *The Medical Repository*, 1807, 141–44.

Doyle, Nora. *Maternal Bodies: Redefining Motherhood in Early America.* Chapel Hill: The University of North Carolina Press, 2018.

Drake, Daniel. "Medical Topography." *Ecletic Repertory and Analytical Review, Medical and Philosphical* 6, no. 2 (1816).

Drennan, William. *A Letter to His Excellency Earl Fitzwilliam Lord Lieutenant, &c. of Ireland.* London: Printed for Richard White, 1795.

Duffy, John. *A History of Public Health in New York City, 1625–1866.* New York: Russel Sage Foundation, 1968.

———. *The Sanitarians: A History of American Public Health.* Urbana, Chicago, and London: University of Illinois Press, 1990.

Dupree, A. Hunter. "The National Pattern of American Learned Societies, 1769–1863." In *The Pursuit of Knowledge in the Early American Republic,* edited by Alexandra Oleson and Sanborn C. Brown, 21–32. Baltimore and London: The Johns Hopkins University Press, 1976.

Dwight, Benjamin W. "Some Remarks on the Origin and Progress of the Malignant Yellow Fever, as It Appeared in the Village of Catskill, State of New-York, during the Summer and Autumn of 1803, in a Letter from Dr. Benjamin W. Dwight to Eneas Monson, M.D. of New-Haven, Connecti." *The Medical Repository* 2, no. 2 (1805): 105–21.

Dyde, Sean. "Cullen, a Cautionary Tale." *Medical History* 59, no. 02 (2015): 222–40.

Eales, Nellie B. "The History of the Lymphatic System, with Special Reference to the Hunter-Monro Controversy." *Journal of the History of Medicine and Allied Sciences* 29, no. 3 (1974): 280–94.

Earle, Rebecca. *The Body of the Conquistador: Food, Race and the Colonial Experience in Spanish America, 1492–1700.* Cambridge and New York: Cambridge University Press, 2012.

Eddy, Matthew Daniel. "The Interactive Notebook: How Students Learned to Keep Notes during the Scottish Enlightenment." *Book History* 19, no. 1 (2016): 86–131. https://doi.org/10.1353/bh.2016.0002.

———. "The Nature of Notebooks: How Enlightenment Schoolchildren Transformed the Tabula Rasa." *Journal of British Studies* 57, no. 2 (2018): 275–307. https://doi.org/10.1017/jbr.2017.239.

Emerson, Roger L. "The Founding of the Edinburgh Medical School." *Journal of the History of Medicine and Allied Sciences* 59, no. 2 (2004): 183–218.

Espinosa, Mariola. "The Question of Racial Immunity to Yellow Fever in History and Historiography." *Social Science History* 38, no. 3–4 (2012): 437–53.

Estes, J. Worth, Billy G. Smith, Sally F. Griffith, Thomas A. Horrocks, Margaret Humphreys, Susan E. Klepp, Phillip Lapsansky, et al. *A Melancholy Scene of Devastation: The Public Response to the 1793 Yellow Fever Epidemic.* Edited by J. Worth Estes and Billy G Smith. Sagamore: Science History Publications/USA, 2013.

Evans, Amos A. "Notes Taken From Dr. Rush's Lectures upon the Institutes and Practice of Medicine and on Clinical Cases, Vol. I." USS Constitution Museum, access via Internet Archive, 1802. http://www.archive.org/details/notestaken-fromdr00evan.

Ewan, Joseph. "The Growth of Learned and Scientific Societies in the Southeastern United States to 1860." In *The Pursuit of Knowledge in the Early American Republic*, edited by Alexandra Oleson and Sanborn C. Brown, 208–18. Baltimore and London: The Johns Hopkins University Press, 1976.

Fenn, Elizabeth A. *Pox Americana: The Great Smallpox Epidemic of 1775–1782.* New York: Hill and Wang, 2001.

Findlen, Paula. *Possessing Nature: Museums, Collecting, and Scientific Culture in Early Modern Italy*, 1994.

Finger, Simon. "An Indissoluble Union: How the American War for Independence Transformed Philadelphia's Medical Community and Created a Public Health Establishment." *Pennsylvania History: A Journal of Mid-Atlantic Studies* 77, no. 1 (2010): 37–72.

———. *Contagious City: The Politics of Public Health in Early Philadelphia.* Ithaca and London: Cornell University Press, 2012.

Fors, Hjalmar. "Medicine and the Making of a City: Spaces of Pharmacy and Scholarly Medicine in Seventeenth-Century Stockholm." *Isis* 107, no. 3 (2016): 473–94.

Forsyth, Gideon E. "Geological, Topographical and Medical Information Concerning the Eastern Part of the State of Ohio; by Dr. Gideon C. Forsyth, of Wheeling; in Two Letters Ot Dr. A.C. Willey, of Block-Island; and by Him Communicated to the Editors." *The Medical Repository*, 1809, 350–58.

Frank, Jason. "Sympathy and Separation: Benjamin Rush and the Contagious Public." *Modern Intellectual History* 6, no. 1 (2009): 27–57.

Fried, Stephen. *Rush: Revolution, Madness, and the Visionary Doctor Who Became a Founding Father.* New York: Crown, 2018.

———. *Rush: Revolution, Madness, and the Visionary Doctor Who Became a Founding Father.* New York: Broadway Books, 2018.

Gates, Warren E. "The Spread of Ibn Khaldûn's Ideas on Climate and Culture." *Source Journal of the History of Ideas Journal of the History of Ideas This* 28, no. 3 (1967): 415–22.

Gelfand, Toby. "The Origins of a Modern Concept of Medical Specialization: John Morgan's Discourse of 1765." *Bulletin of the History of Medicine* 50, no. 4 (1976): 511–35.

Gerbi, Antonello, and Jeremy Moyle. *The Dispute of the New World: The History of a Polemic, 1750–1900.* Pittsburgh, PA: University of Pittsburgh Press, 1973.

Gibson, William. "Remarks on Bronchocele or Goitre." *The Philadelphia Journal of the Medical and Physical Sciences* 1, no. 1 (1820): 44.

Glacken, Clarence J. *Traces on the Rhodian Shore: Nature and Culture in Western Thought from Ancienct Times to the End of the Eighteenth Century*. Berkeley: University of California Press, 1967.

Golinski, Jan. "Debating the Atmospheric Constitution: Yellow Fever and the American Climate." *Eighteenth-Century Studies* 49, no. 2 (2016): 149–65.

———. *Science as Public Culture: Chemistry and Enlightenment in Britain, 1760–1820*. Cambridge and New York: Cambridge University Press, 1992.

Graham, Jenny. "Revolutionary in Exile: The Emigration of Joseph Priestley to America 1794–1804." *Transactions of the American Philosophical Society* 85, no. 2 (1995): 1–213.

Greene, Jack P. *Peripheries and Center: Constitutional Development in the Extended Polities of the British Empire and the United States, 1607–1788*. Athens and London: University of Georgia Press, 1986.

Greene, John C. *American Science in the Age of Jefferson*. Ames: Iowa State University Press, 1984.

Greenwald, Isidor. "Observations on the History of Goiter in Ohio and in West Virginia." *Journal of the History of Medicine and Allied Sciences* 10, no. 3 (1955): 277–89.

Gregory, John. *A Father's Legacy to His Daughters*. Dublin: Thomas Ewing and Caleb Jenkin, 1774.

———. *Observations on the Duties and Offices of a Physician and on the Method of Prosecuting Enquiries in Philosophy*. London: Printed for W. Strahan and T. Cadell, 1770.

Greifenstein, Charles. "Benjamin Rush and the Medical Theorists of the 18th Century." Philadelphia, n.d.

Griffin, Patrick. *America's Revolution*. Oxford and New York: Oxford University Press, 2012.

———. "Introduction: Imagining an American Imperial-Revolutionary History." In *Experiencing Empire: Power, People, and Revolution in Early America*, 1–24. Charlottesville: University of Virginia Press, 2017.

Gronim, Sara Stidstone. "Imagining Inoculation: Smallpox, the Body, and Social Relations of Healing in the Eighteenth Century." *Bulletin of the History of Medicine* 80, no. 2 (2006): 247–68. https://doi.org/10.1353/bhm.2006.0057.

Gross, Samuel. *Lives of Eminent American Physicians and Surgeons of the Nineteenth Century*. Philadelphia: Lindsay & Blakiston, 1861.

Grove, Richard H. *Green Imperialism: Colonial Expansion, Tropical Island Edens and the Origins of Environmentalism, 1600–1860*. Cambridge: Cambridge University Press, 1995.

Guerrini, Anita. "Archibald Pitcairne and Newtonian Medicine." *Medical History* 31 (1987): 70–83.

————. *Obesity and Depression in the Enlightenment: The Life and Times of George Cheyne*. Norman, OK: University of Oklahoma Press, 2000.

Gunther-Canada, Wendy. "Cultivating Virtue: Catherine Macaulay and Mary Wollstonecraft on Civic Education." *Women & Politics* 25, no. 3 (2003): 47–70.

Haakonssen, Lisbeth. *Medicine and Morals in the Enlightenment: John Gregory, Thomas Percival, and Benjamin Rush*. Amsterdam and Atlanta: Rodopi, 1997.

Hall, Thomas S. *History of General Physiology: 600 B.C. to A.D. 1900*, 1969.

Hamlin, Christopher. "Commentary: Ackerknecht and 'Anticontagionism': A Tale of Two Dichotomies." *International Journal of Epidemiology* 38, no. 1 (2009): 22–27.

————. *More Than Hot: A Short History of Fever*. Baltimore and London: The Johns Hopkins University Press, 2014.

————. "Predisposing Causes and Public Health in Early Nineteenth Century Medical Thought." *Social History of Medicine* 5, no. 1992 (1992): 43–70.

————. "William Pulteney Alison, the Scottish Philosophy, and the Making of a Political Medicine." *Journal of the History of Medicine and Allied Sciences* 61, no. 2 (2006): 144–86.

Hare, Edward. "The History of 'Nervous Disorders' from 1600 to 1840, and a Comparison with Modern Views." *British Journal of Psychiatry* 159 (1991): 37–45.

Harrison, M. "'The Tender Frame of Man': Disease, Climate, and Racial Difference in India and the West Indies, 1760–1860." *Bulletin of the History of Medicine* 70, no. 1 (1996): 68–93.

Harrison, Mark. "The Evils of Quarantine." In *Contagion*, 2013.

————. *Climates and Constitutions: Health, Race, Environment and British Imperialism in India, 1600–1850*. New York: Oxford University Press, 1999.

————. *Medicine in an Age of Commerce and Empire: Britian and Its Tropical Colonies*. Oxford: Oxford University Press, 2010.

Hartley, David. *Hartley's Theory of the Human Mind, on the Principle of the Association of Ideas*. London: Printed for J. Johnson, 1775.

————. *Observations on Man, His Frame, His Duty, and His Expectations: In Two Parts. Part the First*. 4th ed. London: Reprinted for J. Johnson, 1801.

————. *Observations on Man, His Frame, His Duty, and His Expectations: In Two Parts. Part the Second: Containing Observation on the Duty and Expectations of Mankind*. 4th ed. London: Reprinted for J. Johnson, 1801.

Hawke, David Freeman. *Benjamin Rush: Revolutionary Gadfly*. Indianapolis and New York: The Bobbs-Merrill Company, Inc., 1971.

Hedges, William L. "Benjamin Rush, Charles Brockden Brown, and the American Plague Year." *Early American Literature* 7, no. 3 (1973): 295–311.

Henderson, Lawrence J. "The Functions of an Environment." *Science* 39, no. 1006 (1914): 524–27.

Herschthal, Eric. "Antislavery Science in the Early Republic: The Case of Dr. Benjamin Rush." *Early American Studies*, no. Spring 2017 (2017): 274–307.

Hillary, William, and Benjamin Rush. *Observations on the Changes of the Air, and the Concomitant Epidemical Diseases in the Island of Barbadoes. To Which Is Added A Treatise on the Putrid Billious Fever, Commonly Called the Yellow Fever; and Such Other Diseases as Are Indigenous or Endemical.* Philadelphia: B. & T. Kite, 1811.

Hindle, Brooke. *The Pursuit of Science in Revolutionary America, 1735–1789.* New York: W.W. Norton and Co., 1956.

———. "The Underside of the Learned Society in New York, 1754–1854." In *The Pursuit of Knowledge in the Early American Republic*, edited by Alexandra Oleson and Sanborn C. Brown, 84–116. Baltimore and London: The Johns Hopkins University Press, 1976.

Hinds, Janie. "Dr. Rush and Mr. Peale: The Figure of the Animal in Late Eighteenth-Century Medical Discourse." *Early American Literature* 48, no. 3 (2013): 641–70. http://muse.jhu.edu/content/crossref/journals/early_american_literature/v048/48.3.hinds.html.

Hogarth, Rana. "A Contemporary Black Perspective on the 1793 Yellow Fever Epidemic in Philadelphia." *American Journal of Public Health* 109, no. 10 (2019): 1337–38. https://doi.org/10.2105/AJPH.2019.305244.

Hughes, Victor. "Rapport fait aux Citoyens Victor Huges et Lebas Agens particulierd du Directoire Executif aux Isles du Vent, par la Commission etablie en vertu de leur Arret du 12eme Vendemiaire, l'an 66eme de la Republic," *The Medical Repository and Review of American Publications*, 3.1. (1800)

Hume, David. "Essay XXIV: Of National Charactes," n.d.

Humphreys, Margaret. *Yellow Fever and the South.* New Brunswick, NJ, and London: Rutgers University Press, 1992.

Irving-Stonebraker, Sarah. "Nature, Knowledge, and Civilization. Connecting the Atlantic and Pacific Worlds in the Enlightenment." *Itinerario* 41, no. 1 (2017): 93–107.

Jackson, Stanley W. "Melancholia and Mechanical Explanation in Eighteenth-Century Medicine." *Journal of the History of Medicine and Allied Sciences* 38, no. 3 (1983): 298–319.

Jardine, L. J. *A Letter from Pennsylvania to a Friend in England: Containing Valuable Information with Respect to America.* Bath: Printed by R. Cruttwell and sold by Silly, London; Lloyd, and Cottle Bristol; and Bull and Co. and Evans, Bath, 1795.

Jefferson, Thomas. *Notes on the State of Virginia.* Philadelphia: R.T. Rawle, 1801.

———. *Notes on the State of Virginia.* Edited by William Peden. Chapel Hill and London: University of North Carolina Press, 1982.

Jepson, Wendy. "Of Soil, Situation, and Salubrity: Medical Topography and Medical Officers in Early Nineteenth-Century British India." *Historical Geography* 32 (2004): 137–55.

Johnson, Mary. "Madame Rivardi's Seminary in the Gothic Mansion." *The Pennsylvania Magazine of History and Biography*, no. January (1980): 3–38.

Johnston, Katherine. "The Constitution of Empire: Place and Bodily Health in the Eighteenth-Century Atlantic." *Atlantic Studies Global Currents* 10, no. 4 (2013): 443–66.

Jones, Abaslom, and Richard Allen. *A Narrative of the Proceedings of the Black People, during the Late Awful Calamity in Philadelphia, in the Year 1793: And a Refutation of Some Censures Thrown upon Them in Some Late Publications*. Philadelphia: Printed for the Authors, by William W. Woodward, At Franklin's Head, 1794.

Jones, Catherine. "Benjamin Rush, Edinburgh Medicine and the Rise of Physician Autobiography." *Clio Medica* 94 (2014): 97–122.

Jones, Colin. "Plague and Its Metaphors in Early Modern France," *Representations*, no. 53 (1 January 1996): 97–127.

Jonsson, Fredrik Albritton. "Climate Change and the Retreat of the Atlantic: The Cameralist Context of Pehr Kalm's Voyage to North America, 1748-51." *William & Mary Quarterly* 72, no. 1 (2015): 99–126.

———. *Enlightenment's Frontier: The Scottish Highlands and the Origins of Environmentalism*. New Haven and London: Yale University Press, 2013.

Judd, Richard W. *The Untilled Garden: Natural History and the Spirit of Conservation in America, 1740–1840*. Cambridge and New York: Cambridge University Press, 2009.

Justice, Benjamin. "Introduction." In *Founding Fathers, Education, and "the Great Contest": The American Philosophical Society Prize of 1797*, edited by Benjamin Justice, 1–20. New York: Palgrave MacMillan, 2013.

———. "'The Great Contest': The American Philosophical Society Education Prize of 1795 and the Problem of American Education." *American Journal of Education* 114 (2008). http://www.journals.uchicago.edu/t-and-c.

Kendi, Ibram X. *Stamped from the Beginning: The Definitive History of Racist Ideas in America*. New York: Bold Type Books, 2016.

Kerber, Linda K. "The Republican Mother: Women and the Enlightenment—An American Perspective." In *Toward and Intellectual History of Women*, 41–62. Chapel Hill and London: University of North Carolina Press, 1997.

Kidd, Colin. *The Forging of Races: Race and Scriptire in the Protestant Atlantic World, 1600–2000*. Cambridge and New York: Cambridge University Press, 2006.

Kilbride, Daniel. "Southern Medical Students in Philadelphia, 1800–1861: Science and Sociability in the 'Republic of Medicine.'" *Journal of Southern History* 65, no. 4 (1999): 697–732.

King, Lester S. *The Medical World of the Eighteenth Century*. Chicago and London: University of Chicago Press, 1958.

King, Martha J. "'Receive the Olive Branch': Benjamin Rush as Reconciler in the Early Republic." *Early American Studies*, no. Spring (2017): 352–81.

Knott, Sarah. "Benjamin Rush's Ferment: Enlightenment Medicine and Female Citizenship in Revolutionary America." In *Women, Gender, and Enlightenment*, edited by Sarah Knott and Barbara Taylor, 649–66. New York: Palgrave MacMillan, 2005.

———. *Sensibility and the American Revolution*. Chapel Hill: University of North Carolina Press, 2009.

———. "Sensibility and the American War for Independence." *The American Historical Review* 109, no. 1 (2004): 19–40.

Kornfeld, Eve. "Crisis in the Capital: The Cultural Significance of Philadelphia's Great Yellow Fever Epidemic." *Pennsylvania History* 51, no. 3 (1984): 189–205.

Kramnick, Isaac. "Eighteenth-Century Science and Radical Social Theory: The Case of Joseph Priestley's Scientific Liberalism." *Journal of British Studies*. Vol. 25, 1986. https://0-www-jstor-org.catalog.sewanee.edu/stable/pdf/175609.pdf?refre qid=excelsior%3A87439b4318914563e693d999228751e8.

Kruschwitz, Peter. "Principiis Obsta: Resist Beginnings!" In *The Petrified Muse*, 2017.

Kupperman, Karen O. "Fear of Hot Climates in the Anglo-American Colonial Experience." *The William and Mary Quarterly* 41, no. 2 (1984): 213–40.

———. "The Puzzle of the American Climate in the Early Colonial Period." *American Historical Review* 87, no. 5 (1982): 1262–89.

Laqueur, Thomas. *Making Sex: Body and Gender from the Greeks to Freud*. Cambridge and London: Harvard University Press, 1990.

———. "Orgasm, Generation, and the Politics of Reproductive Biology." *Representations*, 1986, 1–41.

Larson, J.L. "Vital Forces: Regulative Principles or Constitutive Agents? A Strategy in German Physiology, 1786–1802." *Isis; an International Review Devoted to the History of Science and Its Cultural Influences* 70, no. 252 (1979): 235–49.

Larson, James L. *Interpreting Nature: The Science of Living Form from Linnaeus to Kant*. Baltimore and London: The Johns Hopkins University Press, 1994.

Lawrence, Christopher. "Medicine as Culture: Edinburgh and the Scottish Enlightenment." University of London, 1984.

———. "Medicine as Culture Edinburgh and the Scottish Enlightenment." University of London, 1984.

Lehman, Christine. "Pierre-Joseph Macquer: Chemistry in the French Enlightenment," 2014.

Leoutsakos, V. "A Short History of the Thyroid Gland." *Hormones* 3, no. 4 (2004): 268–71. https://doi.org/10.14310/horm.2002.11137.

Lepore, Jill. *A Is for American: Letters and Other Characters in the Newly United States*. New York: Vintage, 2002.

Lettsom, John Coakley. *Recollections of Dr. Rush*. London: Printed by J. Nichols, Son, and Bentley, Red Lion Passage, Fleet Street., 1815.

Lyons, Jonathan. *The Society for Useful Knoweldge: How Benjamin Franklin and Friends Brought the Enlightenment in America*. New York and London: Blooms-bury Press, 2013.

Macquer, Pierre Joseph. *Dictionnaire de Chyie, Tome Premiere*. Paris: Chez Lacombe, 1766.

———. *Dictionnaire de Chymie, Tome Second*. Paris: Chez Lacombe, 1766.

Macrery, Joseph. "A Description of the Hot Springs and Volcanic Appearances near the Washita, or Black River, in Louisiana," *The Medical Repository and Review of American Publications*, 3.1 (1806)

Magaw, Samuel. "Address Delivered in the Young Ladies' Academy, at Philadelphia, on February 8th, 1787, at the Close of a Public Examination," *The American Museum or Repository of Ancient and Modern Fugitive Pieces, Prose and Poetical*, 3.2 (Philadelphia: Mathew Carey, 1788), 25–28.

Manion, Jennifer. *Liberty's Prisoners: Carceral Culture in Early America*. Philadelphia: University of Pennsylvania, 2015.

Markoff, Lewis. "Yellow Fever Outbreak in Sudan." *The New England Journal of Medicine*, 2013, 689–91.

Marks, Geoffrey, and William K. Beatty. *The Story of Medicine in America*. New York: Charles Scribner's Sons, 1973.

Martin, Alexander M. "Sewage and the City: Filth, Smell, and Representations of Urban Life in Moscow, 1770–1880." *The Russian Review* 67, no. 2 (2008): 243–74.

May, Henry F. *The Enlightenment in America*. New York and Oxford: Oxford University Press, 1976.

McConville, Brendan. *The King's Three Faces: The Rise and Fall of Royal America, 1688–1776*. Chapel Hill: University of North Carolina Press, 2006.

McCosh, James. *The Scottish Philosophy, Biographical, Expository, Critical, From Hutcheson to Hamilton*. New York: Robert Carter and Brothers, 1874.

McCullough, L B. "Hume's Influence on John Gregory and the History of Medical Ethics." *The Journal of Medicine and Philosophy* 24, no. 4 (1999): 376–95. https://doi.org/10.1076/jmep.24.4.376.5979.

McMahon, Lucia. *Mere Equals: The Paradox of Educated Women in the Early American Republic*. Ithaca and London: Cornell University Press, 2012.

McNair, James B. "Thomas Horsfield—American Naturalist and Explorer." *Torreya* 42, no. 1 (1942): 1–9.

Mease, James. "Review: Geological Account of the United States," *The Medical Repository and Review of American Publications*. 5.1 (1808).

Meigs, Charles D. *Females and Their Diseases: A Series of Letters to His Class*. Philadelphia: Lea and Blanchard, 1848.

Mendelsohn, Evertt. *Heat and Life: The Development of the Theory of Animal Heat*. Cambridge: Harvard University Press, 1964.

Meranze, Michael. *Laboratories of Virtue: Punishment, Revolution, and Authority in Philadelphia, 1760-1835.* Chapel Hill and London: University of North Carolina Press, 1996.

Meyer, William B. "Why Did Syracuse Manufacture Solar Salt?" *Source New York History* 86, no. 2 (2005): 195–209.

Miller, Ian. *A Modern History of the Stomach: Gastric Illness, Medicine and British Society, 1800–1950.* London: Pickering & Chatto, 2011.

Minter, Catherine J. "The Concept of Irritability and the Critique of Sensibility in Eighteenth-Century Germany." *The Modern Language Review* 106, no. 2 (2011): 463–76.

Miranda, Francisco de. *The New Democracy in America: Travels of Francisco de Miranda in the United States, 1783–84.* Edited by John S. Ezell and Judson P. Wood, trans. Norman, OK: University of Oklahoma Press, 1963.

Mitchell, S. Weir. *Historical Notes of Dr. Benjamin Rush 1777.* Philadelphia, 1903.

Mitchell, Thomas D. *The Character of Rush, an Introductory to the Course on the Theory and Practice of Medicine in the Philadelphia College of Medicine.* Philadelphia: John H. Gihon, 1848.

Mitman, Gregg. "In Search of Health: Landscape and Disease in American Environmental History." *Environmental History* 10, no. 2 (2005): 184–210.

Monro, Alexander. *A State of Facts Concerning The First Proposal of Performing the Paracentesis of the Thorax, on Account of Air Effused from the Lungs into the Cavities of the Pleurae; and Concerning The Discovery of the Lymphatic Valvular Absorbent System of Vessels in O.* Edinburgh: Printed by Balfour, Auld, and Smellie, 1770.

Montesquieu, Charles de Secondat, baron de. *The Spirit of Laws.* London: Printed for J. Nourse, and P. Vaillant, in the Strand, 1766.

Moran, Mary Catherine. "Between the Savage and the Civil: Dr John Gregory's Natural History of Femininity." In *Women, Gender, and Enlightenment.* New York: Palgrave MacMillan, 2005.

Morgan, John. *A Discourse upon the Institution of Medical Schools in America.* Philadelphia: Printed and sold by William Bradford, 1765.

Morman, Edward T. "Guarding Against Alien Impurities: The Philadelphia Lazaretto 1854–1893." *The Pennsylvania Magazine of History and Biography* 108, no. 2 (1984): 131–51.

Moseley, Benjamin. *Medical Tracts.* 2nd ed. London: Printed by John Nichols, 1800.

Myrsiades, Linda. *Medical Culture in Revolutionary America: Feuds, Duels, and a Court-Martial.* Madison and Teaneck: Fairleigh Dickinson University Press, 2009.

Naramore, Sarah E. "Making Endemic Goiter an American Disease, 1800–1820." *Journal Of The History Of Medicine And Allied Sciences* 76, no. 3 (2021): 239–63. https://doi.org/10.1093/jhmas/jrab018.

————. "'My Master and Friend': Social Networks and Professional Identity in American Medicine, 1789–1815." *Social History of Medicine* 0, no. 0 (2020): 1–24. https://doi.org/10.1093/shm/hkaa016.

Naramore, Sarah Elizabeth. "Recommended for 'Frequent Perusal' and 'Improving the Science of Medicine': Benjamin Rush's American Editions and the Circulation of Medical Knowledge in the Early Republic." *Endeavour* 45, no. 1–2 (2021): 100765. https://doi.org/10.1016/j.endeavour.2021.100765.

Nash, Linda. *Inescapable Ecologies: A History of Environment, Disease, and Knowledge.* Berkeley, Los Angles, and London: University of California Press, 2006.

Nash, Margaret A. "Rethinking Republican Motherhood: Benjamin Rush and the Young Ladies' Academy of Philadelphia." *Journal of the Early Republic* 17, no. 2 (1997): 171–91.

Neubauer, John. "Dr. John Brown (1735–1788) and Early German Romanticism." *Journal of the History of Ideas* 28, no. 3 (1967): 367–82.

Newman, Paul Douglas. *Fries's Rebellion: The Enduring Struggle for the American Revolution.* Philadelphia: University of Pennsylvania, 2012.

"News, February 19, 1787." *The Daily Advertiser.* February 19, 1787.

Niazi, Asfandyar Khan, Sanjay Kaira, Awais Irfan, and Aliya Islam. "Thyroidology over the Ages." *Indian Journal of Endocrinology and Metabolism* 17, no. 1 (2011): 95–100. https://doi.org/10.4103/2230.

Noll, Mark. *America's God: From Jonathan Edwards to Abraham Lincoln.* Oxford and New York: Oxford University Press, 2002.

Noll, Mark A. "Common Sense Traditions and American Evangelical Thought." *American Quarterly* 37, no. 2 (1985): 216–38.

Norton, Mary Beth. *Liberty's Daughters: The Revolutionary Experience of American Women, 1750–1800.* Ithaca and London: Cornell University Press, 1980.

————. *Separated by Their Sex: Women in Public and Private in the Colonial Atlantic World.* Ithaca and London: Cornell University Press, 2011.

Noyes, Russell. "The Transformation of Hypochondriasis in British Medicine, 1680—1830." *Social History of Medicine* 24, no. 2 (2011): 281–98.

Ogden, Emily. "Mesmer's Demon: Fiction, Falsehood, and the Mechanical Imagination." *Early American Literature* 47, no. 1 (2012): 143–70.

Onuf, Peter S. "Liberty, Development, and Union: Visions of the West in the 1780s." *The William and Mary Quarterly* 43, no. 2 (1986): 179–213.

Osman, W.A. "Alessandro Volta and the Inflammable-Air Eudiometer." *Annals of Science,* 1958, 215–42.

Ovid. "Remedia Amoris." In *Love Poems, Letters, and Remedies of Ovid,* edited by David R. Slavitt and Michael Dirda, 320–52. Cambridge and London: Harvard University Press, 2011.

Park, Benjamin. "The Bonds of Union: Benjamin Rush, Noah Webster, and Defining the Nation in the Early Republic." *Early American Studies,* no. Spring 2017 (2017): 382–408.

Paules, Catharine I., and Anthony S. Fauci. "Yellow Fever—Once Again on the Radar Screen in the Americas." *The New England Journal of Medicine*, 2017, 1397–99.

Pencak, William. "Free Health Care for the Poor: The Philadelphia Dispensary." *The Pennsylvania Magazine of History and Biography* 136, no. 1 (2012): 25–52.

Pernick, Martin S. "Politics, Parties, and Pestilence: Epidemic Yellow Fever in Philadelphia and the Rise of the First Party System Epidemic Yellow Fever in Philadelphia and the Rise of the First Party System." *The William and Mary Quarterly* 29, no. 4 (1972): 559–86.

Phillips, Denise. *Acolytes of Nature: Defining Natural Science in Germany*. Chicago and London: University of Chicago Press, 2012.

Plummer, Betty L., and James Durham. "Letters of James Durham to Benjamin Rush." *The Journal of Negro History* 65, no. 3 (1980): 261–69.

Ponzio, Paolo. "The Articulation of the Idea of Experience in the 16th and 17th Centuries." *Quaestio* 4 (2004): 175–95.

Porter, Dorothy. *The History of Public Health and the Modern State*. Amsterdam and Atlanta: Rodopi, 1994.

Powell, J.M. *Bring Out Your Dead: The Great Plague of Yellow Fever in Philadelphia in 1793*. 2nd ed. Philadelphia: University of Pennsylvania, 1993.

Priestley, Joseph. *Hartley's Theory of the Human Mind, on the Principle of the Association of Ideas; with Essays Relating to the Subject of It*. London: Printed for J. Johnson, 1775.

Pringle, John, and Benjamin Rush. *Observations on the Diseases of the Army*. Philadelphia: Edward Earle, 1810.

Ramsay, David. "A Case of Extra-Uterine Foetus, with Some Observations on the Subject Generally." *The Medical Repository, and Review of American Publications on Medicine, Surgery, and the Auxiliary Branches of Science* I, no. 3 (1804): 221–28.

———. "Extracts from an Address delivered before the Medical Society of South-Carolina," *The Medical Repository and Review of American Publications* 4 (1801).

Ratcliff, Jessica. "The East India Company, the Company's Museum, and the Political Economy of Natural History in the Early Nineteenth Century." *Isis* 107, no. 3 (2016): 495–517.

Reid-Maroney, Nina. *Philadelphia's Enlightenment, 1740–1800*. Westport and London: Greenwood, 2001.

Reid, Thomas. *Essays on the Powers of the Human Mind*. Edinburgh: Printed Bell & Bradfute, 1803.

Reill, Peter Hanns. *Vitalizing Nature in the Enlightenment*. Berkeley and Los Angeles: University of California Press, 2005.

Reiss, Benjamin. *Theaters of Madness: Insane Asylums and Nineteenth-Century American Culture*. Chicago and London: University of Chicago Press, 2008.

Riley, James C. *The Eighteenth-Century Campaign to Avoid Disease*. New York: St. Martin's Press, 1987.

Risse, G. B. "Schelling, 'Naturphilosophie' and John Brown's System of Medicine." *Bulletin of the History of Medicine* 50, no. 3 (1976): 321–34.

Rockman, Marcy. "New World with a New Sky: Climatic Variability, Environmental Expectations, and the Historical Period Colonization of Eastern North America." *ear* 44, no. 3 (2010): 4–20.

Roe, Shirley A. *Matter, Life, and Generation: Eighteenth-Century Embryology and the Haller-Wolff Debate*. Cambridge and New York: Cambridge University Press, 1981.

Roger, Jacques, and Keith Rodney Benson. "The New Scientific Mentality." In *The Life Sciences in Eighteenth-Century French Thought*, 133–204. Stanford University Press, 1997.

Roney, Jessica Choppin. "1776, Viewed from the West." *Journal of the Early Republic* 37, no. 4 (2017): 41. https://doi.org/10.1353/jer.2017.0067.

Rosenberg, Charles E. *In the Care of Strangers: The Rise of America's Hospital System*. Baltimore and London: The Johns Hopkins University Press, 1987.

———. *Our Present Complaint: American Medicine, Then and Now*. Baltimore and London: The Johns Hopkins University Press, 2007.

Rosenfeld, Sophia. "Benjamin Rush's Common Sense." *Early American Studies*, no. Spring (2017): 252–73.

Rosner, Lisa. "Thistle on the Delaware: Edinburgh Medical Education and Philadelphia Practice, 1800-1825." *Social History of Medicine* 5, no. 1 (1992): 19–42.

Rothman, Sheila A. *Living in the Shadow of Death: Tuberculosis and the Social Experience of Illness in American History*. New York: Basic Books, 1994.

Rush, Benjamin. "'A Defense of the Use of the Bible as a School Book. Addressed to the Rev. Jeremy Belknap of Boston.'" In *Essays, Literary, Moral and Philosophical*, edited by 2nd, 92–113. Philadelphia: Thomas and William Bradford, 1806.

———. *A Letter by Dr. Benjamin Rush Describing the Consecration of the German College at Lancaster in June, 1787: Printed, with an Introduction, from a Newly Discovered Manuscript, Now in the Fackenthal Library at Franklin and Marshall College*. Edited by L.H. Butterfield. Lancaster, PA: Franklin and Marshall College, 1947.

———. "A Plan for Establishing Public Schools in Pennsylvania, and for Conducting Education Agreeably to a Republican Form of Government. Addressed to the Legislature and Citizens of Pennsylvania, in the Year 1786." In *Essays, Literary, Moral and Philosophical*, 2nd ed., 1–5. Philadelphia: Thomas and William Bradford, 1806.

———. "An Account of the Bilious Remitting Yellow Fever, as It Appeared in Philadelphia in the Year 1793." In *Medical Inquiries and Observations, Volume III*, 2nd ed. Philadelphia: J. Conrad & Co., 1805.

————. *An Account of the Bilious Remitting Yellow Fever, as It Appeared in the City of Philadelphia, in the Year 1793*. Philadelphia: Printed by Thomas Dobson, 1794.

————. *An Account of the Bilious Remitting Yellow Fever as It Appeared in the City of Philadelphia in the Year 1793*. Philadelphia: Thomas Dobson, 1794.

————. "An Account of the Climate of Pennsylvania, and Its Influence upon the Human Body." In *Medical Inquiries and Observations*, 2nd ed., 69–114. Philadelphia: J. Conrad & Co., 1805.

————. "An Account of the Influence of the Military and Political Events of the American Revolution upon the Human Body." In *Medical Inquiries and Observations*, 2nd ed., 277–94. Philadelphia: J. Conrad & Co., 1805.

————. *An Account of the Manners of the German Inhabitants of Pennsylvania*. Philadelphia, 1875.

————. *An Address to the Inhabitants of the British Settlements, on the Slavery of the Negroes in America, the Second Edition*. 2nd ed. Philadelphia: Printed and Sold by John Dunlap, 1773.

————. "An Enquiry into the Effects of Public Punishments upon Criminals, and upon Society. Read in the Society for Promoting Political Enquiries, Convened at the Hosue of Benjamin Franklin, Esq. in Philadelphia, March 9th, 1787." In *Essays, Literary, Moral and Philosophical*, 2nd ed., 136–63. Philadelphia: Printed by Thomas and William Bradford, 1806.

————. *An Enquiry into the Effects of Public Punishments upon Criminals and upon Society: Read in the Society for Promoting Political Enquiries, Convened at the House of His Excellency Benjamin Franklin, Esquire in Philadelphia, March 9th, 1787*. Philadelphia: Printed by Joseph James, in Chestnut-Street, 1787.

————. "An Inquiry into the Cause of Animal Life." In *Medical Inquiries and Observations, Volume II*, 2nd ed., 369. Philadelphia: J. Conrad & Co., 1805.

————. "An Inquiry into the Functions of the Spleen, Liver, Pancreas, and Thyroid Gland." *The Philadelphia Medical Museum* 3 (1807): 9–29.

————. *An Inquiry into the Influence of Physical Causes upon the Moral Faculty: Delivered before a Meeting of the American Philosophical Society, Held at Philadelphia, on the Twenty-Seventh of February, 1786*. Edited by George Combe. Philadelphia: Haswell, Barrington, and Haswell, 1839.

————. *An Inquiry Into the Influence of Physical Causes Upon the Moral Faculty: Delivered Before a Meeting of the American Philosophical Society, Held at Philadelphia, on the Twenty-Seventh of February, 1786*. Philadelphia: Haswell, Barrington, and Haswell, 1786.

————. "An Inquiry into the Influence of Physical Causes upon the Moral Faculty." In *Medical Inquiries and Observations, Volume II*, 2nd ed., 1–58. Philadelphia: J. Conrad & Co., 1805.

————. "An Inquiry into the Natural History of Medicine among the Indians of North-America; and a Comparative View of Their Diseases and Remedies with Those of Civilized Nations." In *Medical Inquiries and Observations, Volume I*, 2nd ed., 1–68. Philadelphia: J. Conrad & Co., 1805.

———. *An Oration, Delivered before the American Philosophical Society: Held in Philadelphia on the 27th of February, 1786; Containing an Enquiry into the Influence of Physical Causes upon the Moral Faculty* . . . Philadelphia: Charles Cist, 1786.

———. *Directions for the Use of the Mineral Water and Cold Bath, at Harrogate near Philadelphia.* Philadelphia: Melchior Steiner, 1786.

———. "Dr. Rush's Directions, for Curing and Preventing the Yellow Fever." *Dunlap's American Daily Advertiser.* September 13, 1793.

———. *Experiments and Observations on the Mineral Waters of Philadelphia, Abington, and Bristol, in the Province of Pennsylvania.* Philadelphia: James Humphreys jr., 1773.

———. *Letters of Benjamin Rush.* Edited by L.H. Butterfield. Princeton, NJ: Published for the American Philosophical Society by Princeton University Press, 1951.

———. *Medical Inquiries and Observations: Volume 3.* 2nd ed. Philadelphia: J. Conrad & Co., 1805.

———. *Medical Inquiries and Observations: Volume 4.* 2nd ed. Philadelphia: J. Conrad & Co., 1805.

———. *Medical Inquiries and Observations Upon the Diseases of the Mind.* 4th ed. Philadelphia: John Grigg, 1830.

———. "Observations upon the Nature and Cure of the Gout." In *Medical Inquiries and Observations, Volume II*, 2nd ed., 224–98. Philadelphia: J. Conrad & Co., 1805.

———. "Observations upon the Study of the Latin and Greek Languages, as a Branch of Liberal Education, with Hints of a Plan of Liberal Instruction, without Them, Accommodated to the Present State of Society, Manners, and Government in the United States." In *Essays, Literary, Moral and Philosophical*, 2nd ed., 21–50. Philadelphia: Thomas and William Bradford, 1806.

———. "Of the Mode of Education Proper in a Republic." In *Essays, Literary, Moral and Philosophical*, 2nd ed., 7–20. Philadelphia: Thomas and William Bradford, 1806.

———. "Pathological and Practical Remarks upon Certain Morbid Affections of the Liver." *The Philadelphia Medical Museum*, 1811, 87–93.

———. *Sermons to the Rich and Studious, on Temperance and Exercise with a Dedication to Dr. Cadogan.* London: Printed for Edward and Charles Dilly, in the Poultry, 1772.

———. *Sixteen Introductory Lectures, to Courses of Lectures upon the Institutes and Practice of Medicine.* Philadelphia: Published by Bradford and Innskeep, 1811.

———. *The Autobiography of Benjamin Rush: His "Travels Through Life" Together with His Commonplace Book for 1789–1813.* Edited by George W. Corner. Princeton, NJ: Princeton University Press, 1948.

———. "The Result of Observations Made upon the Diseases Which Occurred in the Military Hospitals of the United States, during the Revolutionary War." In *Medical Inquiries and Observations*, 2nd ed., 267–76. Philadelphia: J. Conrad & Co., 1805.

———. "Thoughts upon Female Education, Accomodated to the Present State of Society, Manners, and Government, in the United States of America. Addressed to the Visitors of the Young Ladies' Academy in Philadelphia, 28th July, 1787, at the Close of the Quarterly E." In *Essays, Literary, Moral and Philosophical*, 2nd ed., 75–92. Philadelphia: Thomas and William Bradford, 1806.

———. "Thoughts upon the Amusements and Punishments Which Are Proper for Schools. Addressed to George Clymer, Esq." In *Essays, Literary, Moral and Philosophical*, 2nd ed., 57–75. Philadelphia: Printed by Thomas and William Bradford, 1806.

———. "To James Currie (Philadelphia, July 26, 1796)." In *Letters of Benjamin Rush, Vol. III*, edited by L.H. Butterfield, 779–80. Princeton, NJ: Princeton University Press, 1951.

———. "To James Rush (Philadelphia, March 19, 1810)." In *Letters of Benjamin Rush, Vol. II*, edited by L.H. Butterfield, 1039. Philadelphia: Princeton University Press, 1951.

———. "To John Adams (Philadelphia, April 10th, 1813)." In *Letters of Benjamin Rush, Vol. II*, edited by L.H. Butterfield, 1191–92. Princeton, NJ: Princeton University Press, 1951.

———. "To John Morgan (Edinburgh, January 20th, 1768)." In *Letters of Benjamin Rush, Vol. I.*, edited by L.H. Butterfield, 49–51. Princeton, NJ: Princeton University Press, 1951.

———. "To the Managers of the Pennsylvania Hospital (September 24, 1810)." In *Letters of Benjamin Rush, Vol. II*, edited by L.H. Butterfield, 1063–66. Princeton, NJ: Princeton University Press, 1951.

———. "To Thomas Jefferson (Philadelphia, March 15th, 1813)." In *Letters of Benjamin Rush, Vol. II*, edited by L.H. Butterfield, 1186–89. Princeton, NJ: Princeton University Press, 1951.

———. "To Thomas Jefferson (Philadelphia, October 6th, 1800)." In *Letters of Benjamin Rush, Vol. II*, edited by L.H. Butterfield, 824–27. Princeton, NJ: Princeton University Press, 1951.

Rush, Benjamin, and Louis Alexander Biddle. *A Memorial Containing Travels Through Life Or Sundry Incidents in the Life of Dr. Benjamin Rush, Born Dec. 24, 1745 (Old Style) Died April 19, 1813*. Edited by Louis Alexander Biddle. Philadelphia, 1905.

Santoro, Lily. "Promoting the Book of Nature: Philadelphia's Role in Popularizing Science for Christian Citizens in the Early Republic." *Pennsylvania History: A Journal of Mid-Atlantic Studies* 84, no. 1 (2017): 30–59.

Saussure, Horace Bénédict. *Voyages Das Les Alpes: Précédés d'un Essai Sur l'histoire Naturelle Des Environs de Geneve*. Geneve: Chez Barde, Manget & Comp., 1786.

Schaffer, Simon. "Measuring Virtue: Eudiometry, Enlightenment and Pneumatic Medicine." In *The Medical Enlightenment of the Eighteenth Century*, edited by Andrew Cunningham and Roger French, 281–318. Cambridge and New York: Cambridge University Press, 1990.

———. "Priestley's Questions: An Historiographic Survey." *History of Science* 22 (1984): 151–83.

Schiebinger, Londa. "Medical Experimentation and Race in the Eighteenth-Century Atlantic World." *Social History of Medicine* 26, no. 3 (2013): 364–82.

———. *Nature's Body: Gender in the Making of Modern Science*. Boston: Beacon Press, 1993.

———. "Skeletons in the Closet: The First Illustrations of the Female Skeleton in Eighteenth—Century Anatomy." *Representations*, 1986, 42–82.

Schiebinger, Londa, Claudia Swan, Daniela Bleichmar, Maire-Noëlle Bourguet, Michael T. Bravo, Jorge Cañizares-Esguerra, Judith Carney, et al. *Colonial Botany: Science, Commerce, and Politics in the Early Modern World*. Edited by Londa Schiebinger and Claudia Swan. Philadelphia: University of Pennsylvania, 2005.

Schofield, Robert E. *Mechanism and Materialism: British Natural Philosophy in An Age of Reaseon*. Princeton, NJ: Princeton University Press, 1970.

Schultz, Christian. "Review: A Memoir Concerning the Disease of Goitre, as It Prevails in the Different Parts of North-America." *Medical Repository of Original Essays and Intelligence Relative to Physic, Surgery, Chemistry, and Natural History* IV, no. 1 (1801): 47–53.

———. "Review: Memoir Concerning the Disease of Goitre." *Medical Repository of Original Essays and Intelligence Relative to Physic, Surgery, Chemistry, and Natural History* IV, no. 2 (1801): 155–63.

Scull, Andrew. *Madness in Civilization: A Cultural History of Insanity from the Bible to Freud, from the Madhouse to Modern Medicine*. London: Thames & Hudson, 2015.

———. *Social Order/Mental Disorder: Anglo-American Psychiatry in Historical Perspective*. Berkeley and Los Angeles: University of California Press, 1989.

Seth, Suman. *Difference and Disease: Medicine, Race, and the Eighteenth-Century British Empire*. Cambridge and New York: Cambridge University Press, 2018.

———. "Materialism, Slavery, and The History of Jamaica." *Isis* 105 (2014): 764–72.

Shryock, Richard Harrison. *Medicine in America: Historical Essays*. Baltimore and London: The Johns Hopkins University Press, 1966.

———. "The Psychiatry of Benjamin Rush," 429–32, 1945.

Slaughter, Thomas P. *The Natures of John and William Bartram*. New York: Alfred A. Knopf, 1996.

Smith-Rosenberg, Carroll, and Charles E. Rosenberg. "The Female Animal: Medical and Biological Views of Woman and Her Role in Nineteenth-Century America." *The Journal of American History* 60, no. 2 (1973): 332–56.

Smith, Billy G. *Ship of Death: A Voyage That Changed the Atlantic World*. New Haven and London: Yale University Press, 2013.

Smith, J. Augustine. "A Case of Extra-Uterine Conception, in Which an Operation Was Performed." *New York Medical and Philosophical Journal and Review1* I, no. 1 (1809): 54–57.

Smith, Samuel Stanhope. *An Essay on the Causes of the Variety of Complexion and Figure in the Human Species*. 2nd ed. New Brunswick, NJ: Published by J. Simpson and Co., 1810.

Spurlin, Paul Merrill. *The French Enlightenment in America: Essays on the Times of the Founding Fathers*. Athens, GA: University of Georgia Press, 1984.

Starr, Paul. *The Social Transformation of American Medicine*. New York: Basic Books, 1982.

Staunton, George. *An Authentic Account of An Embassy from the King of Great Britain to the Emperor of China . . . Vol. I*. Vol. I. London: Printed by W. Blumer and Co., 1797.

Stoll, Mark. *Protestantism, Capitalism, and Nature in America*. Albuquerque: University of New Mexico Press, 1997.

Strang, Cameron B. *Frontiers of Science: Imperialism and Natural Knowledge in the Gulf South Borderlands, 1500–1850*. Chapel Hill: University of North Carolina Press, 2018.

———. "Perpetual War and Natural Knowledge in the United States, 1775–1860." *Journal of the Early Republic* 38, no. 3 (2018): 387–413. https://doi.org/10.1353/jer.2018.0045.

Sydenham, Thomas. *The Entire Works of Dr. Thomas Sydenham: Newly Made English from the Originals: Wherein the History of Acute and Chronic Diseases, and the Safest and Most Effectual Methods of Treating Them, Are Faithfully, Clearly, and Accurately Delivered*. Edited by John Swan, 1742.

———. *Thomae Sydenham, M.D. Opera Universa: In Quibus Non Solummodo Morborum Acutorum Historiae & Curationes, Nova & Exquisita Methodo, Diligentissime Traduntur; Verum Etiam Morborum Fere Omnium Chronicorum Curatio Brevissima, Pariter Ac Fidelissima, in Publici*. Lugduni Batavorum: Apud Joannem Heyligert, et Gaultherum Leffen, 1754.

Sydenham, Thomas, and Benjamin Rush. *The Works of Thomas Sydenham, M.D., on Acute and Chronic Diseases: With Their Histories and Modes of Cure*. Philadelphia: B. & T. Kite, 1809.

Sydenham, Thomas, and George Wallis. *The Works of Thomas Sydenham, M.D. on Acute and Chronic Diseases; Wherein There Histories and Modes of Cure, as Recited by Him, Are Delivered with Accuracy and Perspicuity. To Which Are Subjoined Notes, Corrective and Explanatory*. London: G.G.J. and J. Robinson, W. Otridge, S. Hayes, and E. Newbery, 1788.

Sykes, Ingrid J. "The Art of Listening: Perceiving Pulse in Eighteenth-Century France." *Journal for Eighteenth-Century Studies*, 2012. https://doi.org/10.1111/j.1754-0208.2012.00534.x.

Taylor, Georgette. "Plummer to Cullen: Novelty in William Cullen's Chemical Pedagogy." In *Cradle of Chemistry*, edited by Robert G.W. Anderson, 59–84. Edinburgh: John Donald Publishers Ltd., 2015.

Thacher, James. *American Medical Biography: Or Memoirs of Eminent Physicians Who Have Flourished in America to Which Is Prefixed a Succinct History of the Medical Science in the United States from the First Settlement of the Country.* Boston: Richardson & Lord and Cottons & Barnard, 1828.

———. "Bond, Thomas, M.D." In *American Medical Biography: Or, Memoirs of Eminent Physicians Who Have Flourished in America. Vol. I.*, 177–78. Richardson & Lord and Cottons & Barnard, 1828.

———. "Waters, Nicholas Baker, M.D." In *American Medical Biography: Or, Memoirs of Eminent Physicians Who Have Flourished in America. Vol. II.*, 170–71. Richardson & Lord and Cottons & Barnard, 1828.

Thiroux d'Arconville, Marie-Genevieve-Charlotte. *Essai Pour Servier a l'histoire de La Putréfaction.* Paris: Chez P. Fr. Didot le jeune, 1766.

Thompson, Peter, Peter S. Onuf, Brian Balogh, Douglas Bradburn, Holly Brewer, John L. Brooke, Max M. Edling, et al. *State and Citizen: British America and the Early United States.* Charlottsville: University of Virginia Press, 2013.

Tomes, Nancy. *The Art of Asylum-Keeping: Thomas Story Kirkbride and the Origins of American Psychiatry.* Philadelphia: University of Pennsylvania, 1994.

———. "The Domesticated Madman: Changing Concepts of Insantiy at the Pennsylvania Hospital, 1780–1830." *The Pennsylvania Magazine of History and Biography* 106, no. 2 (1982): 271–86.

Ulrich, Laurel Thatcher. *A Midwife's Tale: The Life of Martha Ballard, Based on Her Diary, 1785–1812.* New York: Alfred A. Knopf, 1991.

Valencius, Conevery Bolton. *The Health of the Country: How American Settlers Understood Themselves and Their Land.* New York: Basic Books, 2002.

———. *The Health of the Country: How American Settlers Understood Themselves and Their Land.* New York: Basic Books, 2002.

Vallee, Eric. "'A Fatal Sympathy': Suicide and the Republic of Abjection in the Writings of Benjamin Rush and Charles Brockden Brown." *Early American Studies* Spring (2017): 332–51.

Valli, Eusebius. *Experiments on Animal Electricity, with Their Application to Physiology and Some Pathological and Medical Observations.* London: Printed for J. Johnson, 1793.

Vaughan, John. *The Valedictory Lecture Delivered Before the Philosophical Society of Delaware.* Wilmington, DE: Printed at the Franklin Press by James Wilson, 1800.

Vermeulen, Han F. "Origins and Institutionalization of Ethnography and Ethnology in Europe and the USA, 1771–1845." In *Fieldwork and Footnotes: Studies in the History of European Anthropology*, 39–59. London and New York: Routledge, 1995.

Vinson, Michael. "The Society for Political Inquiries: The Limits of Republican Discourse in Philadelphia on the Eve of the Constitutional Convention." *The Pennsylvania Magazine of History and Biography* 113, no. 2 (1989): 185–205.

Vogel, Brant. "The Letter from Dublin: Climate Change, Colonialism, and the Royal Society in the Seventeenth Century." *Osiris* 26, no. 1 (2011): 111–28.

Volney, Constantin-François. *Travels Through Egypt and Syria, in the Years 1783, 1784, & 1785: Containing the Present Natural and Political State of Those Countries; Their Productions, Arts, Manufactures & Commerce; with Observations on the Manners, Customs and Government of the Turks.* New York: John Tiebout, 1798.

———. *View of the Climate and Soil of the United States of America: To Which Are Annexed Some Accounts of Florida, the French Colony on the Scioto, Certain Canadian Colonies, and the Savages or Natives.* London: Printed for J. Johnson, 1804.

Waring, Joseph Ioor. "The Influence of Benjamin Rush on the Practice of Bleeding in South Carolina." *Bulletin of the History of Medicine* 35 (1961): 230–37.

Warner, John Harley. *Against the Spirit of System: The French Impulse in Nineteenth-Century American Medicine.* Princeton, NJ: Princeton University Press, 1998.

———. *The Therapeutic Perspective: Medical Practice, Knowledge, and Identity in America, 1820-1885.* Cambridge and London: Harvard University Press, 1986.

Warner, Sam Bass. *The Private City: Philadelphia in Three Periods of Its Growth.* Philadelphia: University of Pennsylvania, 1968.

Waserman, Manfred J., and Virginia Kay Mayfield. "Nicolas Chervin's Yellow Fever Survey, 1820–1822." *Journal of the History of Medicine and Allied Sciences* 26, no. 1 (1971): 40–51.

Webster, Elizabeth E. "American Science and the Pursuit of 'Useful Knowledge' in the Polite Eighteenth Century, 1750–1806." University of Notre Dame, 2010.

Webster, Noah. *Collection of Papers On the Subject of Bilious Fevers, Prevalent in the United States for a Few Years Past.* New York: Printed by Hopkins, Webb and Co. No. 40, Pine-Street, 1796.

———. *Noah Webster: Letters on Yellow Fever Addressed to Dr. William Currie.* Baltimore: The Johns Hopkins University Press, 1947.

———. "On the Connection of Earthquakes with Epidemic Diseases and on the Succession of Epidemics," *The Medical Repository and Review of American Publications* 4.4 (1801)

Weidenhammer, Erich. "Patronage and Enlightened Medicine in the Eighteenth-Century British Military: The Rise and Fall of Dr John Pringle, 1707–1787." *Social History of Medicine* 29, no. 1 (2016): 21–43.

Weimerskirch, P.J. "Benjamin Rush and John Minson Galt, II. Pioneers of Bibliotherapy in America." *Bulletin of the Medical Library Association* 53, no. 4 (1965): 510–26.

Weiner, Dora B., and Michael J Sauter. "The City of Paris and the Rise of Clinical Medicine." *Osiris* 18 (2003): 23–42.

White, Sam. "Unpuzzling American Climate: New World Experience and the Foundations of a New Science." *Isis* 106, no. 3 (2015): 544–66.

Whytt, Robert. *Observations on the Nature, Causes, and Cure of Those Disorders Which Have Been Commonly Called Nervous Hypochondirac, or Hysteric: To Which Are Prefixed Some Remarks on the Sympathy of the Nerves.* Edinburgh and London: Printed for T. Becket, and P. Du Hondt, London; and J. Balfour, Edinburgh, 1765.

Wild, Wayne. *Medicine-by-Post: The Changing Voice of Illness in Eighteenth-Century British Consultation Letters and Literature.* Amsterdam and New York: Rodopi, 2006.

Williams, Elizabeth A. *A Cultural History of Medical Vitalism in Enlightenment Montpellier.* Aldershot, Engl and Burlington, VT: Ashgate, 2003.

———. "Neuroses of the Stomach: Eating, Gender, and Psychopathology in French Medicine, 1800–1870." *Isis* 98, no. 1 (2007): 54–79.

———. "Stomach and Psyche: Eating, Digestion, and Mental Illness in the Medicine of Philippe Pinel." *Bulletin of the History of Medicine* 84, no. 3 (2010): 358–86.

Williams, R. B. "Discovered in Philadelphia: A Third Set of Thomas Horsfield's Nature Prints of Plants from Java." *Archives of Natural History* 39, no. 38 (2014): 169–71.

Willoughby, Christopher D. "'His Native, Hot Country': Racial Science and Environment in Antebellum American Medical Thought." *Journal of the History of Medicine and Allied Sciences*, 2017, 1–24.

Wilmer, Benjamin. *Cases and Remarks in Surgery: To Which Is Subjoined, An Appendix, Containing the Method of Curing the Bronchocele in Coventry.* London: Printed for T. Longman, 1779.

Wilson, David B. *Seeking Nature's Logic: Natural Philosophy in the Scottish Enlightenment.* University Park, PA: The Pennsylvania State University Press, 2009.

Wilson, Leonard G. "Fevers and Science in Early Nineteenth Century Medicine." *Journal of the History of Medicine and Allied Sciences* 33, no. 3 (1978): 386–407.

Winterer, Caroline. *American Enlightenments: Pursuing Happiness in the Age of Reason.* New Haven and London: Yale University Press, 2016.

———. *The Culture of Classicism: Ancient Greece and Rome in American Intellectual Life, 1780–1910.* Baltimore: The Johns Hopkins University Press, 2002.

Wolf, Edwin. "Medical Books in Colonial Philadelphia." In *Centenary of Index Medicus, 1879–1979*, edited by John B. Blake, 72–92. Bethesda, MD: U.S. Dept. of Health and Human Services, Public Health Service, National Institutes of Health, National Library of Medicine, 1980.

Wolloch, Nathaniel. "The Civilizing Process, Nature, and Stadial Theory." *Eighteenth-Century Studies (Article) Eighteenth-Century Studies* 44, no. 2 (2011): 245–59.

Wollstonecraft, Mary. *Thoughts on the Education of Daughters: With Reflections on Female Conduct, in the More Important Duties of Life.* London: Printed for J. Johnson, 1787.

Wood, Gordon S. *The Americanization of Benjamin Franklin*. New York: Penguin Press, 2004.

Wood, P.B. "The Natural History of Man in the Scottish Enlightenment." *History of Science* XXVII (1989): 89–123.

Woodbury, Frank. "Benjamin Rush: Patriot, Physician and Psychiator." *Transactions of the American Medico-Psychological Association* 20 (1913): 427–30.

Wulf, Karin A. *Not All Wives: Women of Colonial Philadelphia*. Ithaca and London: Cornell University Press, 2000.

Wynes, Charles E. "Dr. James Durham, Mysterious Eighteenth-Century Black Physician: Man or Myth?" *The Pennsylvania Magazine of History and Biography* 103, no. July (1979): 325–33.

Yokota, Kariann A. "Not Written in Black and White: American National Identity and the Curious Color Transformation of Henry Moss." *Common-Place.Org* 4, no. 2 (2004): 1–6.

Yokota, Kariann Akemi. *Unbecoming British: How Revolutionary America Became a Postcolonial Nation*. Oxford and New York: Oxford University Press, 2011.

Zagarri, Rosemarie. "Morals, Manners, and the Republican Mother." *American Quarterly* 44, no. 2 (1992): 192–215.

———. "The Rights of Man and Woman in Post-Revolutionary America." *The William and Mary Quarterly* 55, no. 2 (1998): 203–30.

Zilberstein, Anya. "Inured to Empire: Wild Rice and Climate Change." *William & Mary Quarterly* 72, no. 1 (2015): 127–58.

Index

Printed in the United States
by Baker & Taylor Publisher Services